Pediatric Pearls
The Handbook of Practical Pediatrics

D0879913

NOTICE

Every effort has been made to ensure that the drug dosage schedules are accurate and in accord with the standards accepted at the time of publication. However, as new research and experience broaden our knowledge, changes in treatment and drug therapy occur. Therefore the reader is advised to check the product information sheet included in the package of each drug he or she plans to administer to be certain that changes have not been made in the recommended dosage or in the contraindications. This is of particular importance in regard to new or infrequently used drugs.

Pediatric Pearls
The Handbook of Practical Pediatrics

Third Edition

BERYL J. ROSENSTEIN, M.D.
Professor of Pediatrics,
The Johns Hopkins University School of Medicine,
Baltimore, Maryland

PATRICIA D. FOSARELLI, M.D.
Assistant Professor of Pediatrics,
The Johns Hopkins University School of Medicine,
Baltimore, Maryland

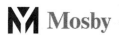 Mosby

St. Louis   Baltimore   Boston
Carlsbad   Chicago   Naples   New York   Philadelphia   Portland
London   Madrid   Mexico City   Singapore   Sydney   Tokyo   Toronto   Wiesbaden

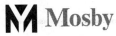
Dedicated to Publishing Excellence

A Times Mirror
Company

Vice President and Publisher:
Anne S. Patterson
Editor: Laura DeYoung
Senior Developmental Editor:
Sandra Clark Brown
Project Manager: Deborah L. Vogel
Production Editor: Jodi M. Willard
Designer: Pati Pye
Manufacturing Supervisor: Linda Ierardi

THIRD EDITION

Copyright © 1997 by Mosby–Year Book, Inc.

Previous editions copyrighted 1993, 1989

Printed in the United States of America
Composition by Graphic World, Inc.
Lithography by Graphic World, Inc.
Printing/binding by Malloy Lithographing, Inc.

Mosby–Year Book, Inc.
11830 Westline Industrial Drive
St. Louis, Missouri 63146

Library of Congress Cataloging-in-Publication Data
Rosenstein, Beryl J.
     Pediatric pearls : the handbook of practical pediatrics / Beryl J.
Rosenstein, Patricia D. Fosarelli. — 3rd ed.
        p.   cm.
     Includes bibliographical references and index.
     ISBN 0–8151–8682–7 (softcover)
     1. Pediatrics—Handbooks, manuals, etc.   I. Fosarelli, Patricia
D.   II. Title.
     [DNLM: 1. Pediatrics—handbooks.   WS 39 R815p 1997]
RJ48.R67   1997
618.92—dc20
DNLM/DLC
for Library of Congress   96–34956
                                                                CIP

97   98   99   00   01/9   8   7   6   5   4   3   2   1

CONTRIBUTORS

M. Douglas Baker, M.D., FAAP
Associate Professor of Pediatrics,
University of Pennsylvania;
Associate Director, Emergency Medicine,
Children's Hospital of Philadelphia,
Philadelphia, Pennsylvania

Paul D. Sponseller, M.D.
Associate Professor, Orthopaedic Surgery,
The Johns Hopkins University School of Medicine;
Chief, Pediatric Orthopaedics,
The Johns Hopkins Hospital,
Baltimore, Maryland

To the house officers of the Harriet Lane Home Service, past and present, who have been our best teachers as well as a constant source of support

PREFACE TO THE THIRD EDITION

When writing new editions of medical books, authors must attempt to make the information as current as possible. In a world in which medical therapies and recommendations can change rapidly, this task is not always easy. Nevertheless, authors must strive to update information through clinical experience, literature review, and discussion with colleagues. This we have done. Chapters have been rewritten, and the resultant products have been submitted to pediatricians who are "expert" in the respective areas. Bibliographies, for the most part, have been updated extensively. Certain sections have been expanded, such as that on HIV infection, and others have been shortened. Two new chapters, Common Behavioral Problems and School Health Issues, have been added to reflect the types of issues that pediatric house officers and practitioners must manage on a daily basis.

We are grateful to all who made the first two editions of *Pediatric Pearls* so successful. We hope this edition will be useful to the students, house officers, and practitioners responsible for the care of young patients, as well as for all the young people who are the recipients of their knowledge, skill, and caring.

ACKNOWLEDGMENTS

We are indebted to all of the chief residents of the Harriet Lane Home Outpatient Department, who nutured this project during its embryonic stages, and to Frank A. Oski, M.D. and Catherine DeAngelis, M.D. for their encouragement and support. We are grateful to a number of our colleagues, who reviewed sections of this edition of the handbook: Hoover Adger, James Casella, Bernard Cohen, Barbara Fivush, John Gearhart, Neal Halsey, Kenton Holden, Nancy Hutton, Alan Lake, Samuel Libber, Carol Marcus, Ambadas Pathak, Leslie Plotnick, Martin Pusic, Michael Repka, Saul Roskes, Peter Rowe, Kenneth Schuberth, Janet Serwint, Charles Shubin, David Tunkel, Eileen Vining, and Michele Wilson. Francine Cheese provided excellent secretarial support. Her ability to decipher and decode our corrections was a source of constant relief and amazement. We thank Michael Johns, M.D., Dean of The Johns Hopkins University School of Medicine, and James Block, M.D., President of The Johns Hopkins Hospital, for allowing us to use The Johns Hopkins Hospital logo on the cover. Last, but certainly not least, we thank Jenny McCartney, Sandra Clark Brown, Laura DeYoung, Jodi Willard, and their colleagues at Mosby–Year Book for their editorial, organizational, and moral support in bringing this project to completion.

Beryl J. Rosenstein, M.D.
Patricia D. Fosarelli, M.D.

CONTENTS

ABBREVIATIONS

ABD	Abdominal
ABG	Arterial blood gas
ABO	Blood groups
ACE	Angiotensin-converting enzyme
ACTH	Adrenocorticotropic hormone
ADD	Attention deficit disorder
ADHD	Attention deficit hyperactivity disorder
AFB	Acid-fast bacilli
AGN	Acute glomerulonephritis
AgNO$_3$	Silver nitrate
ALT	Alanine transferase (SGOT)
ALTE	Apparent life-threatening event
AN	Anorexia nervosa
ANA	Antinuclear antibody
ANC	Absolute neutrophil count
AOM	Acute otitis media
AP	Anteroposterior
ASA	Acetylsalicylic acid
ASAP	As soon as possible
ASO	Antistreptolysin-O
AST	Aspartate transferase
A-V	Atrioventricular
AV	Arteriovenous
AZT	Zidovudine
BAL	Dimercaprol
BC	Blood culture
bid	Twice a day
BM	Bowel movement
BN	Bulimia nervosa
BP	Blood pressure
BPD	Bronchopulmonary dysplasia
bpm	Beats per minute
BRATS	Banana, rice, applesauce, toast, saltines

BUN	Blood urea nitrogen
C	Centigrade
C3	Serum complement
Ca	Calcium
Ca:Cr	Calcium:creatinine
Calcium EDTA	Calcium disodium edetate
CBC	Complete blood count
cc	Cubic centimeter
CCB	Calcium channel blocker
CDC	Centers for Disease Control and Prevention
CF	Cystic fibrosis
CFU	Colony-forming unit
CHD	Congenital heart disease
CHF	Congestive heart failure
CIE	Counterimmunoelectrophoresis
cm	Centimeter
CMV	Cytomegalovirus
CNS	Central nervous system
CO	Carbon monoxide
CO$_2$	Carbon dioxide
Col	Colonies
CPAP	Continuous positive airway pressure
CPK	Creatine phosphokinase
CPR	Cardiopulmonary resuscitation
Cr	Creatinine
CRP	C-reactive protein
C&S	Culture and sensitivity
CSF	Cerebrospinal fluid
C-spine	Cervical spine
CT	Computed tomography
CV	Cardiovascular
CVA	Costovertebral angle
c/w	compared with
CXR	Chest x-ray
d	Day
D/C	Discontinue
DDAVP	Desmopressin
DDH	Developmental dysplasia of the hip
ddI	Dideoxyinosine
DEA	Drug Enforcement Agency
DIC	Disseminated intravascular coagulation

diff	Differential
DKA	Diabetic ketoacidosis
dL	Deciliter
DMSA	2,3-Dimercaptosuccinic acid
DMT	Dimethyltryptamine
DNA	Deoxyribonucleic acid
DNR	Do not resuscitate
DTaP	Diphtheria–tetanus–acellular pertussis
DTP	Diphtheria-tetanus-pertussis
DTR	Deep tendon reflex
D$_5$W	5% dextrose in water
D$_{25}$W	25% dextrose in water
Dx	Diagnosis
EBV	Epstein-Barr virus
ECG	Electrocardiogram
ECHO	Echocardiogram
ED	Emergency department
EDTA	Ethylenediaminetetraacetic acid
EEG	Electroencephalogram
ELISA	Enzyme-linked immunosorbent assay
EM	Erythema multiforme
ENT	Ear, nose, and throat
EOS	Eosinophils
EP	Erythrocyte protoporphyrin
ESR	Erythrocyte sedimentation rate
ET	Endotracheal
ETT	Endotracheal tube
F	Fahrenheit
FB	Foreign body
FDA	Food and Drug Administration
Fe	Iron
FEP	Free erythroctye protoporphyrin
FEV$_1$	Forced expiratory volume in 1 second
FHx	Family history
FSH	Follicle-stimulating hormone
FTA-ABS	Fluorescent treponemal antibody absorption (test)
FTT	Failure to thrive
F/U	Follow-up
Fx	Fracture
g	Gram
G−	Gram negative

GABHS	Group A β-hemolytic streptococcus
GC	Gonococcal
G-CSF	Granulocyte colony-stimulating factor
GE	Gastroenteritis
GER	Gastroesophageal reflux
GGT	Gamma-glutamyltransferase
GI	Gastrointestinal
GnRH	Gonadotropin-releasing hormone
G-6-PD	Glucose-6-phosphate dehydrogenase
gt	drop
gtt	drops
GU	Genitourinary
GYN	Gynecology
h	Hour
Hb A$_{1c}$	Glycosylated forms of hemoglobin that can be separated from the main Hgb fractions Hb A$_1$ and Hb A$_2$
HbCV	*Haemophilus influenzae* b conjugate vaccine
HBIG	Hepatitis B immune globulin
HBsAg	Hepatitis B surface antigen
HBV	Hepatitis B virus
HC	Head circumference
hCG	Human chorionic gonadotropin
HCO$_3$	Bicarbonate
Hct	Hematocrit
HDCV	Human diploid cell vaccine
HDL	High-density lipoprotein
HEENT	Head, eyes, ears, nose, and throat
Hg	Mercury
Hgb	Hemoglobin
HIB	*Haemophilus influenzae* type B
HIV	Human immunodeficiency virus
H/O	History of
H$_2$O$_2$	Hydrogen peroxide
H&P	History and physical
HPF	High-power field
HPV	Human papilloma virus
hr	Hour
HR	Heart rate
hs	At bedtime
HSP	Henoch-Schönlein purpura
HSV	Herpes simplex virus

HUS	Hemolytic-uremic syndrome
Hx	History
IBD	Inflammatory bowel disease
ICP	Intracranial pressure
I&D	Incision and drainage
IDDM	Insulin-dependent diabetes mellitus
IFA	Immunofluorescent antibody
IgA	Immunoglobulin A
IgG	Immunoglobulin G
IgM	Immunoglobulin M
IM	Intramuscular
INH	Isoniazid
IO	Intraosseus
I&O	Intake and output
IPV	Inactivated polio vaccine (Salk)
ITP	Immune thrombocytopenic purpura
IU	International unit
IUD	Intrauterine device
IV	Intravenous
IVIG	Intravenous immune globulin
IVP	Intravenous pyelogram
JRA	Juvenile rheumatoid arthritis
K	Potassium
Kcal	Kilocalories
KCl	Potassium chloride
KD	Kawasaki disease
KOH	Potassium hydroxide
KPO$_4$	Potassium phosphate
KS	Ketosteroid
kV	Kilovolt
LATS	Long-acting thyroid-stimulating hormone
LDH	Lactic (acid) dehydrogenase
LDL	Low-density lipoprotein
LET	Lidocaine, epinephrine, tetracaine
LFTs	Liver function tests
LH	Luteinizing hormone
LP	Lumbar puncture
LSD	Lysergic acid diethylamide
LTB	Laryngotracheobronchitis
max	Maximum
MCHC	Mean corpuscular hemoglobin concentration
MCV	Mean corpuscular volume

MDA	Methylenedioxyamphetamine
MDI	Metered dose inhaler
mEq	Milliequivalent
μg	Microgram
mg	Milligram
Mg	Magnesium
min	Minute
mm	Millimeter
MMR	Measles-mumps-rubella
mo	Month
Monos	Mononuclear cells
MRI	Magnetic resonance imaging
Na	Sodium
NAC	N-acetyl-L-cysteine
NaHCO$_3$	Sodium bicarbonate
Neg	Negative
NF	Neurofibromatosis
NG	Nasogastric
NH$_3$	Ammonia
NH$_4$	Ammonium
NIDDM	Non–insulin-dependent diabetes mellitus
NP	Nasopharyngeal
NPO	Nothing by mouth
NSAID	Nonsteroidal antiinflammatory drug
NTM	Nontuberculous mycobacteria
O$_2$	Oxygen
OCD	Obsessive-compulsive disorder
OGES	Oral glucose-electrolyte solution
25-OH-D	25-Hydroxyvitamin D
OM	Otitis media
OME	Otitis media with effusion
OPV	Oral polio vaccine (Sabin)
OR	Operating room
OTC	Over-the-counter (drug)
oz	Ounce
P	Phosphorus
PA	Posteroanterior
Pb	Lead
PCA	Patient-controlled analgesia
Pco$_2$	Partial pressure of carbon dioxide
PCP	Phencyclidine

PCR	Polymerase chain reaction
PE	Physical examination
PEFR	Peak expiratory flow rate
PET	Positron emission topography
PID	Pelvic inflammatory disease (salpingitis)
PMI	Point of maximal impulse
PMNs	Polymorphonuclear cells
PO	By mouth
PO$_2$	Partial pressure of oxygen
PO$_4$	Phosphate
PPD	Purified protein derivative
PPD-B	Purified protein derivative–Battey
prn	As needed
PTSD	Post–traumatic stress disorder
pt	Patient
PT	Prothrombin time
PTT	Partial thromboplastin time
PUD	Peptic ulcer disease
PVC	Premature ventricular contraction
q	Every
qd	Once a day
qid	Four times a day
qxh	Every "x" hours
RA	Rheumatoid arthritis
RAIU	Radioactive iodine uptake
RAST	Radioallergosorbent test
RBC	Red blood cell
RDW	Red cell distribution width
RE	Racemic epinephrine
REM	Rapid eye movement
RF	Rheumatic fever
RIA	Radioimmunoassay
RIG	Rabies immune globulin
RLQ	Right lower quadrant
RMSF	Rocky Mountain spotted fever
R/O	Rule out
RPR	Rapid plasma reagin
RR	Respiratory rate
RSV	Respiratory syncytial virus
RTA	Renal tubular acidosis
RUQ	Right upper quadrant

RVA	Rabies vaccine adsorbed
Rx	Prescription, drugs, medication
SaO$_2$	Oxygen percent saturation (arterial)
SBE	Subacute bacterial endocarditis
SBI	Serious bacterial infection
SCFE	Slipped capital femoral epiphysis
SIADH	Syndrome of inappropriate antidiuretic hormone
SIDS	Sudden infant death syndrome
Sig	Directions
SJS	Stevens-Johnson syndrome
SLE	Systemic lupus erythematosus
SMA	Sequential multiple analyzer
SOB	Shortness of breath
SOM	Serous otitis media
S/P	Status post
spec. gr.	Specific gravity
SQ	Subcutaneous
SS	Sickle cell
S&S	Signs/symptoms
SSD	Sickle-cell disease
STD	Sexually transmitted disease
STS	Serologic test for syphillis
Sx	Symptoms
T	Temperature
T$_3$	Triiodothyronine
T$_4$	Free thyroxine
T&A	Tonsillectomy and adenoidectomy
TAC	Tetracine, adrenaline, and cocaine
TAR	Thrombocytopenia, absent radii
TB	Tuberculosis
TC	Throat culture
3TC	Lamivudine
TCA	Tricyclic antidepressant
TEF	Tracheoesophaeal fistula
THC	Tetrahydrocannabinol
TIBC	Total iron-binding capacity
tid	Three times a day
TM	Tympanic membrane
TMP/SMZ	Trimethoprim-sulfamethoxazole
TORCH	Toxoplasmosis, other (viruses), rubella, cytomegalovirus, herpes simplex virus

TPN	Total parenteral nutrition
TRH	Thyroid-releasing hormone
Trich	*Trichomonas*
TSH	Thyroid-stimulating hormone
tsp	Teaspoon
Tx	Treatment
U	Unit
U/A	Urinalysis
URI	Upper respiratory infection
US	Ultrasound
UTI	Urinary tract infection
VCUG	Voiding cystourethrogram
VDRL	Venereal Disease Research Laboratory
VGE	Viral gastroenteritis
VP	Ventriculoperitoneal
vs	Versus
VZIG	Varicella-zoster immune globulin
WBC	White blood cell
WHO	World Health Organization
w/u	Work-up
yr	Year
ZnPP	Zinc protoporphyrin
1°	Primary
2°	Secondary
$\approx$	Approximately
$\geq$	Equal to or greater than
$\leq$	Equal to or less than

GENERAL APPROACH TO THE PATIENT

1

A. HISTORY

1. A careful, pertinent, and thorough history is an essential first step in understanding any patient's problem(s). In addition to the chief complaint and the present illness, explore the patient's past medical history, past and current medications (including nonprescription medications), immunizations, hospitalizations, prior surgery, transfusions, previous major illnesses and accidents, recent exposures, family history, social situation, and sources of medical care. Record this information so that it is both available and useful in the future. Be sure to talk to the person most knowledgeable about the patient's history.
2. Be alert for "the hidden diagnosis"; the patient's or family's complaint may have little or nothing to do with the actual problem. Try to determine what is really troubling the patient and/or the family; open-ended questions may be especially helpful.

EXAMPLE: Chief complaint: Stomach pains
Actual diagnosis: School phobia or sexual abuse

3. Also include the following in the history:
   a. Patient's address and phone number (or nearest phone)
   b. Parent's or guardian's name
   c. Names and addresses of other physicians from whom and clinics in which the patient receives medical care

B. PHYSICAL EXAMINATION

1. Obtain weight, length, and vital signs (temperature, HR, respiratory rate; BP in children and adolescents); determine head circumference, if appropriate (e.g., in an infant or toddler).
2. The PE should include pertinent positive and negative findings. Do not limit the exam to the organ system that is the basis for the chief complaint. Carefully observe the child to ascertain the degree of discomfort (if any) experienced during the exam. Ascertaining the

degree of discomfort is especially important when the diagnosis is uncertain or when the chronicity/reported severity of the child's symptoms does not match the physical appearance of the child. Be sure to describe the child's appearance in your charting. Terms such as "well-developed, well-nourished white female" might not completely describe the child's "true" appearance. For example, was she happy or sad? Did she look her age or older? Younger? Was she cooperative with you? With her parent? Did she seem to understand your directives during the exam? Was she clean or soiled? Remember, your description might be of great use to the *next* person who examines the child; therefore be as complete as possible.

Depending on a child's degree of emotional or physical discomfort, examining a child is sometimes quite difficult. Therefore it is important to explain what you will be doing as you proceed or in response to questions. In the long run, a hurried attitude hurts the examiner, the patient, and the parent. Sometimes children need to be distracted during the exam so that they do not "help" (e.g., during the assessment of the patellar tendon reflex) or "hinder" (e.g., during the examination of the lungs or heart when silence is needed). Patience and a gentle explanation of what is needed usually secure better conditions for true assessments, especially with children older than toddlers. For the child to relax sufficiently, the exam at times needs to be performed while the child is sitting on a parent's lap or while holding the child's hand; so be it. If the child starts to cry during the course of the exam or feels uncomfortable with what is happening, that part of the exam should not be forced at that time *unless it is truly an emergency.*

The child's feelings and concerns should always be heard and respected. There might be major reasons (of which you are unaware) why the child does not want a certain procedure to be performed. For example, a child who screams and cries when the examiner attempts to visualize the genitalia might be reliving an abusive situation. Therefore be sensitive to what is communicated both verbally and nonverbally. Do not be afraid to back off or to get assistance when needed.

The older child and adolescent should be asked if he or she prefers the parent to be in or out of the room during the exam. Respect the patient's wishes. If the parent is not in the room, a chaperon should be present when the genitalia are being examined, regardless of whether the patient is male or female.

C. LABORATORY

1. Order only those tests that will affect patient management. A costly work-up is not indicated every time a diagnosis is uncertain. It is imperative to follow up on the results. Failure to do so is not good medical practice and may leave the examiner open to legal action if a test result dictates a certain action that is not taken because the examiner is unaware of the result.
2. In this book the suggested laboratory tests for each discussed entity are presented. If you promise to notify the parent (or patient) of the test results, make sure that you do so in a timely fashion, and document the communication.

MEDICAL ASSESSMENT BY TELEPHONE

A. GENERAL PRINCIPLES

1. Identify yourself.
2. Request identification of the child, the caller, and the caller's relationship to the child.
3. Ascertain the child's age and approximate weight.
4. Listen to the parent's story.
5. When asking questions, wait for the answer to one question before going on to the next one.
6. Remain courteous and calm (even if the parent is neither).
7. Avoid using ambiguous or medical terms that might confuse the parent.
8. Identify the child's problem to your satisfaction before rendering advice; plainly state what you believe the problem to be.
9. If the child does not need to be seen, explain why not and give the parent specific therapies to try; give advice on what to do if these measures fail.
10. Instruct the parent on the symptoms that are part of the natural course of the illness and those that warn of a worsening condition. Indicate which symptoms warrant medical attention.
11. Ask the parent to repeat any instructions you have given, and ask whether there are any questions.
12. Encourage the parent to call back if he or she has questions or if the child's condition changes.
13. Follow up on any child who has symptoms that concern you (do not depend on the parent to call back). If the family has no phone, obtain the phone number of a relative or friend.

14. It is advisable to briefly document the content of all calls, but it is imperative to document calls when a medication (prescription or OTC) is ordered or when the parent is urged to bring the child to medical attention.

B. SPECIAL PRINCIPLES FOR THE MOST COMMON PROBLEMS PRESENTING BY PHONE

(Modified from DeAngelis C: *Pediatric primary care,* ed 3, Boston, 1984, Little, Brown.)

1. Respiratory complaints
   a. Does the child have a cold? Is it getting better or worse? In what way?
   b. Has the child been febrile? How high was his or her temperature?
   c. What medications (how much, for how long, and how often) have been used for the fever and the cold?
   d. Does the child have a cough? Is there vomiting with it?
   e. Does the child have a runny nose? What color is the nasal discharge?
   f. Does the child seem to breathe more noisily than usual?
   g. When the child breathes, can you see his or her ribs?
   h. Is any area of the body blue?
   i. Do the nostrils move with each breath?
   j. Can the parent count the child's breaths? (If the parent does not have a watch with a second hand, he or she can count out loud while you time the breaths.)
   k. Is there a hoarse cry or barky cough?
   l. Is there a rash?
   m. Is the child vomiting or having diarrhea?
   n. How is the child's appetite, sleeping, and activity?
   o. What is the child doing now?
2. Fever
   a. Did the parent take the child's temperature, or did he or she just feel warm?
   b. What was the temperature? Rectal, oral, axillary, or aural?
   c. Has the child been given medicine to reduce the temperature? Which one, how much, and how often? When was the last dose?
   d. Does the temperature seem to come down with the medicine?
   e. What else have you tried to make the child better?
   f. What other signs of illness are there (e.g., respiratory problems, rash)?
   g. How is the child acting, sleeping, and eating?

    h. Has the child received a shot? What type? When?

    i. Does the child seem to be in pain? How so?

    j. Are any of the child's contacts ill?

3. Dermatologic problems

    a. How long has the child had the rash, and where did it first appear?

    b. Where is the rash now? Is it on the palms and soles?

    c. What color is the rash, and how large are the individual spots?

    d. Can the parent feel the rash as well as see it?

    e. Does it disappear with pressure?

    f. Does any part of the rash have blisters or crusts?

    g. Does the rash itch, burn, or hurt?

    h. Has the child had a similar rash in the past?

    i. Has he or she been around anyone else with a similar rash?

    j. What other signs of illness does the child have?

    k. How is he or she eating, sleeping, and playing?

    l. Does he or she have a high temperature?

    m. Has the child recently taken or is the child currently taking any medications? Which ones?

4. Trauma

    a. What type of injury did the child sustain (e.g., fall, laceration, burn, bite)? How and when did it occur? To which body part was the injury sustained?

    b. If the child struck his or her head, did he or she lose consciousness, vomit, or have a seizure after the episode? How is the child acting now? If another body part was injured, is he or she using it normally now? What has the parent done?

    c. If the child sustained a laceration, is he or she still bleeding? How large is the laceration? Is the blood bright red and spurting? What has the parent done to stop the bleeding? What is the child doing now? When was the child's last tetanus shot?

    d. If the child was burned, what part of the body was burned? How large an area is involved? Is there an area of redness or are there blisters? Have the blisters broken? Does the child complain of pain at the burn site? What has the parent done for the burn? How is the child acting? When was the child's last tetanus shot?

    e. If the child was bitten, what bit the child? If the bite is from a dog, is the dog known to the family? Has it been behaving abnormally? Has it had its shots? Was the dog provoked? If the bite is from a wild animal, what type of animal was it? When was the child's last tetanus shot? What has the parent done? How does the area look? How is the child acting? Has the animal been captured?

5. Gastrointestinal complaints
   a. Is the child experiencing diarrhea, vomiting, or both?
   b. How long have these symptoms been occurring?
   c. If the child is vomiting, is he or she merely coughing up phlegm, spitting up after feeding, or actually vomiting?
   d. When does the vomiting occur in relation to meals?
   e. Can the child eat certain foods without vomiting? Which ones?
   f. Can the child drink anything without vomiting?
   g. Could the child have accidentally ingested a household product or medication?
   h. Does the vomiting occur forcefully or effortlessly?
   i. Does the child seem hungry or in pain?
   j. How many bowel movements has the child had today? Yesterday?
   k. How many times has the child vomited today? Yesterday?
   l. Is the vomitus or stool red or green?
   m. What does the stool look like? Does it have any formed elements in it?
   n. Is the child taking any medication?
   o. What has the parent done for the illness, including dietary and medicinal regimens?
   p. Is the illness getting better or worse?
   q. Is the child's mouth wet?
   r. Has the child been urinating the usual number of times and in the usual amounts?
   s. What other signs of illness are present (e.g., rash, respiratory symptoms)?
   t. Has the child had a fever? How high was the temperature?
   u. How well is the child sleeping?
   v. How is the child's appetite for foods and liquids?
   w. What liquids and foods has the parent given to the child today? How were they tolerated?
   x. How is the child's activity?
   y. Do any of the child's contacts have similar complaints?
   z. What is the child doing now?

THERAPEUTICS

A. MEDICATIONS
1. Consider the following: whether the drug is really indicated, what therapeutic effects to expect, side effects (may differ according to age of patient), half-life, dosage, cost (use the generic form when

possible), interactions with other drugs (e.g., erythromycin and
theophylline), and the risk of poisoning.
2. Consider the most appropriate form of administration (e.g., tablet,
   capsule, liquid, suppository).
3. Consider frequency and periodicity of administration (qid generally
   means 8 AM, noon, 4 PM, and 8 PM; q6h is 8 AM, 2 PM, 8 PM, and 2 AM).
   Simplify regimens as much as possible and make them convenient
   with school, sleep, and other activities.
4. Arrange to follow blood levels when necessary (e.g., anticonvulsant
   and theophylline).
5. Consider compliance of the patient and family. Compliance decreases
   as the number of medications increases and when specified times for
   administration are inconvenient.
6. Teach the parent or patient about the indications, effects, and side
   effects of the medication; how to administer and accurately measure
   it; and how to prevent inadvertent overdosing.
   a. Have the patient or parent repeat what you have stated.
   b. Special instructions should always be written.
   c. Explain to the parent that the medication must be taken for the full
      course, even if the symptoms disappear in several days.
7. Document that you have explained to the parent or patient the action
   and any common side effects of the drug. In addition, document any
   adverse drug effects reported by the parent or patient and report them,
   if applicable, to the FDA.

B. PRESCRIPTIONS
1. Be sure that the patient is able (i.e., has the money, time, or
   transportation) to get the prescription filled.
2. Write legibly. Not only is it inconsiderate to write illegibly, it is also
   potentially dangerous if prescriptions are filled incorrectly. If you
   cannot write well, print. Use only standard abbreviations.
3. Include all pertinent information.
   a. Patient's name, address, age
   b. Name and form of the drug (e.g., tablet, liquid, capsule); dosage or
      concentration (e.g., 500 mg tablet, 500 mg/5 ml, 250 mg/5 ml)
   c. The amount to dispense, such as the number of tablets, amount
      of liquid. Remember, some medications come in "standard"
      amounts (e.g., 150 ml); it might cost the parent *more* if the
      pharmacist must "break" the bottle to comply with your prescrip-
      tion (e.g., the medication comes in a standard size of 150 ml and
      you prescribe 130 ml). Pharmacists' policies seem to vary in this

     regard; know what the pharmacists in your area do in such situations.

    d. Directions (Sig) such as amount, frequency, route, and duration (e.g., 5 ml q4h PO × 7 days). Do not use teaspoon measures.

    e. Whether a refill is necessary (and how many times) or no refill

    f. Do not forget signature and DEA number if a controlled substance is prescribed.

4. Include all prescription data (name of drug, form, dosing regimen, and amount dispensed) in the patient's medical record.

C. COUNSELING PATIENT AND FAMILY

1. Counseling is *essential* for physician and patient rapport. It improves communication and understanding of the illness, improves compliance with follow-up and medication, alleviates fears and misconceptions, and prevents mismanagement at home. The patient and family will also know what to expect and when to return if certain signs or symptoms develop. Nurses can teach temperature measurement/management and review the physician's instructions with the patient or parent.

2. In general it is better to contact the family for telephone follow-up than to expect them to call you. Arrange a time when and a number where they can be reached. Keep track of patients in need of telephone contact so that such patients do not fall through the cracks.

D. DOCUMENTATION

1. Be sure to document adequately and legibly the results of the history and PE, the laboratory tests ordered, the test results, clinical impression(s), the therapeutic modalities suggested, and medications prescribed or OTC medications recommended. Also document when a return visit or telephone follow-up is necessary.

2. Although documentation seems like a great deal of work (it is), it assists the next person who sees the patient and can be a saving grace if litigation is threatened.

BIBLIOGRAPHY

Jellinik M et al: The difficult parent—and the difficult physician, *Contemp Pediatr,* 8:118, Jan 1991.
Jellinik M et al: Coping with the truly difficult parent, *Contemp Pediatr,* 8:19, Feb 1991.

Katz H: *Telephone manual of pediatric care,* New York, 1982, John Wiley & Sons.

Korsch B: What do patients and parents want to know? What do they need to know? *Pediatrics* 74(suppl):917, 1984.

Korsch B: Do you know these patients: high-risk pediatric encounters, *Pediatr Rev* 10:101, 1988.

Schmitt B: *Pediatric telephone advice,* Boston, 1980, Little, Brown.

CARDIOPULMONARY RESUSCITATION

2

M. Douglas Baker

A. ALPHABET OF RESUSCITATION (ABCDE)

NOTE: Most pediatric arrests are primarily pulmonary events.

1. **A**irway: Airway obstruction is commonly the precipitating event in a pediatric cardiopulmonary arrest. Clear the oropharynx of secretions and vomitus (use large-bore suctioning); this procedure should not be done blindly. Open the airway using the chin-lift or jaw-thrust technique. In general and especially in the traumatized child, maintain in-line C-spine; *do not* hyperextend the neck. An oral or nasal airway may be inserted to prevent the tongue from obstructing the airway. The tip of the oral airway should just approximate the angle of the mandible. The preferred nasal airway should measure in length from the nostril to the tragus of the ear.

2. **B**reathing: With the exception of total airway obstruction (which occurs with foreign body aspiration and some anatomic abnormalities), any child may be effectively ventilated via the bag-valve-mask technique. This technique should be used until the placement of an ETT is feasible. ETT size approximates the width of the patient's little fingernail (Table 2-1).

   Watch the chest for good expansion; note any improvement in perfusion and pulses. The patient's trachea should be intubated if the bag-valve-mask technique is insufficient or if adequate and spontaneous respirations cannot be maintained. Muscle relaxants may be needed to intubate and are discussed later in this chapter. Assess the lungs after intubation for equal breath sounds bilaterally, and assess the adequacy of ventilation and perfusion. Pulse oximetry can be very helpful.

TABLE 2-1.
Endotracheal Tube Size

Newborn, 3.0–3.5 mm (internal diameter)

$$\text{Tube diameter (mm)} = \frac{\text{age (yr)} + 16}{4}$$

TABLE 2-2.
Guidelines for Cardiopulmonary Resuscitation

	Newborn	Child	Adult
Compression (rate/min)	120	100	80
Depth of compression (in)	½–1	1–1½	1½–2
Ventilation (rate/min)	20	16	12

3. Circulation (Table 2-2)
   a. Make sure a firm board is under the chest for effective closed-chest cardiac massage.
   b. Give one breath per 4-5 compressions (ratio remains the same regardless of age or size).
   c. The time of compression = time uncompressed for best cardiac output.
   d. Synchronize compressions with respirations (ventilate as compression is released).
   e. Compressions should be applied evenly over the midsternum; the proper placement for compressions is one fingerbreadth below where the transnipple line intersects the sternum.
   f. Check the efficacy of CPR. Palpate peripheral pulses (femoral, brachial, carotid) while pumping. Assess perfusion (capillary refill should be <2 seconds). Assess ventilation. Assess pupil reactivity.
4. Drugs
   a. It is essential to know the indications, effects, and dosages of a few first-line resuscitation drugs. These drugs are listed in Table 2-3 and in *The Harriet Lane Handbook*, ed. 14. You do not need to wait for an ECG or arterial blood gas results before giving drugs. Establish good vascular access as soon as possible. Peripheral access remains the first-line approach. However, in the sickest patients such access might be difficult to achieve. If a percutaneous venous line cannot be established quickly (within 2 minutes), consider alternate routes

TABLE 2-3.
First-Line Resuscitation Drugs

Drug	Indication	Effect	Dose
Epinephrine	Asystole, ventricular fibrillation, bradycardia, normovolemic hypotension	+ Inotropic, + chronotropic; may convert fine ventricular fibrillation to coarse ventricular fibrillation; may enhance chance of successful cardioversion; less effective in presence of severe metabolic acidosis	For asystole: First IV/IO dose: 0.01 mg/kg (0.1 ml/kg of 1:10,000) Subsequent IV/IO doses: 0.1 mg/kg (0.1 ml/kg of 1:1000) All ET doses: 0.1 mg/kg (0.1 ml/kg of 1:1000) For bradycardia: First IV/IO dose: 0.01 mg/kg (0.1 ml/kg of 1:10,000) Subsequent IV/IO doses: May repeat first dose, double, or increase All ET doses: 0.1 mg/kg (0.1 ml/kg of 1:1000)
$NaHCO_3$	Metabolic acidosis	↑ pH (with adequate ventilation); ↑ P_{CO_2} (with inadequate ventilation)	1 mEq/kg IV slowly (1 ml/kg);dilute standard 1 mEq/ml solution in half in newborn; give only after establishing adequate ventilation **Adult dose:** 1–2 amp (44 mEq/ amp); NOTE: be sure to clear IV line of $NaHCO_3$ because epinephrine and calcium are inactivated in alkaline solutions; do *not* give via endotracheal tube

Continued.

TABLE 2-3. (cont.)

Drug	Indication	Effect	Dose
Calcium (10% calcium chloride)	Hypocalcemia, hyperkalemia, hypermagnesemia, calcium channel blocker excess	↑ Myocardial contractility, counteracts K toxic effects, bradycardia	10–20 mg/kg or 0.1–0.25 ml/kg IV *slowly* (preferably through central line) **Adult dose:** 10 ml; remember to clear IV line of $NaHCO_3$ ($NaHCO_3$ + Ca = chalk)
Atropine	Sinus bradycardia, atrioventricular block, preintubation	Decreases vagal tone, increases conduction through AV node	0.02 mg/kg, min dose 0.1 mg, max dose 2 mg or 0.04 mg/kg (whichever is smaller); NOTE: insufficient dose may cause paradoxical bradycardia; may be given by endotracheal tube at same IV dose
Lidocaine	Ventricular fibrillation, ventricular tachycardia, premature ventricular contractions	↓ Automaticity and ectopic pacemakers	Concentration 2% (20 mg/ml) 1.0 mg/kg bolus IV (0.05 ml/kg) followed by continuous infusion of 10–50 μg/kg/min; may be given by endotracheal tube at same IV bolus dose

NOTE: All drugs given IV may be given intraosseously (IO) at the same doses.

(e.g., intraosseous [proximal tibial], central line via the Seldinger technique, central line via cutdown).

NOTE: The following four drugs may be given via an ETT:

    Lidocaine   Naloxone
    Atropine   Epinephrine

NOTE: Endotracheal doses of lidocaine, atropine, and naloxone are the same as IV/intraosseous doses. However, the ET dose of epinephrine is 10 times the IV/intraosseous dose.

b. Other drugs
   1) Glucose: Indicated for documented hypoglycemia; best administered as a 5 ml/kg bolus of 10% dextrose. A bolus of D_{25} (2 ml/kg) can be used but may result in rebound hypoglycemia if not followed by glucose infusion.
   2) Naloxone (Narcan): Narcotic antidote; dosage is 0.1 mg/kg/ dose q2-3min. Many physicians give a standard 1-2 mg dose to all ages. Drug may be given endotracheally at the same dose.
   3) Dopamine: Has many effects that are dose dependent (see the following points). Before using dopamine, expand intravascular volume in shock states secondary to hypovolemia.
      a) Dosage
         (1) Low dosage: 1-7 µg/kg/min; increases renal blood flow
         (2) Moderate dosage: 7-20 µg/kg/min; promotes vasoconstriction; increases cardiac output and blood pressure
         (3) High dosage: 20-30 µg/kg/min; systemic vasoconstriction; decreases renal blood flow
      b) Toxicity: Minimal at reasonable dosages
         (1) Tachyarrhythmias and excessively high BP occur.
         (2) Avoid extravasation and resultant local vasoconstriction.
         (3) Do not administer in alkaline solutions.
   4) Isoproterenol infusion
      a) Indications
         (1) Status asthmaticus unresponsive to other measures
         (2) Bradycardia unresponsive to other measures; preferred drug for patients with bradycardia accompanied by heart block
      b) Effects of isoproterenol on CV system: ↑ HR, ↑ myocardial contractility (resulting in ↑ myocardial oxygen demand), ↑ arterial and venous vasodilation; contraindicated in ischemic heart disease (including aortic stenosis) and in patients with hypovolemia
      c) Dosage
         (1) Starting dosage: 0.1 µg/kg/min, titrated to 1.0 µg/kg/min
         (2) Dosage may be further increased by 0.1 µg/kg/min q15min until improvement or toxicity; usual maximum dosage 1.5 µg/kg/min
      d) Caution: Establish two IV lines when initiating isoproterenol infusions in patients with asthma. The abrupt cessation of this drug (such as occurs with IV malfunction) may result in a

quick return of severe bronchospasm. Isoproterenol also increases myocardial oxygen consumption, which may be dangerous if Po_2 <60.

    e) Toxicity: HR exceeds baseline by 40 bpm; arrhythmia or ST-segment changes are present.

   5) Bretylium and dobutamine: Refer to *The Harriet Lane Handbook*, ed. 14, and to *Pediatr Clin North Am* 27(3):495, 1980.

5. ECG: Observe rhythms and complexes.

   a. Defibrillation: Use in ventricular fibrillation. Place one paddle to the right of the upper sternum and below the clavicle; place the other paddle to the left of the left nipple in the anterior axillary line; or place the paddles on the chest and back directly over the heart.

   b. Dosage: If <50 kg, 2 W/sec/kg; if >50 kg, 200 W/sec. If a single shock is not effective, continue cardiac massage, then repeat the shock at double power. If not effective, give three shocks in succession, then epinephrine, shock, lidocaine, shock, bretylium, shock, bretylium, shock, lidocaine.

   c. Cardioversion: This technique is the same as defibrillation but in a synchronized mode and with reduced dosage (0.5-1 W/sec/kg).

B. ORGANIZATION

1. One person to direct and monitor (oversees entire procedure)
2. One person to oxygenate and ventilate; establish and maintain airway/nasogastric tube
3. One person for cardiac massage
4. One or two people to establish venous access and draw blood studies
5. One person to prepare medications
6. One person to record medications, procedures, and pertinent occurrences
7. One person to get equipment, supplies, and other personnel if needed
8. Total of seven or eight on arrest team. *Keep unnecessary people out of the way.*

C. MUSCLE RELAXANTS

1. Indications: Need to intubate in the face of increased muscle tone, seizures, or a struggling patient with respiratory failure
2. Drugs: First atropine 0.02 mg/kg (minimum 0.15 mg) to block vagal effects of succinylcholine, then succinylcholine 1-2 mg/kg

   a. Fasciculation with paralysis occurs within 30 seconds and lasts for a few minutes.

b. If worried about aspiration during fasciculation (e.g., recent meal), give a desfasciculating dosage of pancuronium (Pavulon) 0.01 mg/kg before administering succinylcholine; apply cricoid pressure while intubating.

c. During elective intubation in a conscious patient, may "obtund" the patient with thiopental 2-4 mg/kg before administering succinylcholine; thiopental should not be given to any patient who is hypotensive.

d. An alternative combination for patients suspected of having intracranial disease includes the following: atropine 0.02 mg/kg, lidocaine 1 mg/kg, thiopental 2-4 mg/kg, vecuronium 0.1 mg/kg. For patients with hypotension, a benzodiazepine can be substituted for thiopental.

WARNING! Succinylcholine is contraindicated in hyperkalemic states (e.g., burns, glaucoma, penetrating ocular injuries) and at times in the presence of severe increased intracranial pressure. Beware of muscle relaxants in patients with an upper airway obstruction.

BIBLIOGRAPHY

Brill JE: Cardiopulmonary resuscitation, *Pediatr Ann* 15:24, 1986.

Holbrook PR et al: Cardiovascular resuscitation drugs for children, *Crit Care Med* 8:588, 1980.

Nugent S et al: Pharmacology and use of muscle relaxants in infants and children, *J Pediatr* 94:481, 1979.

Orlowski JP: Cardiopulmonary resuscitation in children, *Pediatr Clin North Am* 27:495, 1980.

Perkin RM, Anas NG: Cardiovascular evaluation and support in the critically ill child, *Pediatr Ann* 15:30, 1986.

Stanksi D, Sheiner L: Pharmacokinetics and dynamics of muscle relaxants, *Anesthesiology* 51:103, 1979.

Stewart RD, Lacovery DC: Administration of endotracheal medications, *Ann Emerg Med* 14:136, 1985.

ABUSE 3

A. CHILD ABUSE

1. Abuse may be active (physical, sexual, psychologic) or passive (physical, emotional, medical, or educational neglect). Physical injury is the easiest to discern; psychologic injury is the hardest.

2. If there is suspicion that a child has been abused, health-care providers are *legally* required to report it to the proper authorities (usually Social Services). Remember, the abused child is being reported to safeguard him or her and other at-risk children from further harm.

3. Always supplement medical input with input from social workers, when available. Social workers have expertise in interviewing skills that permits them to discover information that might otherwise remain hidden.

4. Approach the person accompanying the child in a nonjudgmental fashion. Ask open, not leading, questions. Do not demonstrate personal prejudices, anger, or disgust. Be as compassionate as possible.

5. If the child has an injury, determine whether the explanation for the injury fits the injury and the child's physical condition and developmental level. If it does, the injury *could* have happened that way; if it does not, the injury *could not* have happened that way.
   a. Was there a delay in seeking medical therapy? Why?
   b. Who was supervising the child at the time of the injury?
   c. Has the child sustained burns, lacerations, head trauma, or fractures in the past? If yes, when and what caused these injuries?

6. Determine the child's health status and the family's living conditions.
   a. Where does the child receive well-child care?
   b. Determine whether the child has a chronic medical condition.
   c. To what support systems does the family have access?
   d. Are the parents employed? Do they have sufficient money for food, clothing, and shelter?
   e. How many persons live with the child?

   f. How many siblings does the child have? What are their ages? Do they live with the child?

7. Determine the child's psychosocial milieu.
   a. Was the child planned?
   b. Who are the child's usual caregivers? Is he or she in day care? If yes, which one?
   c. What is the child's best characteristic? Worst characteristic?
   d. What does the child do that merits discipline? How is he or she usually disciplined?
   e. Does domestic violence occur? Against whom?
   f. Do any family members have difficulty with alcohol or drug abuse? Who?
   g. If the child is older than 2 years of age, is he or she toilet trained? If yes, does he or she ever have accidents? If yes, how is he or she treated after such episodes?

NOTE: Many children are abused in conjunction with toilet training, incontinence, meal battles, and sleep problems.

8. While performing the PE, look for both overt and subtle signs of abuse.
   a. Is the child clean or dirty?
   b. Fearful or calm?
   c. Clingy or aggressive?
   d. Verbal or silent?
   e. Does the child make eye contact with his or her parent? With the examiner?
   f. Does the child want to be held by the parent, or does the child prefer to go to the examiner? How does the parent react to the child's cries or requests?

NOTE: Psychologically abused children may be timid or may be aggressive; both behaviors relate to their poor self-image. Neglected children may actually prefer the examiner to their parents.

9. A *thorough* PE is performed; particular attention should be given to the following:
   a. Skin markings: Lacerations, burns, ecchymoses, linear contusions (could have been made with items such as belts or straps), contusions with definite shapes (e.g., coat hangers, belt buckles), circular contusions on trunk or limbs (may indicate finger pressure points), bites, and other markings
   b. Oral trauma: Torn frenulum (often a result of forced bottle feeding or pacifier insertion in an infant or toddler), contused gums, loose teeth (could result from a blow to the mouth)

c. Nasal trauma

d. Ear trauma

e. Eye trauma: Hyphema, periorbital hematomas, hemorrhage. Check fundi for retinal hemorrhages.

f. Chest injuries

g. Blunt abdominal trauma

h. Genital trauma (see Section B)

i. Limb trauma: Asymmetries, fractures, dislocations, inability to walk, and other signs of trauma

j. Head trauma: Hematomas, lacerations, deformities. Document positive and negative findings.

k. Growth parameters (plot on growth curves)

10. Laboratory tests should be dictated by the history and physical findings.

    a. A U/A is indicated if there is evidence of acute genital, abdominal, or back trauma.

    b. Evidence of active bleeding, ecchymoses, or blunt abdominal trauma suggests a CBC with platelets and clotting studies.

    c. Deformed or tender limbs, tender ribs, and abdominal, head, or chest trauma dictate x-ray examinations. Trauma surveys (to determine past or occult fractures) are useful mainly in preverbal children and mentally limited patients and should be performed in children younger than 3 years of age who have suspected physical abuse.

11. Photographs (labeled with the date, patient name, and photographer name) of suspicious skin markings should be obtained and included in the medical record.

12. The child's disposition should be based on both medical and social concerns.

    a. Children with moderate-to-severe injuries, unstable neurologic or cardiovascular exam results, or acute psychologic disturbances should be admitted.

    b. When a child is not admitted, a decision must be made regarding where he or she may be discharged. If the suspected abuser lives with the child, the child might be sent to another relative or to foster care. If the suspected abuser does not live with the child, the child might be sent home with the parent. Immediate placement is made by the social service agency; ultimate placement is at the discretion of the judicial system.

    c. Siblings and other children exposed to the alleged abuser should also be promptly examined and removed from the home, if necessary; in such a case, solicit social service and/or police assistance.

B. SEXUAL ABUSE

1. Sexual abuse entails actively or passively engaging a child in masturbation, fondling, voyeurism, pornography, or oral, anal, or genital intercourse. The use of bribes, gifts, or compliments to engage a young child in sexual acts should be regarded as forced sexual abuse.

2. A social worker should always be involved at the onset of the evaluation. Some communities have designated sexual assault and rape centers. If the patient is in no other medical distress and if the rape, genital trauma, or sexual assault is recent (<72 hours), he or she should go to one of these centers under a police escort for evaluation. If the patient is too unstable for referral, perform a complete evaluation and therapy at the hospital.

3. Careful documentation is mandatory and includes a detailed history of the event written as quotations of the parent or, if appropriate, in the patient's words.
   a. Who is the alleged assailant?
   b. When and where did the episode occur?
   c. Did penile or other penetration occur?
   d. Did other trauma occur? What was it?
   e. Who (name and relationship) is now accompanying the patient?
   f. Obtaining an accurate history may be difficult, and disclosure might not be immediate. Children may be afraid to reveal the details or the assailant's name.

4. A complete PE is necessary. Place special emphasis on the oral, perineal, and anal areas for signs of old or new trauma, pharyngitis, mouth lesions, urethral or vaginal discharge, patulous anus, anal discharge or lesions, or a tender rectum. A careful skin exam is also necessary.
   a. Document positive findings with properly labeled photographs or drawings.
   b. Record the appearance of the hymenal opening in a prepubertal child. Applying toluidine blue dye may facilitate the detection of hymenal ring defects or small perineal lacerations, especially if done within 24 hours of the assault. Do not force an exam in a frightened or uncooperative patient; consider the use of sedation or referral.

c. An exam by an experienced examiner (perhaps with the child under sedation or anesthesia) may be necessary, especially if active bleeding is present.

5. If very recent (<72 hours) sexual abuse is suspected, obtain the following specimens when possible and place in the appropriate containers (forensic kit if available). Alternatively and preferably, send the patient to a sexual assault center, if available; such centers are specially equipped to collect the following specimens, which are sent to a forensic laboratory for processing:

a. Hair, if any, combed from the pubic area

b. Vaginal fluid: wet mount of material examined immediately for motile sperm

c. Gonococcus culture (throat or mouth, rectum, cervix/vagina, penile urethra) as appropriate

d. Chlamydia cultures of genital secretions as appropriate

e. Swab of vaginal secretions mixed in a test tube with 2 ml normal saline solution. The sample is sent on ice immediately to the laboratory for an acid phosphatase test for semen. The laboratory may also be able to test sperm for DNA pattern. This test may be available only through a police laboratory via a sexual assault center.

f. Scrape from skin or clothing any areas that may represent dried semen for acid phosphatase testing or DNA typing.

g. Obtain blood and urine tests as follows:

1) Serologic test for syphilis (repeat in 4-6 weeks). Keep in mind that young children might remember the "blood test" most vividly; therefore be as selective and gentle as possible.

2) Toxicology screen if appropriate

3) Pregnancy test as appropriate. Pregnancy can be detected as early as 9 days after fertilization.

4) U/A

5) A baseline HIV test is also suggested by some investigators.

6. If sexual activity occurred at least several days before, perform the following:

a. A complete PE plus an external genital exam with specific regard to the vaginal introitus and rectum. If appropriate, diagram abnormal findings on the patient's record.

b. A gonococcus culture from the vagina, throat, and rectum. Obtain specimens to test for syphilis and chlamydia.

c. Pregnancy test if appropriate

   d. U/A

   e. Baseline HIV test

   f. If there are *any* questions, obtain a consultation from a knowl-
     edgeable consultant.

7. Arrange appropriate follow-up for the child and family. A social
   worker can arrange shelter if needed. Prompt individual or group
   psychologic counseling can be very reassuring to the victim and can
   assist in a more complete healing.

8. Parents/foster parents/guardians should be counseled to not make a
   bad situation worse by using such terms as "ruined," "violated," or
   "dirty" around the child. A child's emotional reaction to sexual abuse
   is magnified by the imposition of adult values and may lead to anxiety,
   feelings of guilt and worthlessness, depression, and suicide ideation
   or attempts by the child. Caretakers can themselves benefit from
   psychologic support and counseling.

BIBLIOGRAPHY

Child abuse

American Academy of Pediatrics—Committee on Child Abuse
   and Neglect: Shaken baby syndrome: inflicted cerebral trauma,
   Pediatrics 92:872, 1993.

American Academy of Pediatrics—Committee on Child Abuse
   and Neglect: Distinguishing sudden infant death syndrome
   from child abuse fatalities, *Pediatrics* 94:124, 1994.

Chadwick D: The diagnosis of inflicted injury in infants and
   young children, *Pediatr Ann* 21:477, 1992.

Cupoli JM: Piecing together the pattern of child abuse, *Contemp
   Pediatr* 4:12, 1987.

Dubowitz H, Bross D: The pediatrician's documentation of child
   maltreatment, *Am J Dis Child* 146:596, 1992.

Feldman K: Patterned abusive bruises of the buttocks and the
   pinnae, *Pediatrics* 90:633, 1992.

Garbarino J: The psychologically battered child: toward a definition, *Pediatr Ann* 18:502, 1989.

Kessler D, Hyden P: Physical, sexual and emotional abuse of
   children, *Ciba Found Symp,* vol 43, 1991.

Kessler D, New M: Emerging trends in child abuse and neglect,
   Pediatr Ann 18:471, 1989.

Kottmeier P: The battered child, *Pediatr Ann* 16:343, 1987.

Leventhal J et al: Fractures in young children, *Am J Dis Child* 147:87, 1993.

McClain P et al: Estimates of fatal child abuse and neglect: US 1979-1988, *Pediatrics* 91:338, 1993.

Sirotnak A, Krugman R: Physical abuse of children: an update, *Pediatr Rev* 15:394, 1994.

Stewart G et al: Trauma in infants less than 3 months of age, *Pediatr Emerg Care* 9:199, 1993.

Thomas S et al: Long-bone fractures in young children: distinguishing accidental injuries from child abuse, *Pediatrics* 88:471, 1991.

Sexual abuse

Adams J et al: Examination findings in legally confirmed child sexual abuse: it's normal to be normal, *Pediatrics* 94:310, 1994.

American Academy of Pediatrics—Committee on Child Abuse and Neglect: Guidelines for the evaluation of sexual abuse of children, *Pediatrics* 87:254, 1991.

Berkowitz C: Child sexual abuse, *Pediatr Rev* 13:443, 1992.

Dubowitz H et al: The diagnosis of child sexual abuse, *Am J Dis Child* 146:688, 1992.

Emans SJ et al: Genital findings in sexually abused, symptomatic and asymptomatic, girls, *Pediatrics* 79:778, 1987.

Gabby T et al: Sexual abuse of children, *Am J Dis Child* 146:700, 1992.

Horowitz DA: Physical examination of sexually abused children and adolescents, *Pediatr Rev* 9:25, 1987.

Jenny C: Sexually transmitted diseases and child abuse, *Pediatr Ann* 21:497, 1992.

Kerns D et al: Concave hymenal variations in suspected child sexual abuse victims, *Pediatrics* 90:265, 1992.

McCann J, Voris J: Perianal injuries resulting from sexual abuse: a longitudinal study, *Pediatrics* 91:390, 1993.

McCann J et al: Genital injuries resulting from sexual abuse: a longitudinal study, *Pediatrics* 89:307, 1992.

McCauley J et al: Toluidine blue in the detection of perineal lacerations in pediatric and adolescent sexual abuse victims, *Pediatrics* 78:1039, 1986.

Seidel J et al: Presentation and evaluation of sexual misuse in the emergency department, *Pediatr Emerg Care* 2:157, 1986.

Sirotnak A: Testing sexually abused children for sexually transmitted diseases: who to test, when to test, and why, *Pediatr Ann* 23:370, 1994.

Spencer M, Dunklee P: Sexual abuse of boys, *Pediatrics* 78:133, 1986.

COMMON BEHAVIORAL PROBLEMS

4

A. AGGRESSIVENESS

1. Children often express frustration through hostility, combativeness, or quarreling. Such behavior usually peaks around age 2 (the "terrible two's") as children kick, stomp, jump up and down, throw themselves on the floor, hold their breath, pull, struggle, throw objects, bite, hit, scream, and cry. Such behavior generally subsides as a child learns how to handle frustration in a more socially acceptable manner.

2. Some children continue these behaviors well beyond the preschool years. Children with the aggressive syndrome exhibit arguing, screaming, temper outbursts, loudness, bullying, threatening comments, cruelty to other people or to animals, fighting, stubbornness, irritability, or mood swings. Approximately 50% of all children with this syndrome show social impairments, psychiatric disorders, or criminal behavior as adults.

3. Hypotheses regarding why certain children are aggressive include a dysfunctional response to frustration (either innate or learned), learned behavior from role models (parents and peers), victimization (i.e., abuse), a biochemical imbalance, and genetic or anatomic "set-ups" such as chromosomal abnormalities or defects in certain areas of the brain.

4. A complete history is mandatory when evaluating a child with aggressive behavior. The aggressiveness must be delineated regarding types of behavior, onset, the settings and situations most likely to elicit aggressiveness, school performance (cognitive limitations), parental response and disciplining style, history of child abuse or substance abuse, persons from whom the child models his or her behavior, and environmental factors fostering the behavior. Children with learning problems or with ADD/ADHD are often aggressive in response to their own frustration and low self-esteem as well as in response to teasing by others.

5. Treatment modalities include parent management training (i.e., the parent learns to handle the child in a more effective manner), cognitive therapy in which the child is taught new coping skills, family therapy, individual counseling, and psychopharmacologic interventions. The earlier the intervention, the more likely it is to be successful. Seriously aggressive children should be managed together with a psychiatrist or a psychologist, especially if drug therapy is used.

B. AUTISM

1. *Autism* is defined as a behavioral syndrome in which there is qualitative impairment in reciprocal social interactions, impaired verbal and nonverbal communication and imaginative activity, and a markedly restricted repertoire of activities and interests. To be classified as autistic, an individual must have been symptomatic since infancy or early childhood. The incidence is 5-15 per 10,000 children; boys outnumber girls 4 to 1.

2. In the area of impaired social interactions, autistic children can be either aloof and unreachable (even to their own family), unaware of others' feelings or social cues (either positive or negative), remote but reachable with a great deal of effort or, on the opposite end of the scale, superficially social (pseudosocial).

3. In the area of impaired communication, autistic children have impaired comprehension and expression of language. They may use nonsense syllables or bits of words from a number of sources that when strung together make no sense. They may demonstrate echolalia, repeating favored expressions repeatedly or answering a question with the same question. They seem to have an inability to use nonverbal gestures when communicating and have no understanding of the nonverbal cues of others. They might speak in a monotone and fail to understand normal variations in speech or, alternatively, they may speak in a sing-song fashion.

4. In the area of restricted activities and interests, autistic children regularly display repetitive movements from which they cannot easily be dissuaded. Such movements include rocking, head banging, staring at an object, singing the same song repeatedly, doing the same activity repeatedly, and twisting hair.

5. Autistic children have IQs that range from mental deficiency to superior intelligence. Although the mean IQ is low, at least 33% of autistic children have IQs higher than 70, and 5% are "autistic savants" with unusual rote memory or visual skills.

6. Autistic children tend to have flat affects and respond little to either praise or punishment. However, some autistic children have very labile affects, even without a discernible external cause.

7. Autistic children might have either a very short or an abnormally long attention span. In the latter, an autistic child might stare at the same object for hours without evidence of boredom.

8. Many autistic children have sensorimotor abnormalities such as clumsiness, drooling, a heightened or absent response to loud noises, a fascination with certain visual stimuli, and insensitivity to pain.

9. Seizures are common.

10. The differential diagnosis is between autism and mental deficiency in low-functioning children, language disorder in younger high-functioning children, and schizophrenia in high-functioning adolescents and young adults.

11. The history should be complete and elicit the presence of the features and behaviors previously described.

12. The PE should be complete and focus on signs of any disease that might otherwise explain the child's symptoms. The examiner should attempt to engage the child in play or conversation to determine his or her responses firsthand.

13. An awake and sleep EEG is indicated; neuroimaging studies are not indicated because the presence of structural abnormalities does not alter the child's therapy.

14. Seizures should be treated with anticonvulsants; ADD/ADHD should be treated appropriately. No drug has demonstrated effectiveness in improving the symptoms of autism. Many autistic children have been overmedicated in an effort to control their behaviors, but such a practice often leads only to a somnolent child, not a treated one.

15. The best treatment currently available is long-term special education. However, the ultimate prognosis is not predictable even when such education is offered continuously and is begun at an early age.

C. COLIC

1. *Colic* describes persistent crying in early infancy (i.e., the first 3 months of life). Although all young infants cry, many cry for prolonged periods each day, which adds another stressor to their parents' lives. Whether an anxious, stressed parent leads to a stressed infant or vice versa, the result is the same: an infant who is experiencing some level of distress and a parent whose self-esteem suffers because of an inability to console the infant.

2. By definition, infants with colic cry inconsolably more than 3 hours

per day at least 3 days per week and for at least 3 weeks. This behavior peaks between ages 6 and 8 weeks and wanes by approximately 3 months. Using this definition, approximately 10% of all infants are colicky. Colic is unrelated to gender, feeding method, or birth weight but is more common in firstborns.

3. The differential diagnosis includes neuromaturational/GI immaturity, a food allergy, GER, difficult temperament, and parental anxiety.

4. Colicky infants typically have bouts of intense crying in which their legs are drawn up to their abdomen; these bouts of crying are often associated with skin color changes and the passage of flatus. Such infants may also be poor sleepers and hypersensitive to external stimuli.

5. The evaluation of a colicky infant should include prenatal, perinatal, medical, family, social, and developmental histories. The timing, duration, and type of symptoms that occur during a crying episode should be noted. Especially important is the feeding history in terms of overfeeding, underfeeding, or maladaptive feeding. Questions regarding formula preparation, timing of feedings, behavior and interest during feedings, position during feedings, frequency of burping, amount taken and the time in which it is taken, and parental reaction to feeding are all important.

6. The PE is usually normal, but a careful search for subtleties that might indicate other reasons for excessive crying (e.g., occult fractures or occult organ trauma) is indicated. Observing a feeding may produce valuable information that was unavailable from the history.

7. Laboratory tests are generally not helpful.

8. Treatment of colic consists of supporting both the parent and infant. Counseling should be provided regarding coping strategies and techniques for calming or feeding the infant and for ameliorating environmental conditions that might exacerbate crying. Dietary manipulations, if used at all, should be held to a minimum; each formula change should be evaluated for 10-14 days before deciding on its role in colic. No drug for colic has been proven effective *and* safe.

D. CONVERSION REACTIONS

1. A conversion reaction is a mechanism by which an unconscious idea or wish is expressed in bodily terms and is experienced as a physical symptom that has specific but unconscious and symbolic meaning to the patient. Any bodily process can serve as the focus of the conversion symptom; the somatic symptoms of relatives or close

friends can also serve this purpose. Although conversion symptoms have no organic basis, their perpetuation may result in biochemical or physiologic changes.

2. A complete history and PE are essential. A clue to the diagnosis of a conversion reaction is the observation that a patient's symptoms do not fit the classic physical, biochemical, or physiologic manifestations of the condition in question. In addition, the patient's reaction to the symptom(s) may be completely inappropriate.

3. Adolescents with conversion reactions are often egocentric, emotionally labile, dramatic, attention-seeking, pseudomature, or sexually provocative. Such adolescents are often overprotected by their parents.

4. Individuals with conversion reactions experience both primary gain (the extent to which the symptom decreases the unpleasant emotion and symbolically communicates the forbidden but unconscious wish) and secondary gain (removal from a conflict or uncomfortable situation).

5. The precipitation of a conversion reaction may result from an acute or long-standing stress such as unresolved grief or anger.

6. The differential diagnosis includes hypochondriasis, malingering, psychosis, and psychophysiologic disorders. In hypochondriasis, the patient is filled with concern when the diagnosis of an organic disease is entertained; a patient with a conversion reaction is indifferent. In malingering, patients *consciously* try to avoid unpleasant situations by attempting to feign illness and are aloof or hostile to physicians. In contrast, individuals with conversion symptoms are interested in seeing a medical provider. In psychosis, bizarre symptoms are reported (e.g., "my brain is shrinking"); plausible symptoms are reported by an individual with a conversion reaction.

7. With psychophysiologic disorders, the patient has an identifiable unpleasant affect that activates the autonomic neuroendocrine system and results in such signs as tachycardia, sweating, or hyperperistalsis. The patient experiences these signs as palpitations, sweating, or diarrhea. Thus the trigger is emotional and the expression of it is clearly organic. Sometimes it is difficult to distinguish between psychophysiologic disorders and conversion reactions.

8. The treatment of conversion reactions may be carried out by the primary medical provider alone (if he or she has the expertise, time, and interest to do so) or together with a mental health professional. It is essential that the primary medical provider conduct the initial

evaluation (history, physical, warranted laboratory tests) and discuss the results with the parent and patient. It is vitally important to state at the onset of the discussion that many physical problems have both physical and emotional causes and that each person's body has a certain physical way of reacting to stress. Such a concurrent physical-psychologic approach better prepares all concerned for any eventual outcome. There are no magical drugs for the treatment of conversion reactions and, in an adolescent, drugs might do more harm than good. The best success follows repeated sessions in which the patient can talk about his or her feelings.

9. Treatment of psychophysiologic symptoms includes relaxation therapy, biofeedback, cognitive therapy (e.g., learning coping skills for times of stress), environmental manipulation (e.g., altering the environment, if possible, to reduce the individual's stress), and individual or family therapy.

E. DEPRESSION

1. The diagnosis of a major depressive illness requires five or more of the following symptoms: depressed mood, loss of interest or pleasure, significant weight loss or gain, failure to make expected weight gains for age, insomnia or hypersomnia, psychomotor agitation or retardation, fatigue or loss of energy, feelings of worthlessness or excessive inappropriate guilt, decreased concentration, and recurrent thoughts of death or suicide (especially with plans).

2. Almost 2% of preschool-age children and 5% of adolescents are clinically depressed; some investigators estimate that almost 10% of all children suffer some form of depression by age 12.

3. Most at risk for depression are children and adolescents who have one or more of the following factors:
   a. Depressed parents
   b. Divorced parents
   c. Hospitalized siblings
   d. ADD/ADHD
   e. Incarceration
   f. Mild mental retardation
   g. Lower socioeconomic status
   h. Chronic illness
   i. Pregnancy or children of their own

4. Although the classic presentation of depression is a sad, weepy child with psychomotor retardation, a depressed child may be hyperactive

and aggressive. Many runaways run because they are depressed about their home situation, peer relationships, or school performance.

5. Children with depression generally look sad, have a negative self-image, lack a sense of fun in their lives, experience pathologic guilt, have few friends or social contacts, are poor students (either an acute onset or a long-standing problem), are chronically fatigued, and have sleep and appetite disturbances, psychomotor retardation, or morbid thoughts.

6. Depressed children have a sense of loss of an object, a person, or their own self-esteem; the latter is especially true of children who fail at school or in peer relations.

7. A meticulous history and PE are indicated for children and adolescents with depression. The history should highlight precipitating episodes, duration and progression of symptoms, family history of depression, school performance, peer relations, and recent traumatic events in the family, neighborhood, school, or peer group. The parents should be asked about other unusual symptoms (e.g., new-onset clumsiness) that might point to an organic process. It is important to talk with the child about the depression and whether he or she has suicidal or homicidal thoughts. The PE should be thorough to rule out an organic process (e.g., a brain tumor) as the cause of the depressive symptoms.

8. Laboratory tests should be kept to a minimum; however, drug testing and a pregnancy test should be considered.

9. Serious depression, especially together with suicidal or homicidal ideation, requires inpatient hospitalization to protect both the child and others. Outpatient therapy is preferable for children and adolescents with mild-to-moderate depression. If the primary medical provider lacks the training, time, or expertise, he or she will want to manage the depressed child or adolescent together with a mental health professional.

10. Psychotherapy has produced good results in treating child and adolescent depression. Also useful are tricyclic antidepressants, monoamine oxidase inhibitors, and lithium carbonate. Drug therapy should be carefully monitored because all of these drugs have potent side effects. Before the initial drug administration, CBC, BUN, electrolytes, thyroid function tests, LFTs, creatinine, and an ECG should be obtained. Because the tricyclics (notably imipramine) have potent cardiac effects, parents and patients should be warned, and resting pulse rates should be monitored periodically. Plasma drug

levels, BP, and ECGs (to look for prolongation of the QRS complex or PR interval) should be monitored.

F. EATING DISORDERS

1. General
   a. Even young children are conscious of their body image; children as young as 8-10 years of age have reported dieting. Children who are obese have fewer friends, which prompts most children to avoid obesity at all costs.
   b. Chronic dieting is particularly common in girls whose body habitus does not match the ideal figure touted by the media. Methods to keep weight down include bulimia (self-induced vomiting) or the use of diet pills, diuretics, ipecac, or laxatives.
   c. Children and adolescents who are chronic dieters often come from families in whom weight and body appearance are of paramount importance. Because there is a genetic component to body habitus, children of parents who are (rightly or wrongly) concerned about their own weight see their parents' attitudes as models for their own.
   d. Risk factors for eating disorders include female gender; menstrual irregularities (interplay of hormones and physical activity); compulsive athletic activities; chronic stress, especially that imposed by perfectionism; and compulsive stereotypic behaviors related to eating (e.g., chewing each bite 100 times).

2. Bulimia nervosa (BN)
   a. BN is a syndrome in which there is binge eating (i.e., rapid ingestion of a large amount of food in a short period of time) at least two times a week and in association with the following:
      1) Self-induced vomiting, severe food restriction, cathartic or laxative abuse, strenuous exercise, and weight fluctuations
      2) Fear of loss of control regarding eating and purging behaviors
      3) A heightened concern with body shape and weight accompanied by dissatisfaction, depression, and self-depreciation
      4) No known physical abnormality to account for these findings
   b. Binge eaters are often unaware of being hungry before eating but cannot stop once they start. It is an addiction. In contrast to those with AN, binge eaters are aware of their feelings.

3. Anorexia nervosa (AN)
   a. AN is a syndrome that includes the following:
      1) A marked fear of fatness, a disturbed perception of body size

(even if underweight), and an obsessional desire to lose increasing amounts of weight

2) Self-starvation with marked weight loss (greater than 15% body weight) or a failure to gain weight

3) Amenorrhea (no bleeding for three or more menstrual cycles) and other physiologic signs associated with starvation

4) Hyperactivity and sleep disturbances

5) Bizarre attitudes regarding food and a denial of illness

6) No known physical cause to account for these findings

b. With AN, hunger may be diminished or increased. Patients with AN often are immature, fearful of growing up, perfectionistic, and lack control in their lives so that all of their efforts are placed on controlling their weight. Such patients are stunted physically, socially, and emotionally.

c. AN and BN are more prevalent in affluent societies in which food is plentiful. Both conditions are more common in female patients (BN—F:M=5:1; AN—F:M=9:1), especially in those who have been sexually abused. At least 10% of individuals with AN engage in bulimic behavior, but those with BN do not usually have symptoms of AN. AN begins earlier (between ages 12 and 16) than BN (between ages 15 and 20).

d. The initial presentation of AN is usually marked weight loss or amenorrhea. Pubertal progression may be arrested. In BN, any symptom might be the presenting one, and sometimes patients seek help of their own accord because they are frightened by their own lack of control.

e. Findings vary by disease.

1) With AN, cachexia is obvious. There may be hypothermia, bradycardia, and hypotension, all of which are signs of physiologic accommodation to starvation. Loss of scalp hair and the presence of lanugo and skin mottling are common. Bones may "stick out," and the thyroid might appear prominent because of the loss of subcutaneous tissue. Abrasions of the palate, buccal mucosa, and the dorsum of the hands indicate self-induced vomiting. Repeated vomiting may also lead to parotid or submandibular gland swelling. Pretibial and ankle edema, mitral valve prolapse, and cardiac arrhythmias may be present. Patients may be hyperactive, restless, and irritable or, alternatively, hypoactive, sluggish, and slow in thinking.

2) With BN, the patient might be underweight, overweight, or of

normal weight. Depending on the severity of illness, physical signs can be minimal or marked. If vomiting is a common occurrence, oral abrasions and salivary gland enlargement are present. Dehydration (with concurrent hypotension and tachycardia) may be present.

3) With AN, laboratory findings include a low WBC, platelet count, and Hct (bone marrow suppression); hypokalemia; low serum Mg and P (late finding); and ECG abnormalities (sinus bradycardia, inverted T waves, A-V block, arrhythmias, low voltage). Electrolytes are otherwise normal unless dehydration, vomiting, and laxative/diuretic abuse are also present. X-ray studies may reveal osteoporosis, gastric distension, and a narrow cardiac silhouette. Cerebral atrophy might be evident on a CT scan.

4) With BN there is often evidence of either hypochloremic alkalosis as a result of repeated vomiting or metabolic acidosis as a result of laxative abuse. Hypokalemia, hypomagnesemia, and hypocalcemia are common. The ECG shows evidence of hypokalemia (arrhythmias, U waves, depressed T waves). X-ray studies show gastric distension and evidence of paralytic ileus.

f. The differential diagnosis includes IBD, achalasia, thyroid disease, adrenal disease, and malignancy (CNS or otherwise).

g. Treatment

1) With AN the patient is terrified of eating, and therefore a sympathetic but firm approach is useful. Expect setbacks; they will occur. Candidates for outpatient management include those whose disease has been in place for no more than 3 or 4 months; those who do not binge, purge, or use laxatives or diuretics; those whose families are relatively well functioning; and those who want help and seem eager to cooperate in their treatment. Indications for hospitalization are severe weight loss, outright starvation, drug use, CHF, metabolic derangements, abnormal ECG, or severe depression. All patients with AN must learn that their disease is controlling them and not the other way around. The disease is also in control of their family, social, and scholastic lives. Regular weigh-ins are mandatory; a weight gain of 0.2 kg/d is desired. Consultation and shared management of the patient with a mental health professional and a nutritionist are necessary.

2) With BN, immediate hospitalization is needed if there are

metabolic or cardiac derangements. The patient should be managed together with a mental health professional and a nutritionist.

4. Overeating

a. A proper diet and activity level are important both to prevent eating disorders and to treat individuals who are overweight or overfat. The term *overweight* refers to individuals whose weight exceeds 120% of that expected for height; this condition may be a function of both body frame and adiposity. Determining whether an individual is overfat is best accomplished by using the triceps skinfold measurement.

b. In the absence of serious physical disease, no child or adult loses weight unless he or she wants to. Therefore the first goal of therapy is to enlist the patient's (and family's) support and cooperation. The medical provider should remind parents that the obese child may be the object of teasing, embarrassment, and self-shame and that all family members need to maximally support the child while he or she is attempting to lose weight.

c. The goal for an actively growing child may be weight maintenance rather than weight loss, especially if the child has only mild-to-moderate obesity. For each 20% increment in excess of ideal weight, 1-2 years of weight maintenance are required to achieve the ideal weight. The loss of 1 pound each month is a reasonable goal when weight loss is required in young children.

d. A food intake diary can be used to identify both problem foods that can be eliminated or reduced and problem times during which eating in the absence of hunger is likely. Reduced fat intake and reduced total calorie intake are important. However, highly restrictive diets should be instituted only when there is a serious medical reason and in consultation with a dietician.

e. Increased activity is important but cannot be the only technique because excess caloric intake is at least as important a factor as insufficient exercise. Children and adolescents should be encouraged to exercise more and to spend less time in sedentary activities such as watching television or videos or playing on the computer.

f. Behavior modification is also important, especially when it focuses on the positive rather than on the negative. For example, the focus can be on the amount of weight that the child has lost, the child's adherence to the diet, or the child's increased physical activity rather than on the amount of weight regained or still left to lose, the child's failure to adhere to the diet, the child's reluctance to become more active, the predictions of the morbidities that the child will experience if he or she fails to lose weight, or the insinuation that the child lacks friends because of his or her weight. In some cases, the eating habits of the entire family should be changed for the health of everyone concerned.

G. FEARS/PHOBIAS/ANXIETY

1. Young children have many fears, which vary by age.
   a. Infants are usually afraid of loud sounds, bright lights, sudden movements, strangers, animals, heights, and separation. All such stimuli represent a threat to the infant, who cannot make sense of them.
   b. In addition to many of the feared items from infancy, toddlers fear new situations, the dark, and water. Because toddlers do not yet understand size relationships, they cannot understand that they cannot be flushed down the toilet or go down a drain. Fear of the dark occurs because children of this age are beginning to develop an imagination, and who knows what lurks in the darkness?
   c. Children between 3 and 5 years of age commonly have night fears and nightmares (a combination of the darkness and imagination), a fear of death, a fear of separation, and phobias (see Point 3).
   d. Children between 6 and 12 years of age develop sophisticated fears about their local and universal world, such as school fears, a fear of new social situations, and a fear of harm to self and to loved ones.
2. Fears are usually transient and diminish over time. However, the following techniques are helpful:
   a. Infants: Avoiding sudden changes in sound or lighting; permitting infants to *gradually* become accustomed to sounds, lights, or persons that will be a part of their lives; urging strangers not to overwhelm infants with kisses and hugs nor to pick them up against their will (to combat stranger anxiety); encouraging infants to be with adults other than the parents for brief periods of time (to combat separation anxiety); *gradually* introducing infants to a potentially scary situation (e.g., a dog) by demonstrating bravery with it (to decrease fear of new objects)
   b. Toddlers: Using a night-light or transitional object to help soothe fear of the dark, encouraging water play to minimize fear of water, permitting toddlers to become accustomed to periods of separation from parents, encouraging toddlers to make-believe they are the feared animal, person, or object

c. Preschool-age children: Using a night-light and gentle bedtime routines to minimize night fears, avoiding stimulating activities or shows before bedtime, talking honestly about death when it comes up in conversation, preparing children for a separation from a parent by talking about it beforehand and even enlisting their help in planning the return

d. School-age children: Communicating with children about their fears and wishes, empathizing with fear about school or peers, appropriately praising them for the good things they can do, minimizing parental pressure to excel academically or socially, acting out dreaded situations to practice different ways of coping, being open and honest about a fear of harm to self or loved ones

3. Phobias are obsessive, persistent, and unrealistic fears that disrupt or distort normal behavior. They may be caused by an adverse experience with the feared object (e.g., being bitten by a dog), having a role model (usually a parent) who is markedly afraid of an object, or hearing about a bad outcome with the feared object.

a. Older children and adults generally recognize that their fear is irrational. However, even the thought of exposure to the feared object (e.g., an escalator) brings on anxiety.

b. There is a preoccupation with and anticipatory anxiety regarding the expectancy of an encounter with the feared object. Usually the child or adult tries to avoid these encounters by any means available.

c. Cajoling and ordering someone to encounter the phobic situation are of no use.

d. Common phobias in childhood and adolescence include animals, toilets (especially public ones), public speaking in class, and social situations.

e. Medications are of little use in simple phobias; psychotherapy, especially desensitization and imaging, is much more successful.

4. Panic attacks differ from phobias. A panic attack is unexpected and not triggered by situations in which the person is the center of attention.

a. Panic attacks are accompanied by at least four of the following symptoms:
   1) Shortness of breath or a sensation of smothering
   2) Dizziness or faintness
   3) Palpitations or a fast heart rate
   4) Trembling or shaking
   5) Sweating
   6) Choking

7) Nausea or abdominal distress
8) Depersonalization or derealization
9) Numbness or tingling
10) Flushes or chills
11) Chest pain or discomfort
12) Fear of dying
13) Fear of going crazy or losing control

b. Diagnostic criteria for a panic attack are four attacks within a 4-week period or one or more attacks followed by 1 month of persistent fear that another will occur.

c. The most common panic reaction is in association with agoraphobia, which is the fear of being in places or situations from which escape might be difficult or embarrassing or in which help might not be available if another panic attack occurs.

d. Although tricyclic antidepressants are used in adults, their efficacy in children and adolescents is less established. Consultation with a mental health professional is needed.

H. GROWING PAINS

1. Growing pains are intermittent limb pains unrelated to the joints; such pains occur late in the day or at night and may be sufficiently intense to wake a child.

2. The pain is unaccompanied by fever, constitutional symptoms, redness, or swelling. If the pain is in the legs (as it usually is), the gait remains normal. Older children generally describe the pain as crampy, especially when it occurs in the muscles of the thighs or calves.

3. There can be symptom-free periods of weeks or months.

4. Growing pains are most likely to begin between ages 3 and 5 years or between ages 8 and 12 years. Girls are more likely to be affected than are boys.

5. The etiology of growing pains is unknown; everything from emotional causes, overuse, inadequate sleep, the weather, and other obscure reasons has been postulated. At one point, a discrepancy in the rate of bone growth vs. tendon/ligament/muscle growth (placing undue traction on these structures) was postulated, but there is no proof for this hypothesis.

6. The history is classic for pains that occur only at night, with a paucity of daytime symptoms and no limitation of activity. The PE and laboratory studies are normal.

7. The differential diagnosis includes hypermobility syndrome (joint

laxity in very active children), intermittent nocturnal leg cramps, patellofemoral pain syndrome (patellar pain in adolescent girls), osteoid osteoma, and somatization syndrome in which the disability is out of proportion to physical findings.

8. There is a benign course; children do "grow out of it." Some investigators have reported that a leg muscle–stretching regimen may successfully decrease symptoms in children who are having frequent episodes.

I. HABITS

1. Many children have habits such as hair twisting or biting, nail chewing, pencil chewing, and nose picking. Although parents may be offended by such habits, they are not done intentionally and in most cases resolve. These habits often are associated with stress, deep concentration, or falling asleep.

2. Other children exhibit stereotypic behaviors such as body rocking, head rolling, or head banging. These behaviors may also be associated with stress or falling asleep. For most children the rhythmic nature of these stereotypies (with the possible exception of head banging) gives some pleasure and may help relieve tension. Head banging is common in temperamentally intense children and often responds to increased holding, rhythmic activation, or medication such as hydroxyzine. If the head banging leads to injury or if there are other behavioral problems, consultation with a mental health professional may be necessary.

3. Habits are not to be confused with tic disorders (see Chapter 14), which are nonrhythmic and do not seem to give the child the degree of pleasure that habits give.

4. The prognosis for habit resolution is good as the child matures.

J. MUNCHAUSEN SYNDROME BY PROXY (POLLE SYNDROME)

1. Munchausen syndrome by proxy (Polle syndrome) is a condition in which parents or guardians purposely and needlessly subject their children, generally of age 6 years or under, to painful and sometimes life-threatening procedures and treatments. There is fabrication of illness and fraudulent reports of chronic or recurring symptoms.

2. The usual perpetrator is a mother, often with some medical background, who appears concerned about her child and is often friendly with and solicitous of the medical staff. She appears calm even when the child is ill. She is the "only one" for whom the child

will comply and seldom leaves the bedside. There is often a pathologic symbiotic relationship between mother and child.

3. Polle syndrome may represent the mother's efforts to keep her child completely dependent on her or may be an attempt to improve poor parental relations as both parents focus on the child. Typically the father is aloof.

4. The child experiences unexplained, prolonged, or extraordinary illnesses, the signs and symptoms of which are witnessed only by the perpetrator and do not make sense clinically. Some children experience life-threatening events. These "illnesses" evoke extensive and painful diagnostic work-ups that are negative and treatments that are ineffective, costly, and sometimes painful.

5. Examples of Polle syndrome include placing the mother's or the child's own blood (from a disconnected IV line) in the child's vomitus, diaper, or ostomy bag; administering poisons, drugs, or abnormal electrolyte solutions; substituting maternal urine for the child's; injecting contaminated materials; and phlebotomizing the child by disconnecting an IV line (which leads to profound anemia).

6. On suspicion of this syndrome, all unnecessary tests and procedures must cease. In addition, the following should occur:
   a. The child should be separated from the mother to see if symptoms occur in her absence.
   b. A psychosocial history of the family should be obtained.
   c. The temporal relationship between the mother's presence and the signs and symptoms of the child's illness should be verified.
   d. Pertinent specimens, both when the mother has been present and when she has been absent, should be obtained.
   e. Signs of the illness should be repeatedly checked and verified.
   f. Video monitoring should be considered.
   g. Psychiatric input is essential.
   h. Child protective services may be needed.

7. The prognosis for children with Polle syndrome is guarded because there is signficant morbidity and mortality. Children may also experience long-term immaturity, separation problems, irritability, aggressiveness, and deception in presenting their own histories.

K. NIGHTMARES/NIGHT TERRORS/SLEEPWALKING/ NIGHT WAKING

1. Nightmares
   a. Dreams occur in all persons and are the way the mind processes the events of the day or life. Dreams occur most often in the early morning hours before awakening.

   b. Toddlers have nightmares about separation issues, preschool-age children about monsters (threat to well-being), and school-age children about dangers and death.
   c. The occurrence of nightmares is strongly influenced by a child's viewing of violence either in real life (parental fighting at home, violence in the neighborhood) or in fantasy (television, videos, movies). Most young children cannot distinguish fantasy from reality, thus making anything plausible in their minds.
   d. Parents should be counseled to calm the child after a nightmare, to permit him or her to talk about it whenever ready to do so, and to limit the amount of violence that a child views either in real life or in fantasy.
   e. If nightmares persist, worsen, or interfere with a child's normal functioning, consultation with a mental health professional is needed.
2. Night terrors
   a. Night terrors are an inherited disorder and affect 2% of all children.
   b. Terrors consist of dream periods (10-30 minutes in duration) from which a child cannot be fully awakened. They generally begin during the first 90 minutes of sleep and can occur in clusters during the same night or in subsequent nights, sometimes for weeks. Even though the child's eyes are open, he or she does not appear to recognize familiar people or objects. The child is frightened, agitated, and might scream or talk incoherently. The episode ends on its own in calm sleep. Afterward, the child has no memory of the event.
   c. Parents should be counseled to refrain from waking a child in the midst of a night terror. They should speak to the child calmly and softly and should hold him or her if doing so does not cause further agitation. Parents should not shake or shout at the child in an effort to "snap him or her out of it"; such actions serve only to agitate the child further.
   d. A cycle of night terrors can be interrupted by waking the child a half hour after he or she falls asleep each night.
   e. Night terrors generally cease by 12 years of age.
3. Sleepwalking
   a. Sleepwalking is an inherited disorder and is seen in 15% of all children.
   b. The sleepwalker has open eyes but a blank look and has coordination that is clumsier than usual. He or she may make repeated stereotypic movements such as buttoning and unbutton-

ing clothes or turning the light on and off. The episode lasts 5-20 minutes, during which time he or she cannot be awakened.

c. Parents should be counseled to gently lead the child back to bed and to protect him or her from injury during the episode.

d. Children should be evaluated further if there are tonic-clonic movements during an episode, or if episodes last longer than 30 minutes, occur during the second half of the night, occur at least two times a week after attempting on seven occasions to awaken the child 15 minutes before the episode begins, or if there are daytime fears or a large amount of family stress.

4. Night waking/crying/feeding

   a. Most young infants awaken at night for a feeding or for a brief episode of crying. By 6 months of age, 50% of children sleep from midnight to 5 AM without awakening; by 12 months of age, 90% do.

   b. For whatever reason, night waking is a problem when it is habitual, prolonged, more for the child's entertainment than for necessity, and interferes with parental functioning.

   c. Some children have difficulty falling asleep and fight bedtime but sleep through the night once they are asleep; other children go to bed easily and sleep through the night but awaken early in the morning.

   d. If a child is an early riser, he or she is probably getting sufficient sleep. Forcing him or her to "sleep" more does not work. Techniques to help a child sleep later include delaying bedtime by an hour and eliminating a nap. Children who continue to rise early despite these measures may simply need less sleep. Older children can be instructed to remain in their room until 6 AM (or whatever time is comfortable for parents) and not call out or come into their parents' room until this time. Until this time these children can play quietly or look at books. Infants should be kept in their crib until 6 AM (or whatever time is comfortable for parents) with a few favorite toys. If the infant cries, the parent can visit the crib but should not remove the infant from the crib. The lights should be off.

   e. Different tactics must be tried if a child fights bedtime, repeatedly comes out of his or her room, or calls to his or her parent to come (or screams if preverbal).

      1) Children should fall asleep in their bed or crib. It is frightening for some children to fall asleep in one room and later awaken in another (dark) room. Being placed in the crib while awake or going to bed awake teaches children

how to fall asleep on their own both at bedtime and during night waking episodes.

2) Many children are afraid of the darkness in their room. If so, a night-light helps. Be sure the parent ensures that the night-light does not cast scary shadows, which can compound a child's fear.

3) Parents should attempt to make the hour or so before bedtime less stimulating so that children gradually unwind. Unfortunately, this situation often does not happen because parents who have been away all day use the middle-to-late evening hours to play actively with their children or to watch television or videos with them. Parents must adjust their habits if children are too "wound up" to go to bed.

4) Children's needs (e.g., bathroom visit, water, hugs) should be provided before they go to bed.

5) Children should be reminded that nighttime is when everyone sleeps—even most animals and birds. A child's fears should be acknowledged, but the parent needs to remain firm about the purpose of the night.

6) If a child is still in a crib, he or she needs to be left in it when he or she cries. The parent can visit at intervals and speak softly to the child, but removing the child from the crib should be avoided on most if not all visits.

7) If an older child will not stay in bed, the parent can permit him or her to quietly play or look at books in his or her room. The child is, however, to remain in his or her room and not disturb others. If the child comes out, he or she should be put back in his or her room without talking to him or her.

8) Children who repeatedly leave their room and enter the parents' room are a challenge. Although some writers advise locking such children in their room (or locking the parents' door), others worry that such a drastic step creates even more fear and separation anxiety. Parents should insist on their need for rest just as such children insist on their need for continued companionship. Beneath the surface of this behavior may lurk psychologic or psychosocial issues that need to be addressed and worked out for both the parents and children. Severe problems may require the services of a mental health professional.

f. Many of the previous suggestions are also applicable to night wakers/criers/feeders. These suggestions include placing the infant in the crib awake, making brief visits to the crib to reassure the infant without providing entertainment and without removing him or her from the crib, and eliminating long daytime naps. Providing a cherished object as the infant's companion during sleep may also be useful.

L. OBSESSIVE-COMPULSIVE DISORDER

1. OCD is marked by repetitive actions that the patient knows are "crazy." There may be repetitive hand-washing, certain rituals that must be performed before going out or going to bed, or certain words that must be uttered before beginning a task.

2. Other patients with OCD have obsessive thoughts that often concern a fear of harm, illness, death, doing wrong or having done wrong, and contamination.

3. The hallmark of OCD is the patient's understanding that the repetitive actions are "crazy" and the repetitive thoughts irrational. This knowledge is in contrast to other psychologic disorders in which the patient is unaware of his or her actions or thinks they are completely rational.

4. Treatment for OCD includes behavior modification, drug therapy, and psychotherapy. Helpful drugs are those that block serotonin reuptake. Other chemicals such as norepinephrine, dopamine, and certain hormones may also play a role in this disorder. PET scan studies of patients with OCD show increased metabolic activity in the frontal lobes and basal ganglia. Although drugs (clomipramine, fluoxetine, and fluvoxamine) have been used in OCD, other treatment modalities may also be useful.

M. POST–TRAUMATIC STRESS DISORDER

1. PTSD is marked by a history of exposure to (an) adverse event(s) that would be markedly distressing to nearly everyone, a trauma that is persistently reexperienced, a desire by the individual to avoid stimuli associated with the trauma, a psychologic numbing of general responsivity, and an increased state of arousal.

2. Initially, PTSD was described among adults who were exposed to combat, concentration camps, bombings, rapes, or other savage attacks. However, PTSD has now been described among children, especially those who have been abused. Such children have difficulty sleeping, nightmares, anxiety, agitation, hypervigilance, and hypersensitivity.

3. PTSD in children can follow one episode or repeated episodes of

abuse, sexual abuse, and witnessed violence, especially if inflicted on loved ones. The presence of more than one of these episodes increases the risk of PTSD, especially if the traumatic event was long-standing. There may also be genetic, gender, perinatal, familial, and early childhood factors that are not yet clear.

4. Treatment for PTSD is best carried out by a mental health professional, usually a child psychiatrist or child psychologist.

N. "SPOILED" CHILD SYNDROME (UNDERCONTROLLING PARENTING)

1. A "spoiled" child is one who is excessively self-centered and immature. This condition results from parental failure to enforce age-appropriate limits. Such a child has a lack of consideration for others, a need to have his or her own way, difficulty in delaying gratification, and temper outbursts. A spoiled child is intrusive, obstructive, manipulative, and negative.

2. Children are not necessarily spoiled by doting parents if parents temper their indulgence with age-appropriate limits and clear expectations.

3. Behaviors that are not indicative of spoiling include the crying spells of young infants, the natural curiosity of toddlers, and the self-assertion of the toddler or 2-year-old who says "no."

4. Children who might be classified as spoiled include trained night feeders and trained night criers (both of whom are seeking attention), children with frequent temper tantrums, and children who demand everything they see in a store, demand constant amusement and attention, or demand that their every need be met immediately.

5. Parents should be counseled to provide age-appropriate limits for their children, to insist that their children cooperate with important rules, and not to give in to tantrums. Children should learn to entertain themselves, to wait their turn (or delay their gratification), and to respect their parents' rights and wishes. Success is more likely if parents and other adults in the home agree on these issues. Further evaluation may be needed if a child does not improve after several months of age-appropriate expectations and limit setting.

O. STUTTERING

1. The term *stuttering* is applied to the repetition of sounds and syllables. This condition occurs in 4% of the population at some time in their lives, and its prevalence is approximately 1% at any given time. There is a male predominance of 3.5:1.

2. Although there may be an inherited predisposition to stuttering, environmental stresses and a child's coping skills also play a role. The likelihood of repetitions and hesitations in speech are increased by anxieties, illness, fatigue, and attempting to speak rapidly. Although these incidents occur with all children, a subgroup never grow out of them. Their speech pattern worsens, which increases their frustration (and hence their stress) and makes it more likely that they will stutter. This fact is particularly true if a parent constantly corrects or shames a child. If left untreated, children who stutter may become reluctant to speak, socially disadvantaged, and eager to avoid situations in which they must communicate.

3. Because stuttering, especially in the early phase, is an intermittent condition, do not be fooled by a child who is reported to stutter but does not do so in your presence.

4. Children between 2 and 5 years of age normally experience hesitations and repetitions in their speech, especially when they are excited and try to talk rapidly. Signs that normal speech *dis*fluencies are becoming *dys*fluencies include part-word repetition (rather than an entire word); multiple rather than single repetitions of the problematic syllable; irregular, rapid, abrupt, or jerky repetitions; a high frequency of *dys*fluency in the speech; and marked facial grimaces while speaking.

5. When the items enumerated in Point 4 are accompanied by stress, frustration, a fear of failure or social situations, and high parental expectations or punitive attitudes, there is a high likelihood that a child will become a chronic stutterer.

6. Children who seem likely to become or who are already chronic stutterers should be referred to a speech pathologist to maximize the chances of a good outcome.

7. Children at low risk to become chronic stutterers are those who have speech *dis*fluencies without tension or embarrassment, very intermittent stuttering, stuttering that occurs most often when excited, and parents who are not overly concerned.

8. In such low-risk cases, a parent can help a stuttering child by encouraging conversation, speaking more slowly and in a more relaxed manner and thus acting as a role model, maintaining a calmness around the house to reduce any sense of hurry that a child might have, giving the child some individual and calm attention each day so that the child does not need to compete with siblings, building self-esteem by appropriate praise and recognition of accomplishments, ceasing to correct or criticize speech, and ceasing to force the

child to repeat what he or she has said. These guidelines are to be followed by parents, siblings, and other adults with whom the child comes into contact. To avoid a self-fulfilling prophecy, a parent should not label the child as a stutterer. Interruptions of others' speech should be forbidden in the home, no matter who is speaking and who is interrupting.

P. TEMPER TANTRUMS

1. Approximately 14% of 1-year-olds, 20% of 2- to 3-year-olds, and 11% of 4-year-olds have temper tantrums. In addition, 5% of 5- to 17-year-olds are reported to have an explosive temper.
2. Tantrums occur when emotions exceed a child's ability to control them, which leads to frustration, rage, or fear. Therefore preverbal toddlers have the most difficulty expressing their emotions except through tantrums. Tantrums decrease once a child is better able to express his or her feelings and is better equipped to understand spoken parental commands or explanations.
3. In trying to master the environment and the self, a child experiences a blow to self-image after a tantrum. This fact is especially true when the child loses a battle of wills between the parent and child. Parents should understand that their handling of the tantrum partly determines the occurrence of future tantrums.
4. Parents should be counseled to use distraction when frustration begins to rise, to present acceptable choices, and to minimize the need to say "no" by keeping children away from potentially explosive situations or tempting environments. Parents should pick their battles carefully. They should not leave younger children alone in the midst of a tantrum and should hold them if that will quickly calm them. Older children should be instructed to go to their room until they calm down. Parents should remain calm, not label the child as "bad," and permit the child to start afresh when the tantrum is over.
5. Many tantrums respond better to being ignored than to any direct intervention. Children have tantrums to attract attention to themselves; when the tantrums fail to produce the desired effect, many children abandon them. In addition, positive reinforcement works well. Giving the child attention when he or she is doing something right (as opposed to when he or she is doing something wrong) is much more effective than giving belittling or negative messages.
6. Problem tantrums may suggest serious underlying problems in the child or parent and include the following:

    a. Age less than 1 year or older than 4 years
    b. Tantrums that occur in school
    c. Tantrums associated with aggression or violent behavior
    d. Associated disturbances in eating, sleep, play, and other activities
    e. Flirtatiousness or heightened modesty (R/O sexual abuse)
    f. Parental sadness, anger, or helplessness about the situation
    g. Parental inability to say positive things about the child

7. Factors contributing to problem tantrums include the following:
    a. Parental overcontrol (thwarting a child's autonomy)
    b. Parental undercontrol (frightening lack of limits)
    c. Parental depression or lack of support
    d. Parental substance abuse
    e. Domestic violence toward adults or children
    f. Parent-child mismatch
    g. Dysfunctional family
    h. Unrealistic environmental restrictions
    i. Child with poor adaptability or an intense temperament
    j. Child with language defects or learning problems
    k. Child with a hearing loss
    l. Child with ADD/ADHD
    m. Child under the influence of medications
    n. Child seeking secondary gain from an unresponsive environment
NOTE: Points h through n increase the likelihood that the child will be frustrated and act out of frustration.

8. Suggested therapies for problem tantrums include those mentioned in Points 4 and 5, behavior modification, time-outs, and extinction techniques. These therapies should be provided with a large dose of positive reinforcement and with empathy directed toward both the parent and child. The parent must understand that not all battles will be eliminated; the parent must also come to terms with the child's degree of development (what can be expected of him or her and what cannot). In severe cases, referral to a mental health professional is necessary.

Q. THUMB-SUCKING

1. The sucking reflex is one of the strongest reflexes that infants have; it is normal for them to suck their thumbs.
2. Many children suck their thumbs well beyond infancy. For some it is simply a habit, whereas for others it is evidence of a behavioral problem.

3. Thumb-sucking occurs in 45% of 3- to 4½-year-olds, 14% of 5-year-olds, and 6% of 6-year-olds. There is a female predominance for this habit.

4. Although thumb-sucking can cause dental malocclusion if it persists into middle childhood, it does not do so in infancy or early childhood. After 6 years of age, thumb-sucking has been associated with flared maxillary incisors, crossbite, open bite, an alteration in the shape of the roof of the mouth, a gap between the upper front teeth, and a flared upper lip.

5. Several aversive methods have been touted as treatments for thumb-sucking but have limited success and are cruel. Placing bitter substances on the thumb to make it less likely that the child will want to put the thumb in his or her mouth works only when the substance is on the thumb. This method cannot be used 24 hours a day, which limits its success. Applying an elastic bandage to the arm nightly (middle arm to forearm) so that there is resistance when the child bends the arm can be done only when the child does not need his or her arms to play, write, or perform other activities. Another technique involves insisting that the child suck all 10 fingers sequentially for an equal amount of time whenever the thumb is sucked, but this technique works only when the child is monitored for compliance. A dental appliance can be used for older children who are experiencing malocclusion and for whom other techniques have been unsuccessful. Hypnosis is useful in motivated older children.

6. Most children stop sucking their thumbs when motivated to do so. Motivation often comes from peer pressure rather than from any aversive technique that a parent has tried. Children who suck their thumbs are less popular than other children, which makes the habit less appealing to a child interested in having friends.

R. VULNERABILITY

1. Early child health problems might significantly affect parental perceptions of child health. Such perceptions can linger and affect subsequent child development.

2. In the vulnerable child syndrome as originally described, severe health problems in infancy leave certain parents with a sense that their child is uniquely vulnerable for future serious medical conditions and needs added protection. Such beliefs might lead to a pathologic parent-child relationship.

3. Vulnerable child syndrome has been described after a number of

conditions, including a complicated pregnancy, prematurity, birth problems, neonatal jaundice, meningitis, cancer, and even the diagnosis of an innocent heart murmur, which is a so-called non-disease.

4. The syndrome has been associated with the development of separation and discipline problems, overprotectiveness, parental obsessions about the child's health, sleep disturbances, hyperactivity (out-of-control child), and an increased use of medical services.

5. Because the parent believes that the child received a reprieve from death, there is a fear that the child will not be as fortunate the next time. The parent's impression of the child's health is easily picked up by the child, which leads the child to have a distorted image of his or her own health.

6. A hurried approach to the parent or child is useless. It may take several visits to learn about the "near brush with death" (real or imagined) in the child or the parent or about the death of another child, relative, or fetus.

7. The parent should be reassured that the child is healthy. The medical provider can empathize with the parent's concerns but can also point out that the parent's reactions contribute to the child's behavior. The parent can learn to set age-appropriate limits and sleeping practices for the child, reduce overprotectiveness, and see illnesses more realistically.

8. A psychologic or psychiatric referral is needed if such counseling is not effective, if the parent is depressed or seriously anxious, or if the child is out of control.

9. For most families, the prognosis is good.

10. To prevent the development or persistence of vulnerable child syndrome, medical providers should avoid hyperbole when describing either a child's condition or any "heroic" efforts to treat him or her.

BIBLIOGRAPHY

Aggressiveness

Alessi N, Wittekindt J: Childhood aggressive behavior, *Pediatr Ann* 18:94, 1989.
Gottlieb S, Friedman S: Conduct disorders in children and adolescents, *Pediatr Rev* 12:218, 1991.

Autism

Rapin I: Autistic children: diagnosis and clinical features, *Pediatrics* 87(suppl):751, 1991.

Colic and crying

Algranati P, Dworkin P: Infant problem behaviors, *Pediatr Rev* 13:16, 1992.

Hewson P et al: Infant colic, distress and crying, *Clin Pediatr* 26:69, 1987.

Conversion reactions/psychosomatic disease

Prazer G: Conversion reactions in adolescents, *Pediatr Rev* 8:279, 1987.

Schecker N: Childhood conversion reactions in the emergency department: Part I, *Pediatr Emerg Care* 3:202, 1987.

Schecker N: Childhood conversion reactions in the emergency department: Part II, *Pediatr Emerg Care* 6:46, 1990.

Stank T, Blum R: Psychosomatic illness in childhood and adolescence, *Clin Pediatr* 25:549, 1986.

Woolston J: A child's reactions to parents' problems, *Pediatr Rev* 8:169, 1986.

Depression

Dolgan J: Depression in children, *Pediatr Ann* 19:45, 1990.

Green M: Maternal depression: bad for children's health, *Contemp Pediatr* 10:28, 1993.

Weller E, Weller R: Pediatric management of depression, *Pediatr Ann* 18:104, 1989.

Eating disorders
Bulimia/anorexia nervosa

Comenci G: Eating disorders in adolescents, *Pediatr Rev* 10:37, 1988.

Harper G: Eating disorders in adolescents, *Pediatr Rev* 15:72, 1994.

Whitaker A: An epidemiological study of anorectic and bulimic symptoms in adolescent girls, *Pediatr Ann* 21:752, 1992.

Dieting/obesity

Dietz W, Robinson T: Assessment and treatment of childhood obesity, *Pediatr Rev,* 14:337, 1993.

Maloney M et al: Dieting behavior and eating attitudes in children, *Pediatrics* 84:482, 1989.

Stony M et al: Demographic and risk factors associated with chronic dieting in adolescents, *Am J Dis Child* 145:994, 1991.

Yates A: Biologic considerations in the etiology of eating disorders, *Pediatr Ann* 21:739, 1992.

Fears/phobias/anxiety

DuPont R: Phobias in children, *J Pediatr* 102:999, 1983.

Mattison R: Pediatric management of anxiety disorders, *Pediatr Ann* 18:114, 1989.

Schowalter J: Fears and phobias, *Pediatr Rev* 15:384, 1994.

Wittmen D, Crouthamel C: Overcoming the common fears of childhood, *Contemp Pediatr* 3:76, 1986.

Growing pains

Sizer I: Are those limb pains "growing" pains? *Contemp Pediatr* 6:143, 1989.

Munchausen syndrome by proxy (Polle syndrome)

Guandolo V: Munchausen syndrome by proxy: an outpatient challenge, *Pediatrics* 75:526, 1985.

McGuire T, Feldman K: Psychologic morbidity of children subjected to Munchausen syndrome by proxy, *Pediatrics* 83:289, 1989.

Meadow R: Munchausen syndrome by proxy: the hinterland of child abuse, *Lancet* 2:343, 1977.

Zitelli B et al: Munchausen syndrome by proxy and its professional participants, *Am J Dis Child* 141:1099, 1987.

Nightmares/night terrors/sleepwalking/night waking

Algranati P, Dworken P: Infancy problem behaviors, *Pediatr Rev* 13:16, 1992.

Ferber R: Sleeplessness, night awakening, and night crying in the infant and toddler, *Pediatr Rev* 9:69, 1987.

Lozoff B, Zuckerman B: Sleep problems in children, *Pediatr Rev* 10:17, 1988.

Schmitt B: Dealing with night terrors and sleepwalking, *Contemp Pediatr* 6:119, 1989.

Schmitt B: When your child has nightmares, *Contemp Pediatr* 6:57, 1989.

Schmitt B: Coping with the early riser, *Contemp Pediatr* 8:67, 1991.

Schmitt B: How to help the trained night crier, *Contemp Pediatr* 9:45, 1992.

Schmitt B: The "two-step" approach to infant sleep problems, *Contemp Pediatr* 9:37, 1992.

Obsessive-compulsive disorder

Sivedo S, Rapoport J: Bad news and good news about obsessive-compulsive disorder, *Contemp Pediatr* 6:130, 1989.

Post–traumatic stress disorder

Famularo R, Fenton T: Early developmental history and pediatric post–traumatic stress disorder, *Arch Pediatr Adolesc Med* 148:1032, 1994.

Famularo R et al: Child maltreatment and the development of post–traumatic stress disorder, *Am J Dis Child* 147:755, 1993.

Spoiled child syndrome

McIntosh B: Spoiled child syndrome, *Pediatrics* 83:108, 1989.

Schmitt B: Preventing spoiled children, *Contemp Pediatr* 9:44, 1992.

Stuttering

Guitar B: Is it stuttering or just normal language development? *Contemp Pediatr* 5:109, 1988.

Guitar B: Stuttering and stammering, *Pediatr Rev* 7:163, 1985.

Schmitt G: Does your child have a stuttering problem? *Contemp Pediatr* 8:83, 1991.

Temperament

Carey W: Temperament, *Contemp Pediatr* 6:139, 1989.

Temper tantrums

Needleman R et al: Temper tantrums: when to worry, *Contemp Pediatr* 6:12, 1989.

Thumb-sucking

Adain S: When thumb-sucking becomes a problem, *Contemp Pediatr* 3:75, 1986.

Friman F et al: Influence of thumb-sucking on peer social acceptance in first-grade children, *Pediatrics* 91:784, 1993.

Heitlen S: Curing thumb-sucking by the book, *Contemp Pediatr* 5:95, 1988.

Vulnerability

Green M: Vulnerable child syndrome and its variants, *Pediatr Rev* 8:75, 1986.
Green M: Vulnerable children, vulnerable mothers, *Contemp Pediatr* 5:102, 1988.
Perrin E et al: Is my child normal yet? Correlates of vulnerability, *Pediatrics* 83:355, 1989.

DERMATOLOGY

5

SPECIFIC CONDITIONS

See Fig. 5-1 for a pattern diagnosis.

A. ACNE

1. Acne results from obstruction of the pilosebaceous unit, enlargement of sebaceous glands, increased sebum production, proliferation of *Propionibacterium acnes,* and secondary inflammatory changes. There is a predilection for the face, chest, and back. Acne usually begins 1-2 years before the onset of puberty.
2. Lesions progress from closed comedones (whiteheads) → open comedones (blackheads) → pustules → papules → nodules (cysts) → atrophic and hypertrophic scars.
3. PE: Assess distribution, morphology, and severity of lesions. The course can be monitored by using a grading system or by obtaining serial photographs.
4. Laboratory evaluation: Not usually helpful. Endocrine evaluation is indicated for patients with signs of androgen excess (R/O adrenal, ovarian disease) and children with severe or persistent disease. Girls with nodulocystic disease may be at increased risk for polycystic ovarian disease.

NOTE: Acneiform eruption secondary to systemic steroid therapy, anticonvulsants, INH, androgens, or closed comedones on the forehead and temples may occur secondary to the use of oil-based hair or scalp preparations (especially in blacks).

5. Treatment needs to be individualized depending on gender, severity, type and distribution of lesions, and therapeutic response.
   a. Mild-to-moderate comedonal or inflammatory acne
      1) Retinoic acid (tretinoin, Retin-A)
         a) Begin by applying 0.025% cream or 0.01% gel every other night; after several weeks, increase to a nightly application, and increase concentration as necessary and as tolerated.
         b) Avoid excess sun exposure; a noncomedogenic sunscreen can be used.

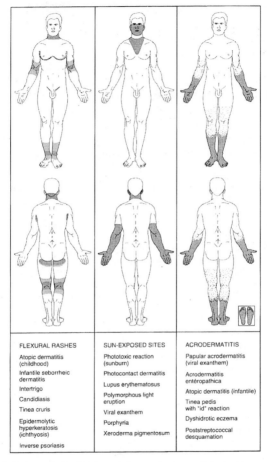

FLEXURAL RASHES

Atopic dermatitis
(childhood)

Infantile seborrheic
dermatitis

Intertrigo

Candidiasis

Tinea cruris

Epidermolytic
hyperkeratosis
(ichthyosis)

Inverse psoriasis

SUN-EXPOSED SITES

Phototoxic reaction
(sunburn)

Photocontact dermatitis

Lupus erythematosus

Polymorphous light
eruption

Viral exanthem

Porphyria

Xeroderma pigmentosum

ACRODERMATITIS

Papular acrodermatitis
(viral exanthem)

Acrodermatitis
enteropathica

Atopic dermatitis (infantile)

Tinea pedis
with "id" reaction

Dyshidrotic eczema

Poststreptococcal
desquamation

FIG 5-1. Pattern distribution of dermatologic conditions. (From Cohen B: *Atlas of Pediatric dermatology,* London, 1993, Mosby-Wolfe.)

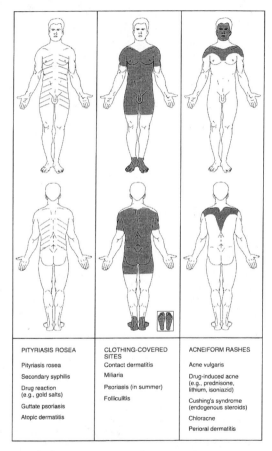

PITYRIASIS ROSEA	CLOTHING-COVERED SITES	ACNEIFORM RASHES
Pityriasis rosea	Contact dermatitis	Acne vulgaris
Secondary syphilis	Miliaria	Drug-induced acne (e.g., prednisone, lithium, isoniazid)
Drug reaction (e.g., gold salts)	Psoriasis (in summer)	Cushing's syndrome (endogenous steroids)
Guttate psoriasis	Folliculitis	Chloracne
Atopic dermatitis		Perioral dermatitis

FIG 5-1, cont'd. For legend see opposite page.

      c) Irritation can be minimized by applying a moisturizer in the morning or by spacing applications to every second or third night.

      d) Lesions may get worse for several weeks before improvement is seen.

  2) Benzoyl peroxide

      a) Begin by applying 2.5% to 5.0% gel or lotion qd or bid. Titrate the concentration against therapeutic and irritant effects.

      b) The typical regimen is to alternate retinoic acid hs with benzoyl peroxide in the morning.

  3) Topical antibiotics

      a) May be used in combination with retinoic acid and/or benzoyl peroxide

      b) Erythromycin solution, gel, or ointment applied bid

      c) Clindamycin 1% solution, gel, or lotion

      d) Tetracycline 1% ointment or solution (2.2 mg/ml)

 b. Systemic antibiotics

  1) Indications for use include the following:

      a) Moderate-to-severe papulopustular inflammatory acne, especially with propensity to scarring

      b) Patient unresponsive to or unable to tolerate topical medication

      c) Acne involving back, shoulders, and trunk

NOTE: A history of severe acne in a first-degree relative is a marker for potentially serious disease.

  2) Tetracycline: 500 mg bid; tapered to maintenance dosage of 250 mg qd. Do *not* administer to pregnant women or children under 12 years of age. Side effects need to be monitored.

  3) Erythromycin: 500 mg bid or 250 mg qid

  4) Clindamycin: Use limited by the risk of pseudomembranous colitis

  5) Minocycline: 100 mg bid for patients unresponsive to tetracycline or erythromycin

NOTE: It may take 4-6 weeks to note a clinical response. Intensify topical medications as systemic therapy is tapered.

 c. Accutane (isotretinoin): Oral systemic analog of vitamin A

  1) Accutane is indicated for patients with severe, recalcitrant, nodulocystic acne that is unresponsive to conventional treatment and especially for patients with a propensity to scarring.

  2) Dosage is 1 mg/kg/d ÷ bid, with adjustments based on efficacy

and side effects; the usual duration of treatment is 4-5 months.

3) Because of teratogenic effects, a negative pregnancy test must be obtained within 2 weeks of initiating treatment, and contraception must be used from 1 month before to 1 month after therapy. Informed consent should be obtained.

4) Monitor for side effects (e.g., dry eyes, chapped lips, epistaxis, pruritus, alopecia, scaling on palms and soles, an inability to wear contact lenses, pseudotumor cerebri).

5) Follow lipid profiles ($\uparrow$ triglycerides, $\uparrow$ LDL, $\downarrow$ HDL), LFTs ($\uparrow$ enzymes), and obtain a pregnancy test.

d. Other therapies (in consultation with dermatologist)

1) Estrogen (in the form of an oral contraceptive) for girls older than 16 years of age who are unresponsive to antibiotics and not candidates for Accutane

2) Low-dose dexamethasone or prednisone for patients with evidence of androgen excess; may use in combination with oral estrogen

3) Intralesional corticosteroid injection of individual lesions

4) Comedo extraction

5) Dermabrasion and laser resurfacing for old scars

B. ATOPIC DERMATITIS (ECZEMA)

1. Eczema is characterized by erythema, edema, papules, and weeping in the active phase. Scales and lichenification may develop later. Paroxysmal and severe pruritus is a hallmark of eczema. If there is no pruritus, the condition is not eczema! Pyoderma (staphylococcus or streptococcus) is often superimposed.

2. Three clinical phases

a. Phase I, infantile eczema (2 months-2 years): Face, neck, scalp, trunk, extensor surfaces of extremities. One third of the patients progress to Phase II.

b. Phase II, childhood eczema (2 years-adolescence): Flexor surfaces are predominantly involved (antecubital, popliteal, neck, wrists, sometimes hands and feet).

1) Atopic dermatitis of the feet appears in some children during this phase and involves the soles of the feet with cracking, erythema, and pain; tinea pedis (athlete's foot) may present as an eczema-like rash on one foot, even in young children.

2) One third of these patients progress to adolescent eczema.

c. Phase III, adolescent eczema: Hands (mostly), eyelids, neck, feet, and flexor areas may be involved.

3. History of asthma or hay fever may be present in patients (30%) and their families (70%).
4. Commonly associated findings include a tendency for dry skin, keratosis pilaris (chicken-skin appearance), increased palmar markings, cheilitis of the upper lip, atopic pleats, lichenification, and ichthyosis vulgaris.
5. Triggers include excessive bathing and hand-washing, occlusive clothing (especially wool), sweating, stress, and a possible food allergy (e.g., eggs, milk, seafood, nuts, wheat, soy).
6. Patients with immunodeficiency may have eczema.
7. Differential diagnosis
   a. Seborrhea
   b. Scabies
   c. Irritant contact dermatitis
   d. Psoriasis
   e. Tinea capitis
   f. Pityriasis rosea
8. Treatment
   a. Educate the family and patient that eczema is a chronic, recurring disorder that cannot be cured but can be controlled with conscientious therapy. The condition usually decreases in severity (and may disappear) with age.
   b. Acute phase
      1) With weeping lesions, use wet compresses (cotton cloth) soaked in aluminum acetate solution (Burow's solution, Domeboro 1 packet/quart cool water). Apply 10-20 minutes, 4-6 × daily × 2-3 days. Plain cool water may also be used as a compress.
      2) Provide systemic antistaphylococcal therapy if superimposed infection is suspected. Local treatment will not work if infection is neglected.
      3) Local steroids: Apply 1% hydrocortisone ointment frequently for maintenance therapy of mild dermatitis of the face and intertriginous areas. A more potent steroid such as triamcinolone 0.1% or even fluocinonide (Lidex) 0.05% may be needed to control flares (e.g., Lidex bid × 4-5 days). *Do not use fluorinated steroids on the face or intertriginous areas.*
      4) Emollients are best for dry, scaling, or fissured eruptions; apply petrolatum, Eucerin, Moisturel, Aquaphor, or Acid Mantle Creme 3-4 × daily.
      5) Baths: Aveeno (oatmeal) bath. Use ½ cup per half tub of tepid

water × 15 minutes. Hot baths and scented soaps are contraindicated. Cleanse bacteria-prone areas with unscented soap.

NOTE: Aveeno (OTC preparation) is expensive, and insurance prescription plans do not cover it.

    6) Antipruritics: Hydroxyzine (Vistaril, Atarax) 1-2 mg/kg may be used hs.

  c. Chronic management: The goal is hydration of the skin and relief of itching.

    1) Avoid irritants (e.g., wool clothing, soaps, excessive bathing, excessive sweating). Keep as much skin covered with cotton clothing as possible.

    2) Use a brief, tepid "drip-dry" bath without soaps (except in groin, anal, axillary areas) followed by the application of a lubricant.

      a) If soap must be used, use a mild nonscented soap (e.g., Dove).

      b) Avoid Ivory, Dial, and Safeguard. With the skin still wet, apply a lubricant (e.g., petrolatum, Eucerin, Keri lotion, Aquaphor) liberally and prn.

NOTE: These preparations are OTC and (except petrolatum) are expensive.

    3) Steroids: Cover involved areas adequately bid.

      a) Use a low-potency steroid (1% hydrocortisone) for long-term use because of the danger of hypopigmentation and systemic absorption.

      b) Attempt to wean the patient from steroids as soon as possible through the liberal use of lubricants several times each day.

    4) Hydroxyzine is sometimes useful for itch relief. Make sure the fingernails are cut short.

    5) Follow-up: Schedule the first visit within 1 week to review therapy. Schedule monthly visits until the patient is using lubricants only; visits q3-6mo then suffice.

    6) Eczema may be seen in systemic disorders (e.g., Wiskott-Aldrich syndrome, severe combined immunodeficiency syndrome).

C. CONTACT DERMATITIS

1. Contact dermatitis involves the acute onset of an intensely pruritic papulovesicular eczematous rash in patches or streaks that are localized to the site of antigen contact. Contact dermatitis can be confused with insect bites, scabies, and eczema. Any dermatitis

localized to one area of skin (e.g., dorsum of feet) is suggestive of contact dermatitis.
2. Contact dermatitis may be allergic or irritant (secondary to toxic chemicals); common causes include the following:
   a. Poison ivy/oak/sumac; usually occur as linear streaks and commonly on face, extremities, and scrotum
   b. Shoe-leather allergy; occurs on sides and dorsum of feet with sparing of interdigital areas and soles; can be confirmed by patch testing
   c. Nickel allergy secondary to poor-quality jewelry
   d. Topical medications
3. Treatment
   a. Avoid further contact with allergen.
   b. Initiate a course (7-10 days) of a topical fluorinated steroid preparation; be cautious with quantity and frequency of application because of the risk of irritation.
   c. An oral antihistamine may be useful to control itching.
   d. If lesions are on the face or genitals, are widespread, or are accompanied by edema (especially with poison ivy), a 10-14–day course of oral prednisone (1 mg/kg/d, max 60 mg) is indicated.
NOTE: Poison ivy is not just a summertime problem.

D. DIAPER RASH
1. Some infants have sensitive skin that is predisposed to diaper dermatitis. Others have seborrheic, psoriatic, or atopic dermatitis, and others may have a candidal rash alone or superimposed on another dermatitis.
2. General guidelines
   a. The most important therapy for any type of diaper rash involves avoiding continuous moisture and excessive heat; change diapers frequently. Avoid plastic pants and occlusive diapers. Keep skin dry (superabsorbent disposable diapers may help), and air-dry the diaper area as much as possible.
   b. Cleanse the diaper area with warm water at each diaper change. If soap is necessary, use a mild one (Dove).
   c. Frequently apply a protective ointment with a petrolatum or zinc oxide base (e.g., A&D ointment, Desitin, zinc oxide).
   d. If pyoderma develops, use wet compresses and a PO antibiotic for streptococcus and staphylococcus coverage. Do not use topical antibiotics because they are very sensitizing.
3. Primary irritant dermatitis results from prolonged contact with urine

and feces and their irritating chemicals and enzymes. It is characterized by erythema, scaling, shallow ulcerations, thickening of skin, and possibly vesicles. It is accentuated on convex areas with sparing of the creases. The peak incidence is between 9 and 12 months of age.

a. Provide treatment as stated under Point 2.

b. If skin is inflamed, initiate a brief course of steroid (1% hydrocortisone) application with each diaper change × 5-7 days. Avoid fluorinated high-potency steroids.

c. Of the diaper rashes that last >4 days, 80% are colonized with *Candida* organisms even before the classic signs of monilial rash appear. Treatment includes alternating topical applications of nystatin, clotrimazole, or ketoconazole cream with 1% steroid ointment bid.

4. Monilial rash (*Candida albicans*): Fiery red, papular lesions with peripheral scaling at times; may also be pustular. Folds and genitals are involved, and satellite lesions are present. It is often difficult to find yeast on KOH. Look for thrush in mouth and perianal lesions.

a. Provide treatment as stated under Point 2.

b. Use topical nystatin, clotrimazole, or ketoconazole. Treatment may be required for as long as 3 weeks.

c. Use oral nystatin for thrush, perianal candidiasis, or chronic/recurrent diaper dermatitis.

E. ERYTHEMA MULTIFORME

1. Clinical features

a. Symmetric distribution of lesions evolving through multiple morphologic stages; erythematous macules, papules, plaques, vesicles, and target (iris) lesions (doughnut-shaped with an erythematous outer border, an inner pale ring, and a purple center). Lesions occur in crops and evolve over days, not hours (hives evolve over hours, not days and usually are not symmetric in distribution).

b. In patients with minor variant EM, lesions tend to occur over the face, dorsum of hands and feet, palms and soles, and extensor surfaces of extremities. The lesions may spread to the trunk and may be associated with burning and itching. There may be shallow mucosal ulcers and lesions, and photoaccentuation is common.

c. Systemic manifestations include fever, malaise, and myalgias.

d. Stevens-Johnson syndrome: Severe form of EM in which there is a prodrome of fever, malaise, myalgias, headache, and diarrhea followed by a sudden onset of high fever, toxicity, skin eruption

(EM), and inflammatory bullous lesions on two or more mucous membranes (oral mucosa, lips, bulbar conjunctiva, and anogenital area). The skin lesions tend to be more monoform, and there may not be neat target lesions.
2. Etiology
   a. Infection: Viral, bacterial, fungal, protozoal, mycoplasma. The most common antecedent illness of recurrent EM is HSV infection.
   b. Reaction to drugs (sulfonamides), foods, immunizations
   c. Connective tissue disorders
   d. Malignancy
3. Management: Work-up should aim at finding the underlying cause.
   a. EM minor: Usually mild and self-limited; complete healing in 3-4 weeks
      1) Oral antihistamines
      2) Moist compresses
      3) Colloidal oatmeal baths
   b. Stevens-Johnson syndrome
      1) Hospitalization with barrier isolation
      2) Fluid and electrolyte support
      3) Treatment of secondary bacterial infection
      4) Moist compresses to bullae, colloidal baths
      5) For mucosal lesions, frequent mouthwashes (diphenhydramine [Benadryl]/Maalox)
      6) There is no good evidence that systemic corticosteroids are effective, but they are usually used in toxic patients.
      7) Obtain an ophthalmology consult. Patients are prone to corneal ulcers, keratitis, uveitis, and panophthalmitis. Eye lesions of HSV infection may mimic EM.

NOTE: Topical acyclovir is not effective in treating herpes-associated EM, but long-term, maintenance oral acyclovir has been effective in *preventing* herpes-associated EM.

F. IMPETIGO
1. Etiology
   a. Bullous lesions: *Staphylococcus aureus*
   b. Nonbullous, crusted, honey-combed lesions: *S. aureus* ± GABHS
   c. A high percentage of *S. aureus* isolates are resistant to penicillin, and 5%-15% are resistant to erythromycin.
2. Treatment
   a. For superficial, localized lesions, topical mupirocin cream (Bac-

troban) applied tid × 7-10 days is the treatment of choice. Bacterial resistance and side effects (transient pruritus and stinging) are rare. There is better compliance than with systemic therapy.

b. For patients with widespread lesions, lymphadenopathy, fever, or lesions around the mouth, treat for 7-10 days with a course of oral cephalexin or cloxacillin. Penicillin is no longer considered adequate treatment for impetigo.

c. Gently cleanse skin; trim nails.

NOTE: Impetigo is highly contagious; check other family members and treat accordingly.

G. PEDICULOSIS

Pediculosis may involve the scalp, pubic area, eyelashes, and body; each type is caused by a specific louse.

1. Pediculosis capitis (head lice)
   a. Scalp pruritus with erythema, excoriations, and crusts; secondary infection is common. Live lice, eggs, and nits may be seen on the hair shaft. Nits fluoresce a pearly color under Wood's lamp.
   b. Head lice are spread by hair-to-hair contact, clothing, brushes, and hair apparel.
   c. Treatment
      1) Wash hair with regular shampoo and apply 1% permethrin cream rinse (Nix) or pyrethrin (RID, A-200). Repeat in 1 week and reexamine for visible lice or viable nits. Nits that are seen at least 10 mm from the scalp can be considered nonviable.
      2) Soak combs and hair apparel in alcohol for 1 hour. Bedding and clothing should be washed in hot water.
      3) Remove nits with a fine-tooth comb.
      4) Examine other family members; notify school.

2. Pediculosis pubis
   a. This condition may infest the pubic and perianal area, thighs, axillae, beard, mustache, and eyelashes; it causes intense pruritus.
   b. It is sexually transmitted in adolescents. Look for other sexually transmitted diseases.
   c. In children, *Pediculus pubis* may infest eyelids and may be a marker of sexual abuse.
   d. Treatment
      1) Shampoo the pubic area for 4 minutes with 1% lindane (Kwell) shampoo *or* apply pyrethrin lotion (RID, A-200) for 10-20 minutes; repeat in 1 week.

     2) Treat all sexual partners.
     3) For eyelid infestation, apply petrolatum 3-5 × daily to asphyxi-
        ate the lice and nits.
3. Pediculosis corporis (body lice) is uncommon in United States but is
  a problem in homeless populations.

H. SCABIES

1. Scabies is caused by the mite *Sarcoptes scabiei;* the mode of
  transmission is usually person-to-person, but it may (rarely) be
  picked up from bedding, clothes, and similar objects.
2. Scabies is characterized by pruritic papules, vesicles, pustules, and
  linear burrows. Secondary bacterial infection is common. Severe
  pruritus, especially at night, may precede skin lesions.
3. In older children and adults, areas of involvement are the webs
  of fingers, axillae, flexures of arms and wrists, belt line, and areas
  around the umbilicus, nipples, genitals, and lower buttocks. In infants, the palms, soles, head, neck, and intergluteal folds may be
  involved.
4. Differential diagnosis: Atopic dermatitis, contact dermatitis, drug
  reaction, insect bites, papular urticaria, acropustulosis
5. Diagnosis: The burrow can be identified by applying topical
  tetracycline and examining skin with a Wood's lamp. Lesions should
  be scraped with a mineral oil–coated scalpel blade and the debris
  placed on a slide and covered. Under low power, look for mites, ova,
  or fecal pellets. The yield with this procedure is low; diagnosis is
  usually based on the clinical appearance and response to treatment.
NOTE: In a family infestation, burrows are most commonly found in
infants and young children.
6. Treatment
  a. Permethrin cream 5% (Elimite) is the drug of choice. Apply from
    the neck down at bedtime and wash off in the morning. In infants
    and young children, the head should also be treated. For severe
    cases, may repeat in 1 week.
  b. An alternate treatment is lindane lotion 1% (Kwell). Apply to cool,
    dry skin at bedtime and wash off after 6-8 hours. The treatment
    should be repeated in 1 week. This treatment is not recommended
    in young infants.
NOTE: Pruritus persists for at least several weeks after adequate
treatment. Additional treatment is warranted only if mites are demonstrated. Antihistamines and topical steroids may help.

    c. Family members should be treated, even if asymptomatic. Permethrin is not approved for use during pregnancy; check with obstetrician.

    d. Clothing and bed linens should be machine washed in hot water (>48.8°C).

    e. Give oral antihistamine for pruritus.

I. SEBORRHEIC DERMATITIS

1. Seborrheic dermatitis is characterized by erythematous, dry, scaling, crusting lesions with or without a greasy, yellowish appearance.

    a. It occurs in areas rich in sebaceous glands (face, scalp, perineum, postauricular and intertriginous areas).

    b. Affected areas are sharply demarcated from uninvolved skin. It is common in infancy (appearing between 2 and 10 weeks of age); it usually resolves by 1 year of age, but a small percentage may go on to adult seborrheic dermatitis.

    c. Scalp lesions (cradle cap) consist of a greasy, salmon-colored, scaly dermatitis.

    d. This condition may be confused with eczema (less itching with seborrhea).

    e. In older children, psoriasis should also be considered in the differential diagnosis.

2. Treatment

    a. Use 1% hydrocortisone cream for dermatitis (not cradle cap).

    b. Keep diaper area dry.

    c. For severe cradle cap, apply baby oil to scalp × 15 minutes, then wash with Sebulex or Head and Shoulders shampoo.

    d. Must often treat for candidal superinfection.

J. TINEA (DERMATOPHYTE INFECTIONS)

1. Essentially three organisms (*Trichophyton, Microsporum, Epidermophyton*) cause tinea infections. Therapy is the same regardless of the organism but differs with the site and extent of infection (topical therapy for localized skin infection; systemic therapy for widespread skin infection and infection of the scalp, hair, or nails).

    a. Clinical appearance: Expanding raised margins, erythema, scaling; may be associated scalp alopecia with visible broken hair stubble; may create a "salt and pepper" appearance with short residual hairs poking above the scalp surface as black dots

    b. Diagnostic procedures

1) Wood's lamp: Fluorescence is seen with skin lesions of tinea versicolor and with *Microsporum* scalp infections. However, *Trichophyton* skin and scalp infections do not fluoresce.
2) Obtain a KOH preparation of scales, nail scrapings, or epilated hairs. Look for spores or hyphae.
3) Send a culture in uncertain cases and in all cases in which oral medication will be used.

2. Tinea corporis (body, "ringworm"), tinea cruris (genitocrural area, "jock itch"), tinea pedis (foot, "athlete's foot")
   a. Treatment: Use topical clotrimazole (Lotrimin), miconazole, or ketoconazole until completely clear, then 1-2 weeks longer. When lesions are multiple and widespread, oral therapy with griseofulvin is indicated.
   b. Erythrasma (caused by *Corynebacterium minutissimum*) is commonly confused with tinea cruris.
      1) Erythrasma is not as inflamed as jock itch and appears as reddish brown, scaly patches in intertriginous areas. Lesions fluoresce coral red under Wood's lamp.
      2) Treat with oral erythromycin 30-50 mg/kg/d × 7 days. It may take weeks to completely resolve.

3. Tinea capitis (scalp and hair)
   a. Treatment: Use micronized griseofulvin 15 mg/kg/d ÷ bid. Severe infections (e.g., kerions) may require 20 mg/kg/d.
      1) Give with whole milk or other foods containing fat to ensure optimal absorption.
      2) At least 8-16 weeks of griseofulvin are required for extensive skin and scalp infections.
      3) Oral ketoconazole should be used only if there is intolerance to griseofulvin.
      4) Adjunct therapy includes antiseborrheic shampoo (selenium sulfide) q2-3d.
   b. It is not necessary to check laboratory tests.

4. Kerion: Circumscribed erythematous, boggy, tender scalp mass with multiple pustules on surface. There may be a low-grade fever and local adenopathy, which represents an immune response to the dermatophyte and may be treated with griseofulvin as previously described.
   a. In some instances, there may be secondary bacterial infection, in which case antibiotics are also required.
   b. Steroids are helpful for severe inflammation. Start prednisone at a dosage of 1 mg/kg/d and taper over a 10-14–day course.

5. Tinea unguium (nails): The most difficult tinea infection to treat. Treatment involves itraconazole.
6. Tinea versicolor: Technically a yeast infection. It is characterized by superficial light tan, red, or white scaly macules that are usually on the neck, upper part of the back, chest, and proximal arms. Lesions are darker than surrounding skin in nonexposed areas and lighter on tanned or black skin.
    a. Diagnosis: A KOH preparation from scale scrapings shows the characteristic grapelike clusters of spores and the curved hyphae of tinea versicolor.
    b. Treatment: Use selenium sulfide solution (Selsun shampoo [OTC]) or propylene glycol 20%-40%. Oral ketoconazole can be used for resistant cases.

K. URTICARIA
1. Intensely pruritic, evanescent wheal and erythema reactions
    a. Lesions are usually circular and well circumscribed but can be of a variable size and pattern.
    b. Angioedema (giant urticaria) consists of transient localized areas of nondependent edema.
    c. Lesions may be localized or generalized. They may be associated with swelling of the tongue, hypopharynx, or larynx.
2. Multiple causes, but often not identified
    a. Drugs: Penicillin, aspirin, NSAIDs
    b. Food: Milk, peanuts, shellfish, egg whites, nuts, food additives
    c. Insect bites
    d. Infection: Bacterial, viral (Epstein-Barr virus, hepatitis), fungal, parasitic
    e. Physical: Heat, cold, exercise, mechanical pressure
    f. Direct skin contact: Medication, chemicals, animal dander
    g. With chronic (>6 weeks) urticaria, think of lymphoma (very rare), collagen disease, or psychogenic disease. Consider a work-up if symptoms suggestive of a systemic condition are present. It may be helpful for the family to keep a symptom diary. Skin tests are helpful only if food, a food additive, or penicillin is the suspected allergen.
3. Treatment
    a. Acute urticaria
        1) Antihistamines
            a) Hydroxyzine (Atarax, Vistaril) 0.5-1.0 mg/kg/dose q4-6h IM; 2 mg/kg/d q6h PO

b) Cyproheptadine (Periactin) 2-4 mg q8-12h or diphenhydramine (Benadryl) 1.25 mg/kg q6h
2) If urticaria is severe, a short course of oral prednisone may be
used but is rarely necessary.
3) Topical steroids are of no benefit.
NOTE: Patients with recurrent acute episodes should keep an EpiPen kit
(0.15-0.30 epinephrine self-injector) handy.
b. Chronic urticaria
1) Try to identify and avoid allergens; identification is possible in
only 20%-30% of cases.
2) Nonsedating antihistamine (terfenadine) may be helpful.
3) Steroids are not indicated.

L. VIRAL RASHES

1. Gianotti-Crosti syndrome (papular acrodermatitis of childhood)
   a. Symmetric distribution of multiple nonpruritic, 5-10–mm,
   pinkish-red papules over the face, arms, legs, buttocks, palms, and
   soles. The lesions fade slowly over 4-10 weeks with mild
   desquamation. There may be generalized lymphadenopathy,
   low-grade fever, mild constitutional symptoms, and hepatomegaly.
   b. In some parts of the world (not the United States), Gianotti-Crosti
   syndrome may be associated with hepatitis B infection.
   c. No treatment is required.
2. Herpes simplex
   a. Cold sores: Grouped vesicles on an erythematous base. They are
   most common on the mucocutaneous border of the lips (usually
   localized to one side) but may occur anywhere on the body. The
   usual culprit is HSV type 1.
   b. Primary gingivostomatitis: Small vesicles on the gingiva, tongue,
   buccal mucosa, and lips. After the vesicle breaks, a ragged shallow
   ulcer with an erythematous base remains and is often covered by
   a yellowish crust. Episodes are often accompanied by fever,
   adenopathy, and irritability and may last 7-10 days.
   c. The diagnosis can be confirmed by a Tzanck preparation or viral
   culture, but such tests are rarely necessary.
   d. In general, treatment is symptomatic.
   1) Use a mouthwash with diphenhydramine (5 ml) or sodium
   bicarbonate (2.5 ml in 250 ml warm water). Viscous lidocaine
   (Xylocaine) should be avoided (risk of seizures or arrhythmias
   secondary to mucosal absorption).
   2) Cold, nonacidic fluids

3) Cool compresses

4) In recurrent disease, the initiation of oral acyclovir at the time of prodromal skin tingling may abort the episode. Long-term suppressive therapy with acyclovir may be indicated in children with recurrent widespread eruptions.

e. Herpetic whitlow: Painful clustered vesicles and crusted lesions of the fingers. This condition may be seen at the time of primary oral herpes infection and is often confused with paronychia. It is common in medical personnel. It may spread following inappropriate incision and drainage. It is often recurrent.

NOTE: Herpes genital infections are uncommon in prepubertal children. Such infections should always raise the suspicion of sexual abuse, but most cases are probably not sexually transmitted.

M. WARTS

1. Common warts: Usually found on dorsum of hands and fingers. They are caused by HPV infection. Local trauma promotes inoculation of the virus, and treatment is as follows:

   a. Benign neglect: Most warts involve over a 2-year period. However, warts that do not resolve often spread to other areas.

   b. Keratolytics (Duofilm—lactic acid and salicylic acid in flexible collodion): Apply each evening; soak for 5 minutes before application, then cover with adhesive tape. Remove in morning. Reapply Duofilm the next evening. Continue until the wart clears.

   c. If Duofilm is unsuccessful, refer to a dermatologist for "CCCCC" (cutting, cautery, carbon dioxide laser, chemical, or cold [liquid nitrogen]).

   d. Rub wart with a potato cut in half, which is then thrown over the right shoulder in the lee of a tree and buried where it lands (Tunnessen, 1985). This must be done at midnight in the light of a full moon!

2. Subungual and periungual warts: Common in children who bite nails or pick at hangnails. Treatment is as follows:

   a. Wrap involved finger with common adhesive tape longitudinally and then circumferentially. Tape is removed for 12 hours every 6½ days and then reapplied. This procedure sounds like voodoo but often works after 3-4 weeks.

   b. If this procedure does not work, refer to a dermatologist for "CCCCC."

3. Plantar warts: Large size may be hidden by a collarette of apparently normal skin. Treatment is as follows:

    a. Pare away superficial thickened skin over the wart. Apply a piece of 40% salicylic acid plaster and cover with tape. Remove the acid plaster every 2-3 days, pare the area, and reapply the plaster. Repeat the procedure until the wart has cleared.

    b. If treatment is unsuccessful, refer to a dermatologist.

4. Anogenital warts (condyloma acuminatum)

    a. Need to consider sexual abuse, but most anogenital warts are acquired at delivery. There may be a long latent period.

    b. Refer to a dermatologist or gynecologist for treatment with podophyllin, cryotherapy, or laser ablation.

NOTE: Patients with immunodeficiency states (AIDS, posttransplant) may develop multiple, resistant warts.

BIBLIOGRAPHY

Acne

Hurwitz S: Acne vulgaris: pathogenesis and management, *Pediatr Rev* 15:47, 1994.

Shalita AR et al: Topical erythromycin vs. clindamycin therapy for acne: multicenter, double-blind comparison, *Arch Dermatol* 120:351, 1984.

Strauss JS et al: Isotretinoin therapy for acne: results of a multi-center dose-response study, *J Am Acad Dermatol* 10:490, 1984.

Winston MH, Shalita AR: Acne vulgaris: pathogenesis and treatment, *Pediatr Clin North Am* 38:899, 1991.

Atopic dermatitis

Fritz KA, Weston WL: Topical glucocorticosteroids, *Ann Allergy* 50:68, 1983.

Hanifen JM: Atopic dermatitis, *Pediatr Clin North Am* 38:763, 1991.

Hurwitz S: Eczematous eruptions in childhood, *Pediatr Rev* 3:23, 1981.

Krowchuk D: Practical aspects of the diagnosis and management of atopic dermatitis, *Pediatr Ann* 16:57, 1987.

Sampson HA, McCaskell CC: Food hypersensitivity and atopic dermatitis, *J Pediatr* 107:669, 1985.

Contact dermatitis

Hogan PA, Weston WL: Allergic contact dermatitis in children, *Pediatr Rev* 14:240, 1993.

Tunnessen WW Jr: Poison ivy, oak and sumac: the three witches of summer, *Contemp Pediatr* 2:24, 1985.

Weston WL, Weston JA: Allergic contact dermatitis in children, *Am J Dis Child* 138:932, 1984.

Diaper rash

Berg RW: Etiology and pathophysiology of diaper dermatitis, *Arch Dermatol* 3:75, 1988.

Jacobs AH: Eruptions in the diaper area, *Pediatr Clin North Am* 25:209, 1978.

Singalavanija S: Diaper dermatitis, *Pediatr Rev* 16:142, 1995.

Weston WL et al: Diaper dermatitis: current concepts, *Pediatrics* 66:532, 1980.

Erythema multiforme

Esterly NB: Special symposium: corticosteroids for erythema multiforme? *Pediatr Dermatol* 6:229, 1989.

Ginsberg CM: Stevens-Johnson syndrome in children, *Pediatr Infect Dis J* 1:155, 1982.

Hurwitz S: Erythema multiforme: a review of its characteristics, diagnostic criteria and management, *Pediatr Rev* 11:217, 1990.

Lemak MA et al: Oral acyclovir for the prevention of herpes-associated erythema multiforme, *J Am Acad Dermatol* 15:50, 1986.

Williams REA, Lever R: Very low–dose acyclovir can be effective as prophylaxis for postherpetic erythema multiforme, *Br J Dermatol* 124:111, 1991.

Impetigo

Demidovich CW et al: Impetigo: current etiology and comparison of penicillin, erythromycin and cephalexin therapies, *Am J Dis Child* 144:1313, 1990.

Leyden JJ: A review of mupirocin ointment in the treatment of impetigo, *Clin Pediatr* 31:549, 1992.

Lookingbill DP: Impetigo, *Pediatr Rev* 7:177, 1985.

Scabies and pediculosis

Carson DS et al: Pyrethins combined with piperonyl butoxide (RID) vs. 1% permethrin (NIX) in the treatment of head lice, *Am J Dis Child* 142:768, 1988.

Hogan DJ et al: Diagnosis and treatment of childhood scabies and pediculosis, *Pediatr Clin North Am* 38:941, 1991.

Lane AT: Scabies and head lice, *Pediatr Ann* 16:51, 1987.
Pruksachatkunakorn C et al: Scabies: how to find and stop the itch, *Postgrad Med* 91:263, 1992.

Seborrheic dermatitis

Allen HB, Honig PJ: Scaling scalp diseases in children, *Clin Pediatr* 22:374, 1983.
Mimouni K et al: Prognosis of infantile seborrheic dermatitis, *J Pediatr* 127:744, 1995.
Williams ML: Differential diagnosis of seborrheic dermatitis, *Pediatr Rev* 7:204, 1986.

Tinea

Frieden IJ: Diagnosis and management of tinea capitis, *Pediatr Ann* 16:39, 1987.
Ginsburg CM et al: Effect of feeding on bioavailability of griseofulvin in children, *J Pediatr* 102:309, 1983.
Krowchuk DP et al: Current status of the identification and management of tinea capitis, *Pediatrics* 72:625, 1983.
Tanz RR et al: Ketoconazole vs. griseofulvin for tinea capitis, *J Pediatr* 112:987, 1988.

Viral rashes

Spear KL, Winkelman RK: Gianotti-Crosti syndrome: a review of ten cases not associated with hepatitis B, *Arch Dermatol* 120:891, 1984.

Warts

Bunney MH et al: An assessment of treating viral warts by comparative treatment trials based on a standard design, *Br J Dermatol* 94:667, 1976.
Cohen BA et al: Anogenital warts in children: clinical and virologic evaluation for sexual abuse, *Arch Dermatol* 126:1575, 1990.
Gellis SS: Warts and molluscum contagiosum in children, *Pediatr Ann* 16:69, 1987.

ENDOCRINOLOGY 6

A. DIABETES

1. Diabetes mellitus is a chronic metabolic disorder in which there is hyperglycemia that is generally secondary to insulin deficiency or, less commonly, to insulin antagonism.
2. There are two major types of primary diabetes: insulin-dependent (type I, IDDM) and noninsulin-dependent (type II, NIDDM).
   a. In IDDM, the insulin-producing capacity of the pancreas is severely limited as a result of the loss of β-cell function.
   b. In NIDDM, which occurs occasionally in children, there is often insulin resistance because of obesity or insulin receptor abnormalities.
3. Secondary diabetes may occur when there is insulin antagonism (excess glucocorticoid, hyperthyroidism, pheochromocytoma, growth hormone excess), unavailable glucose (glycogen storage disease), or the use of certain drugs (thiazide diuretics).
4. Important historical information includes the presence of weight loss, polydypsia, polyphagia, polyuria (especially nocturia or nocturnal enuresis), general health (physical and emotional), school performance, and a family history of diabetes.
5. Unless there has been weight loss or there is marked obesity (NIDDM), results of the PE usually are normal, except when the patient is in diabetic ketoacidosis (see Section B).
6. Laboratory tests include assessment of fasting blood glucose concentrations (suggestive: fasting level >120 mg/dL) or 2-hour postprandial concentrations (>180 mg/dL) on two separate occasions. Consider a glucose tolerance test if elevated glucose concentrations are discovered coincidentally during a well-child or acute-illness visit. The child is given 1.75 g/kg (max 75 g) of glucose in an oral solution after a 3-day preparation during which the child should take in at least 50% of the calories as carbohydrates. Both insulin and glucose concentrations are measured at the onset and at 30, 60, 90, 120, 180, and 240 minutes.
7. Treatment

a. Insulin: The child newly diagnosed with diabetes usually requires 0.5-1.0 U/kg/d of insulin, whereas the adolescent requires 1-1.2 U/kg/d. Insulin requirements are lower during the "honeymoon" or remission period; therefore individual monitoring is always essential.

1) Control is usually achieved with two daily doses of insulin; approximately two thirds of the daily dose is usually given in the morning, and one third is given in the late afternoon before dinner.

2) The doses are usually split from one-third regular and two-thirds intermediate to one-half regular and one-half intermediate. Both types are drawn into the same syringe and injected SQ.

3) If hyperglycemia is present between breakfast and lunch, the amount of AM regular insulin may be increased. If hyperglycemia is present later in the day, the amount of AM intermediate insulin may be increased.

4) Insulin dosages >1.5-2 U/kg/d might worsen diabetic control and produce widely variable blood glucose values. Rebound hyperglycemia following hypoglycemia (Somogyi phenomenon) results from the release of counterregulatory hormones (catecholamines, cortisol, glucagon, growth hormone) in response to hypoglycemia.

5) Increases or decreases in insulin dosage should be on the order of 10% at a time.

6) Blood glucose concentrations are assessed via glucose meters or strips before meals, before snacks, at bedtime and, if evening intermediate-acting insulin is used, in the middle of the night. Fasting and preprandial blood glucose levels in the 70-150 mg/dL range, postprandial levels below 180-200 mg/dL, and middle-of-the-night values above 65-70 mg/dL indicate good control.

7) Additional insulin may be needed during times of medical, surgical, or emotional stress.

8) Measuring Hb A_{1C} levels approximately every 3 months gives a picture of the quality of glucose control during the previous 3-4 months. Acceptable values are generally below 10%, depending on each laboratory's normal range.

9) Urinary ketones should be monitored periodically, especially if blood glucose levels are above 250-300 mg/dL or if the child is sick.

10) Blood lipids should also be assessed.

b. Diet: A child with diabetes requires the proper calories and nutrients to control his or her disease and to promote adequate growth.
   1) Before puberty, total intake usually approximates 1000 calories + (100 calories × age in years).
   2) The diet should be composed of approximately 55%-60% carbohydrates (starches rather than simple sugars), 25%-30% fat (polyunsaturated, vegetable sources), and approximately 15%-20% protein.
   3) Twenty percent of the calories should be consumed at breakfast, 20% at lunch, 30% at dinner, and 30% divided into three snacks, but these percentages depend on each individual's activity level. Meals should be timed on a regular basis.
c. Exercise: The child with diabetes needs adequate exercise. He or she should always carry a simple sugar in case he or she becomes hypoglycemic during exercise. If this condition occurs repeatedly, the diet should be adjusted or the insulin dose decreased.
d. Hypoglycemia: The symptoms of hypoglycemia result from catecholamine release (trembling, sweating, tachycardia) and from cerebral glucopenia (sleepiness, confusion, mood changes, seizures, coma).
   1) Causes include excess insulin, decreased oral intake, and exercise without a concomitant increase in calories.
   2) The child and family should be educated in depth about hypoglycemic episodes. If alert, the child with hypoglycemia may ingest a carbohydrate snack to stop the attack. Instant glucose or cake icing can be applied between the teeth and cheek in children who are vomiting or unable to eat on their own.
   3) The child who is having seizures, is stuporous, or is vomiting intractably should receive IV glucose and/or 1.0 mg glucagon IM.
e. Psychologic support is needed for both patients and parents to assist in coping with the impact of a chronic condition on their daily lives.
f. Diabetes should be managed in conjunction with an endocrinologist and diabetes management team.

B. DIABETIC KETOACIDOSIS

1. DKA is a state of metabolic derangement in which the patient is acidotic, has an elevated serum glucose level, and has serum ketones present; the acidosis is secondary to the ketosis. DKA occurs at times

of physical or emotional stress, infectious illness, and noncompliance with insulin therapy. The first presentation of new-onset diabetes is often DKA.

2. Important historical information includes whether the patient is known to have diabetes, the usual (and most recent) insulin dose, diet in the previous 24 hours, and whether the child is physically or emotionally ill or stressed (and the symptoms thereof).

3. The PE of the patient with DKA often reveals him or her to be weak, sleepy, lethargic, or frankly comatose. The patient may be severely dehydrated. If awake, the patient may have abdominal pain, nausea, or vomiting. There may be a fruity odor (ketosis) to the breath, and Kussmaul's respirations may be present.

4. For a patient in whom DKA is suspected, the following baseline studies should be performed immediately:
   a. Dextrostix/Chemstrip: Glucose elevated
   b. Serum acetone: Positive
   c. Serum glucose: Elevated
   d. Venous pH: Low
   e. Serum CO_2: Low
   f. Serum BUN: Normal or high
   g. Serum PO_4: Low
   h. Serum K: Low, normal, or high
   i. Serum Ca: Low to normal
   j. Urine glucose/ketones: Elevated

5. DKA constitutes a medical emergency. Begin treatment immediately.
   a. Fluids
      1) Assess hydration; the patient with DKA *will* be dehydrated.
      2) Administer normal saline (or Ringer's) solution at 20 ml/kg/h × 1-2 hours. In children whose serum osmolality is high, a normal saline infusion is continued until serum osmolality decreases toward normal.
      3) Administer half-normal saline solution to replace the deficit plus maintenance and ongoing losses over 24 hours. Various recommendations have been made for the rate of this fluid replacement; a common rate is 50% of the deficit replaced in the first 8-10 hours, with the remaining 50% replaced in the next 14-16 hours (ongoing losses would need to be added to the amount of fluids replaced). Fluids can be given before insulin administration.

NOTE: To minimize the risk of cerebral edema, be careful not to administer fluids too quickly.

b. Insulin
  1) Administer regular insulin 0.1 U/kg by IV bolus *after* the blood glucose level is known. Some endocrinologists recommend administering 1 hour of IV fluid before giving any insulin.
  2) Follow with a regular insulin drip of 0.1 U/kg/h piggybacked into the IV line (e.g., 50 U insulin/250 ml saline solution). An insulin drip is preferable to repeated boluses to maintain finer control of the serum glucose level. If acidosis does not improve within 2 hours, the IV insulin rate may be increased to 0.15-0.20 U/kg/h.

NOTE: To maintain potency, insulin infusates should be discarded every 6 hours and are preferably administered through a constant infusion pump. Never delay starting an insulin drip because the patient has had a recent dose of insulin.

c. Glucose
  1) Measure Dextrostix/Chemstrip qh.
  2) Measure serum glucose q3-4h (more frequently early in therapy).
  3) Rate of glucose fall should be 75-100 mg/dL/h. A drop that is too rapid may precipitate CNS dysfunction.
    a) If glucose falls <50 mg/dL/h, consider increasing the insulin rate.
    b) If glucose falls >100 mg/dL/h, continue insulin drip (0.1 U/kg/h) and add D_5W to the IV.
  4) When serum glucose approaches 250-300 mg/dL, add D_5W to the IV, even if early in therapy.
  5) When serum glucose is <200-250 mg/dL and if ketonemia is still present, continue insulin drip and add more IV glucose until ketosis is cleared.

d. Acidosis
  1) Administer bicarbonate *only if* pH <7.10, serum HCO_3 <5 mEq/L. The dosage is 1-2 mEq/kg $NaHCO_3$ IV over 1-2 hours *or* added to the first bottle of half-normal saline solution. Administer only enough bicarbonate to raise the pH to a maximum of 7.20.
  2) Follow venous pH and HCO_3 30 minutes after the infusion and then q2-4h.

e. Serum ketones
  1) Consider initially measuring serum ketones along with serum glucose.
  2) β-Hydroxybutyrate is not measured by Acetest tablets, but as

therapy progresses it converts to a measurable ketone, acetoac-
etate. This phenomenon can give the false impression that
ketosis is worsening.

NOTE: Because ABG results are now available so rapidly, serum
ketones are not usually measured.

    f. Electrolytes
      1) Follow serum electrolytes q3-4h.
      2) Phosphate
        a) Phosphate is depleted in DKA and is further depleted with
          therapy.
        b) Replace with potassium phosphate (see the following point).
      3) Potassium
        a) K is depleted in DKA even though serum K can be "normal,"
          high, or low.
        b) ECG can be used to approximate serum K.
        c) Withhold K at the beginning of therapy if the serum K level
          is elevated or if the patient is anuric.
        d) Administer maintenance plus deficit K over 24 hours.
          Replace K, half as KCl and half as KPO_4 for the first 8 hr,
          then as all KCl. A general guide is to give 40 mEq/L if initial
          K is less than normal. In severe hypokalemia, large K inputs
          are necessary. However, if the K level is elevated at the onset
          of treatment, K should not be added to the IV fluids until the
          serum K has fallen into the normal range. Depending on the
          dose infused, patients may require cardiac monitoring while
          receiving K.
    g. Monitor vital signs, fluid intake, and output.

C. HYPOGLYCEMIA

1. Hypoglycemia is defined by a low serum glucose concentration
(premature infant ≤25 mg/dL; term infant 1-3 days old ≤35 mg/dL;
infant ≤40 mg/dL; children ≤50 mg/dL).
2. Hypoglycemia may result from prolonged or excessive insulin
secretion or from disturbances in gluconeogenesis or glycogenolysis,
which occur when there are excessive body needs (e.g., sick
premature infants).
3. Symptoms of hypoglycemia are caused by catecholamine release
(tachycardia, diaphoresis, flushing, anxiety, weakness, hunger) and
by cerebral glucopenia (confusion, behavior changes, stupor, seizures, coma).

   a. If severe and prolonged, hypoglycemia may cause brain damage.
   b. In the neonate, symptoms include jitteriness, pallor, diaphoresis, hypothermia, weakness, poor feeding, apathy, seizures, and apnea/tachypnea.
4. Important historical information includes the presence of the aforementioned symptoms, their timing and frequency, the possibility of drug or toxin ingestion, the patient's growth and general health, and a family history of similar episodes.
5. The PE should be complete.
6. Causes of hypoglycemia
   a. Neonatal hypoglycemia: Secondary to hepatic enzyme immaturity, reduced hepatic glycogen stores resulting from in-utero malnutrition, sepsis, severe systemic illness, hyperinsulinism resulting from maternal diabetes, or hyperplasia/increased secretion (nesidioblastosis) of β cells or islet cells
   b. Postprandial hypoglycemia: Postprandial hypersecretion of insulin or heightened tissue response to normal insulin levels
   c. Fasting (hyperinsulinism)
   d. Deficiency of hormones regulating serum glucose levels: Growth hormone, ACTH/cortisol, catecholamines, thyroid hormone, glucagon
   e. Defective liver enzymes that control gluconeogenesis/glycogenolysis: Glycogen storage disease, galactosemia, maple syrup–urine disease, fructose metabolism disorders, fatty acid degradation defects
   f. Adrenal disease: Insufficiency, congenital adrenal hypoplasia
   g. Hepatic disease: Insults resulting from tumors, leukemia, hepatitis, toxins
   h. Ketotic hypoglycemia: Thought to be secondary to endogenous gluconeogenic amino acids (notably alanine). Attacks occur in the morning; are associated with stress, fasting, or infection; and respond rapidly to glucose administration. Such children are normal between attacks.
   i. Early stages of NIDDM: Erratic insulin secretion, exercise-induced hypoglycemia in diabetes, insulin overdose
   j. Miscellaneous: Drugs (e.g., insulin, alcohol, salicylates, oral hypoglycemic agents, propranolol), kwashiorkor, Reye's syndrome
7. Laboratory tests are dictated by the findings of the history and PE. A 5-hour glucose tolerance test and glucagon tolerance test, which challenges the liver's glycogenolysis potential, may be useful,

especially if the child has no reactive symptoms. A work-up for hyperinsulinism, hormonal deficiencies, and metabolic defects is very important.

8. Short-term treatment of hypoglycemia includes PO or IV glucose administration.

   a. If the child is alert, he or she should be encouraged to drink carbohydrate solutions; if incapable of taking oral fluids, he or she should receive IV glucose (10%-25% dextrose solution).

   b. Glucagon (1.0 mg IM) may also terminate the hypoglycemic attack but is useful only in children with hyperinsulinemia. Blood glucose and insulin levels should be followed.

   c. Long-term management is tailored to the underlying disorder causing the attacks. Children with ketotic hypoglycemia should be fed frequently; those with hormonal deficiencies may respond to exogenous replacement; those with enzyme deficiencies should receive the appropriate diet; those with hyperinsulinism may improve with diazoxide.

9. Both patients and parents require psychologic support to assist them in coping with the impact of this condition on their lives.

10. The patient with hypoglycemia should be managed by an endocrinologist.

D. HYPERTHYROIDISM

1. Hyperthyroidism results from the excessive secretion of thyroid hormone.

   a. There is a neonatal variant of hyperthyroidism (usually secondary to maternal hyperthyroidism) and the more common acquired type. A diffuse goiter is generally present. Hyperthyroidism usually is considered a manifestation of an autoimmune disease.

   b. The sex ratio is equal in the congenital variant; in the acquired variant, the female-to-male ratio is 5:1.

2. Important historical information includes the child's appetite (usually voracious with weight loss or little or no weight gain), mental state (restless, irritable, hyperactive, anxious), presence of tremors, proptosis (uncommon in children), excessive sweating, and increased stool frequency. The older patient may complain of palpitations.

3. The PE should be complete, with particular attention given to vital signs (elevated HR and widened pulse pressure), ocular signs (proptosis), cardiac assessment (decompensation may occur, especially in infants), and thyroid (size, appearance, consistency, presence of a bruit).

4. In thyroid "storm" (malignant hyperthyroidism, which is rare in pediatric patients), the patient may have hyperthermia, tachycardia, delirium, or coma; such an episode may be fatal.
5. Laboratory tests include measurement of thyroxine (T_4) and triiodothyronine (T_3) by RIA; both T_3 and T_4, as well as the T_3 resin uptake, are elevated. Antithyroglobulin and TSH receptor–stimulating antibodies may be present.
6. Treatment modalities include surgical and medical approaches, but surgery is usually performed *only* if medical therapy is unsuccessful or not feasible.
   a. Medical therapy of congenital hyperthyroidism consists of Lugol's solution (1 gt q8h) and propylthiouracil (5-10 mg/kg/d ÷ q8h). Propranolol might also be needed to control tachycardia (1-2 mg/kg/d PO ÷ q6h).
   b. Parenteral fluids, digoxin, and propranolol may be necessary if the infant is ill (especially cardiac decompensation).
   c. Medical therapy for acquired hyperthyroidism consists of propylthiouracil (5-10 mg/kg/d ÷ q8h) or methimazole (0.5-0.7 mg/kg/d qd or bid); the drug dosage is carefully titrated to the child's response because excess medication can precipitate hypothyroidism. The CBC should be followed to look for agranulocytosis. Treatment continues for at least 2 years and should be tapered slowly before discontinuation.
   d. Hyperthyroidism should be managed in conjunction with an endocrinologist.

E. HYPOTHYROIDISM

1. Hypothyroidism results from deficient production of thyroid hormones. There is a congenital variant and an acquired type.
2. Congenital form (cretinism): Early (first weeks of life) signs/symptoms include prolonged neonatal jaundice, poor appetite and suck (large tongue), choking or dyspnea with feeding, constipation, infrequent cry, sluggishness, hypothermia, and bradycardia.
   a. If the condition remains uncorrected for the first 3-6 months of life, the infant will likely display linear growth retardation, large fontanelles, hypertelorism with periorbital puffiness, a flat nose, a gaping mouth with a protruding and enlarged tongue, a hoarse cry, a short neck, sparse hair, hypotonicity, and apathy.
   b. If untreated, mental development is permanently retarded.
3. Acquired form: The patient may have apathy, dry skin, hypothermia, and constipation.

   a. Depending on age and the duration of symptoms, physical growth and development may be affected to a greater or lesser degree.
   b. The thyroid gland may be enlarged or small.
   c. In lymphocytic thyroiditis, the gland is nodular, firm, and nontender. In suppurative thyroiditis, which is a rare cause of hypothyroidism, the gland is tender, large, and warm, with redness of the overlying skin.
4. Causes of hypothyroidism
   a. Pituitary disease (global)
   b. Deficiency of TSH or TRH
   c. Thyroid gland dysgenesis: Absence, hypoplasia, ectopia
   d. Thyroid gland dysfunction/enzyme deficiencies: Defects in iodide trapping, oxidation, or incorporation into hormones; defects in thyroglobulin synthesis, hormone production, storage, or release
   e. Suppurative thyroiditis: Secondary to infection or trauma; rare cause of hypothyroidism
   f. Autoimmune thyroiditis (Hashimoto's disease): Most common form of acquired hypothyroidism with female-to-male ratio of 4-7:1. The gland is infiltrated by lymphocytes and plasma cells. At least half of all affected patients have antithyroid antibodies. Familial clustering occurs. This condition is associated with other autoimmune diseases, Down syndrome, and Turner's syndrome.
   g. Lack of dietary iodine (rare)
   h. S/P subtotal thyroidectomy
   i. Antithyroid (i.e., RAI) medication overdose
   j. Maternal ingestion of iodides or antithyroid medications during pregnancy
5. The history and PE should elicit signs and symptoms as listed under Points 2 and 3.
6. Laboratory tests include measurement of T_4 (low or borderline), T_3 resin uptake (low), and TSH (high if defect in thyroid, low if defect in pituitary or hypothalamus).
7. Neonatal screening identifies the majority of patients with congenital hypothyroidism.
8. Treatment of congenital hypothyroidism must be prompt if mental retardation is to be avoided.
   a. Because a good portion of T_3 is derived from T_4, the patient with hypothyroidism may be treated with oral sodium-L-thyroxine (neonates: initially 8-10 µg/kg/d; 0-12 months: 7-15 µg/kg/d; 1-5 years: 5-7 µg/kg/d; 5-10 years: 3-5 µg/kg/d; 10-20 years: 2-4 µg/kg/d).

b. The patient with suppurative thyroiditis merits I&D of the gland with appropriate antibiotic therapy.

c. Patients with hypothyroidism should be managed in conjunction with an endocrinologist.

F. SHORT STATURE

1. In infants, short stature may be associated with an overall failure to thrive. In older children and adolescents, short stature may be an isolated finding.

2. Short stature may result from growth failure or marked deceleration of growth so that the individual "falls" from his or her prior height percentile.

3. Important historical information includes prenatal and birth histories, growth pattern, presence of chronic disease, long-term medication use, developmental milestones, and the heights and pubertal patterns of parents and siblings.

4. A thorough PE is mandatory; however, most individuals with short stature have a normal exam.

5. The causes of short stature are numerous.

a. Genetic or familial (heights of relatives are useful)

b. Constitutional delay: Normal growth in early infancy with deceleration of growth by late infancy, early toddlerhood, or early childhood years; puberty, height, and bone age delayed by 2-4 years; adult height usually normal

c. Small for gestational age

d. Malnutrition or malabsorption (lack of calories for growth)

e. Chronic debilitating disease, especially inflammatory bowel disease

f. Emotional deprivation (hypothalamic suppression?)

g. Medications such as glucocorticoids, methylphenidate (Ritalin), pemoline (Cylert), and dextroamphetamine (Dexedrine)

h. Endogenous cortisol excess (Cushing's syndrome): Other associated signs are moon facies, hirsutism, buffalo hump, striae, hypertension, fatigue, voice deepening, obesity, and amenorrhea.

i. Cartilage or skeletal dysplasia (short extremities with normal-size head and trunk)

j. Turner's syndrome (genotype 45, XO, and related forms): Other associated signs are webbed neck, small jaw, prominent ears, epicanthal folds, low posterior hairline, a broad chest, and cardiac defects.

k. Pituitary dysgenesis/dysfunction: Growth may be normal initially, but by 1-2 years of age, growth is usually retarded and the body habitus is infantile. Other signs of pituitary dysfunction may be evident.

　　l. Hypothyroidism

　　m. Miscellaneous: Hypoparathyroidism, pseudohypoparathyroidism, and rickets

6. Laboratory tests are dictated by the history and PE. Bone age should be assessed.

7. Treatment includes reassurance when the work-up is negative and height velocity is normal; the provision of adequate calories for growth and the proper control of chronic illnesses are mandatory. Growth hormone and/or thyroid hormone is used in *appropriate* individuals and always in consultation with an endocrinologist.

G. GYNECOMASTIA

1. Gynecomastia in the male adolescent refers to unilateral or bilateral breast enlargement and is usually a result of a transient estrogen/ testosterone imbalance.

　　a. Gynecomastia usually begins at Tanner stage II or III, lasts for several months, and gradually disappears within 1-2 years.

　　b. The most common finding is a small, tender, round subareolar mass between 2 and 3 cm in diameter. The mass is not fixed, and there is no overlying skin dimpling.

　　c. Massive gynecomastia may indicate a major endocrine abnormality, perhaps in association with other abnormalities of sexual maturation.

2. Important historical information includes the duration of breast enlargement, breast symptoms, and pubertal progression.

3. A complete PE usually reveals only the breast enlargement, with the remainder of the exam being normal. However, the testes must be palpated because gynecomastia may be a first sign of a testicular tumor or Klinefelter's syndrome.

4. Common causes of gynecomastia

　　a. Normal variant: Adolescent gynecomastia

　　b. Pseudogynecomastia: "Swelling" not a result of breast tissue but a result of obesity or increased muscle mass

　　c. Klinefelter's syndrome: Karyotype, XXY

　　d. Drug use: Estrogen, chorionic gonadotropin, steroid, tricyclic antidepressant, methadone, marijuana, amphetamine, digitalis, cimetidine

　　e. Testicular tumor, liver cancer

5. Treatment consists of reassuring the patient; in most cases discontinuation of causative medications may help. Surgical correction may be required.

H. PREMATURE THELARCHE
1. Premature thelarche is isolated breast development in girls. It might (rarely) result from exogenous estrogen (not "true" premature thelarche) or from a slight increase in endogenous estrogen release.
2. The condition usually appears in girls between 1 and 4 years of age. Breast buds of 2-4 cm are evident without nipple or areola involvement. The child may complain of breast tenderness, and one breast may be more involved than the other. No growth acceleration is noted.
3. Important historical information includes the growth pattern and the use of medications or creams containing estrogen.
4. The PE should be complete. Note the appearance and size of the breasts, the appearance of the vaginal mucosa, and whether genital hair is present. A rectal exam should be done to detect any ovarian or uterine enlargement.
5. Laboratory tests
   a. Laboratory tests *may* include a bone-age assessment (normal in premature thelarche), a vaginal smear for estrogen effect, a pelvic ultrasound (to R/O organ enlargement, masses), and serum concentrations of LH, FSH, and estradiol-17β.
   b. In many cases no laboratory tests are indicated.
6. Treatment consists of close follow-up to detect other signs of puberty, discontinuation of any estrogen preparation (if used), and reassurance. Breast development may regress or stay the same. The onset of puberty usually occurs at the normal age. Follow-up is extremely important.

I. PREMATURE ADRENARCHE
1. Premature adrenarche is the isolated appearance of sexual hair (with or without axillary hair) before 8 years of age in girls and 9 years of age in boys without estrogen effects or other androgenic signs.
2. The condition probably results from increased hormonal production by the adrenal gland. Urinary 17-ketosteroid levels are generally slightly elevated for the patient's age.
3. Important historical information includes that obtained for precocious puberty (see Section J).
4. A complete PE is mandatory, including a careful genital exam. Breast

enlargement is usually absent; no estrogen effects are evident. Virilization is absent. Growth velocity and clitoral size should be normal.

5. Laboratory tests include bone-age assessment (usually normal or only slightly advanced), vaginal smear (should be prepubertal pattern), and serum androgen levels (rarely needed).

6. The patient and family should be reassured. The patient should be carefully followed to note any progression of development, especially height or bone-age acceleration. If virilization occurs, adrenal hypersecretion or an ovarian or adrenal tumor should be suspected.

J. PRECOCIOUS PUBERTY

1. Precocious puberty is present when pubertal development begins before 8 years of age in girls and 9 years of age in boys.
   a. Isosexual precocious puberty refers to development appropriate to gender, whereas heterosexual precocious puberty refers to development appropriate to the opposite sex.

2. Important historical information includes the following:
   a. Prenatal and birth histories
   b. Age of attainment of developmental milestones
   c. Growth pattern
   d. The presence of chronic medical conditions; long-term use of medications
   e. A history of encephalitis, seizures, head trauma, hydrocephalus, headaches, visual symptoms, behavior changes, abdominal pain, and genitourinary symptoms
   f. A family history of neurofibromatosis, tuberous sclerosis, or McCune-Albright syndrome
   g. If the patient is a boy, information on the ages of pubertal attainment of the father and brothers is necessary.
   h. If the patient is a girl, the ages of menarche for sisters, mother, and grandmothers should be elicited.

3. The PE must be complete. Emphasis should be placed on the neurologic exam, the ophthalmologic evaluation (fundoscopic and visual fields assessment), and the genital exam (Tanner staging of pubic hair, genitals, and breasts). A rectal exam should be performed in girls to exclude the possibility of an ovarian mass.

4. Causes of precocious puberty
   a. Idiopathic (central): Premature activation of hypothalamic-pituitary axis for unknown reasons. 80% of girls and <50% of boys

with precocious puberty have this diagnosis. The diagnosis is confirmed by demonstrating pubertal levels of LH after the IV or SQ administration of GnRH.

b. Central pituitary/hypothalamic disease: Postinjury, hemorrhage, tumor, hydrocephalus, postinfectious

c. Neurofibromatosis, tuberous sclerosis, McCune-Albright (café au lait spots, fibrous dysplasia, bone cysts)

d. Gonadotropin-secreting tumors: Teratoma, hepatoblastoma, chorioepithelioma

e. Ovarian tumors: Granulosa cell tumor, arrhenoblastoma, lipid cell tumor, thecoma, dysgerminoma, cyst

f. Testicular tumors: Leydig's cell tumor, seminoma

g. Adrenal tumor or hyperplasia

h. Exogenous estrogen therapy

i. Anabolic steroid therapy

j. Androgen therapy

k. Hypothyroidism (severe and prolonged)

5. Useful laboratory tests include the following:

a. GnRH stimulation test: Either a traditional multisample IV test or a newer single sample SQ test can give a reliable LH level.

b. Head MRI or CT scan: To determine an intracranial lesion in the hypothalamus

c. Bone-age assessment: Advanced in precocious puberty; delayed in hypothyroidism

d. Serum gonadotropins: May be useful as a screen for puberty. However, low levels do not rule out central precocious puberty.

e. Serum estradiol-17β concentration: Elevated to levels consistent with the stage of puberty

f. Serum hCG concentration to exclude pregnancy or a gonadotropin-secreting tumor

g. Serum dihydroepiandrosterone sulfate concentration as a measure of adrenal function

6. If an ovarian tumor is suspected by PE or if serum gonadotropin levels are prepubertal, an abdominal ultrasound or CT scan should be obtained.

a. Depending on the type of ovarian tumor, various hormones are elevated in the serum (e.g., estradiol with granulosa cell tumors, progesterone with thecomas).

b. A vaginal smear to determine the amount of estrogen or progesterone effect may be useful.

7. If adrenal pathology is suspected (e.g., heterosexual precocious puberty in a girl), an abdominal CT or MRI scan is useful.
8. Treatment
   a. The first rule of treatment is to reassure and support the child. Parents should be encouraged to treat the child in an age-appropriate manner.
   b. Tumors should be removed, if possible, or otherwise treated medically.
   c. Congenital adrenal hyperplasia is treated with glucocorticoid therapy.
   d. In girls, idiopathic and several variants of central precocious puberty may be treated with a GnRH analog (*only* under an endocrinologist's direction).

K. RICKETS

1. Rickets is a defect in the mineralization of bone and growth-plate cartilage. There are three stages (↓ intestinal Ca transport, compensatory hyperparathyroidism, and inadequate parathyroid response).
2. The causes of rickets can be dietary (↓ intake, especially in vegetarians, premature infants on TPN, or breast-fed infants), a sequela of prematurity (↓ Ca, ↓ PO_4 intake, vitamin D deficiency), a side effect of certain drugs (furosemide, phenobarbital, phenytoin, antacids), renal/liver disease, malabsorption, or hypophosphatasia. Breast-fed infants who do not receive supplemental vitamin D are a newly recognized risk group.
3. The history should include details about the birth, diet, vitamin supplementation, medications, suspicion about renal/liver disease, stool appearance and pattern, history of bone pain, delayed growth, anorexia, bowed legs, or muscle weakness.
4. The PE should be complete. Look for splayed wrists, rachitic rosary (enlarged costochondral junctions), craniotabes, and bowed legs.
5. If rickets is suspected, a urine Ca:Cr ratio; urine P and Mg; urine pH (to R/O RTA); serum Ca, P, Mg; and total CO_2 should be obtained. Depending on the history, levels of alkaline phosphatase, BUN, Cr, 25-hydroxyvitamin D (25-OH-D), and 1,25-OH-D might also be useful. Also helpful are x-ray studies of the ribs (ends are cupped and appear farther from sternum than usual) and long bones (indistinct or widened epiphyseal plates, concave and widened ends of bones, ↑ distance from mineralized area of shafts to epiphyseal plates, osteopenia, irregular bone margins).

6. With vitamin D deficiency, serum Ca is normal or ↓, P is ↓ (without excess urine P), alkaline phosphatase is ↓, and 25-OH-D is ↓. In rickets resulting from P wasting, urine P is ↑ with a ↓ serum P; alkaline phosphatase is ↑, but serum Ca and 25-OH-D are normal.
7. Treatment of rickets depends entirely on the cause. Ca deficiency requires diet modification to include 500 mg/d of Ca, supplemental Ca, or vitamin D. For premature infants with rickets, supplement the diet with Ca glubionate (60 mg elemental Ca/kg/d) and KPO_4 (30 mg elemental K/kg/d). In infants, vitamin D deficiency is treated with 1000-4000 IU/d of cholecalciferol (vitamin D_3) PO; when the rickets has healed, the dosage can be lowered to 400 IU/d. RTA is treated with 2-3 mEq/kg/d of $NaHCO_3$ or sodium citrate. Rickets resulting from P wasting is treated with P supplements q4h PO in conjunction with 1,25-OH-D. Vitamin D deficiency associated with malabsorption/liver disease and renal disease requires joint management with a gastroenterologist and nephrologist, respectively, an endocrinologist, and a nutritionist.

BIBLIOGRAPHY

Diabetes

Plotnick L: Insulin-dependent diabetes mellitus, *Pediatr Rev* 15:137, 1994.

Reynolds J: Nutritional management of children and adolescents with insulin-dependent diabetes mellitus, *Pediatr Rev* 9:155, 1987.

Schiffrin A: Management of childhood diabetes, *Pediatr Ann* 16:694, 1987.

Skyler JS, Rabinovitch A: Etiology and pathogenesis of insulin-dependent diabetes mellitus, *Pediatr Ann* 16:682, 1987.

Diabetic ketoacidosis

Chase HP, Gary SK, Jelley DH: Diabetic ketoacidosis in children and the role of outpatient management, *Pediatr Rev* 11:297, 1990.

Plotnick L: Insulin-dependent diabetes mellitus, *Pediatr Rev* 15:137, 1994.

Schiffer A: Management of childhood diabetes, *Pediatr Ann* 16:694, 1987.

Hypoglycemia

Gruppuso P, Schwartz R: Hypoglycemia in infancy, *Pediatr Rev* 11:117, 1989.

Schatz D: Hypoglycemia in childhood diabetes, *Pediatr Ann* 23:289, 1994.

Hyperthyroidism

Behrman R, Vaughan V: The endocrine system: disorders of the thyroid gland. In *Nelson textbook of pediatrics,* ed 13, Philadelphia, 1987, WB Saunders.

Sills I: Hyperthyroidism, *Pediatr Rev* 15:417, 1994.

Hypothyroidism

Behrman R, Vaughan V: The endocrine system: disorders of the thyroid gland. In *Nelson textbook of pediatrics,* ed 13, Philadelphia, 1987, WB Saunders.

Fisher D: Hypothyroidism, *Pediatr Rev* 15:227, 1994.

Gruthers A: Congenital hypothyroidism, *Pediatr Ann* 21:15, 1992.

Short stature

LaFranchi S et al: Constitutional delay of growth, *Pediatrics* 81:82, 1991.

Root A et al: Short stature: when is growth hormone indicated? *Contemp Pediatr* 4:26, 1987.

Sandberg D et al: Short stature: a psychological burden requiring growth hormone therapy? *Pediatrics* 94:832, 1994.

Gynecomastia

Neinstein LS: Gynecomastia. In *Adolescent health care,* ed 2, Baltimore, 1991, Urban & Schwarzenberg.

Premature thelarche/premature adrenarche/ precocious puberty

Eckert KL et al: A single-sample, subcutaneous gonadotropin-releasing hormone test for central precocious puberty, *Pediatrics* 97:517, 1996.

Laue L, Cutler G: Unusual presentation: precocious puberty, *Contemp Pediatr* 10:102, 1993.

Lee P: Laboratory monitoring of children with precocious puberty, *Arch Pediatr Adolesc Med* 148:369, 1994.

Pescovitz OH: Precocious puberty, *Pediatr Rev* 11:229, 1990.

Rosenfield RL: Androgen disorders in children: too much, too early, too little, or too late, *Pediatr Rev* 5:147, 1983.

Schwartz D, Root A: Puberty in girls: normal or delayed? *Contemp Pediatr* 6:83, 1989.

Schwartz D, Root A: Puberty in girls: early, incomplete, or precocious? *Contemp Pediatr* 7:147, 1990.

Rickets

Bergstron W: Twenty ways to get rickets in the 1990s, *Contemp Pediatr,* 8:92, 1991.

Graef J, editor: *Manual of pediatric therapeutics,* ed 4, Boston, 1988, Little, Brown.

Markel H et al: *The portable pediatrician,* St Louis, 1992, Mosby.

FEVER

7

A. DEFINITION
1. Fever is defined as a rectal temperature greater than 38°C.
2. Rectal temperature is approximately 0.6°C higher than oral temperature, 1.1°C higher than axillary temperature, and equivalent to aural temperature.

B. DETECTION
1. Mothers can identify a high temperature in most young children without the use of a thermometer. A mother is almost always correct when she says that her child does *not* have fever on the basis of subjective criteria.
2. Liquid-crystal forehead temperature strips are associated with false-negative results and are not reliable.
3. Rectal temperature is the gold standard and is more reliable than oral, axillary, or aural temperature. Aural temperature devices may not be highly sensitive in young infants.
4. Fever may result from overbundling a small infant. When this condition is suspected, the child should be unbundled and the temperature retaken in 15-30 minutes; if normal, the infant may be considered to be afebrile.

C. CONSEQUENCES
1. Fever is an important physiologic sign of illness and is valuable in following the course of an illness and the response to therapy.
2. Effects of fever include the following:
   a. Increased HR, increased cardiac output
   b. Antiinfection properties or effects
   c. Malaise, discomfort, irritability (a result of disease or fever?)

D. NOT ALL FEVERS NEED TREATMENT
1. Why is symptomatic treatment possibly indicated?
   a. May reduce discomfort
   b. May reduce risk of a febrile seizure

c. May decrease energy expenditure in patients with cardiovascular compromise (e.g., CHD or sickle-cell disease)
2. Determine when symptomatic treatment is indicated, and advise parents accordingly.
   a. Educate parents that the temperature "won't keep going up" if no treatment is given (>41°C is rare) and that a temperature <41°C does not cause damage.
   b. Treat the patient, not the number.

E. TREATMENT
1. Remove excess clothing and blankets. Hydrate the patient with cool oral liquids.
2. Antipyretics
   a. Acetaminophen 10-15 mg/kg/dose q4-6h or 60-80 mg/kg/24h per year of age up to 5 years. Be sure parents understand the difference in concentration of acetaminophen in drops vs. elixir (1 tsp elixir = 80, 120, 160, or 325 mg; 1 tsp drops = 240 or 500 mg). Acetaminophen preparations include the following:
      1) Drops = 48, 100 mg/ml
      2) Elixir = 80, 120, 160, 325 mg/5 ml
      3) Chewable tablets = 80, 120, 160 mg
      4) Tablets = 120, 325, 500, 650 mg
      5) Suppositories = 80, 120, 125, 300, 325, 600 mg each
   b. Ibuprofen, a nonsteroidal antiinflammatory drug, at a dosage of 5-10 mg/kg q6-8h is as effective an antipyretic as acetaminophen.
   c. Aspirin is contraindicated as an antipyretic in children because of the risk of Reye's syndrome.
   d. The slight additional temperature reduction achieved with tepid-water sponging does not justify the added inconvenience or time.

F. EVALUATION OF THE FEBRILE INFANT <3 MONTHS OF AGE
1. Signs and symptoms of serious bacterial infection (SBI) can be subtle and nonspecific, and it is difficult to accurately identify all febrile infants who have SBI.
2. In general, the appearance of the infant is the most sensitive predictor of SBI. The most important factors in the global assessment include the following:
   a. Feeding pattern
   b. Irritability
   c. Responsiveness

   d. Level of activity

   e. Ability to be consoled

NOTE: Clinical appearance and observation scales may not be reliable in infants <3 months of age, even if performed by experienced physicians.

3. Neonates (<4 weeks of age) who have a history of *tactile* fever but are afebrile on presentation should receive a complete evaluation for possible SBI. However, the risk of SBI is very low if the patient appears well, has no focal findings, and has reassuring laboratory values. The neonate who has a history of an elevated *rectal* temperature and is afebrile on presentation *is* at increased risk of SBI.

4. The rate of SBI increases with an increasing degree of fever; 10% of all children with a temperature >40.5°C have bacteremia.

5. The response of febrile infants to an antipyretic is not clinically useful in detecting those with SBI or in differentiating a viral vs. bacterial infection.

6. The Rochester criteria can be used to identify those infants at *low risk* for SBI. If a febrile infant fulfills these criteria, the negative predictive value is approximately 99% for SBI or bacteremia. These criteria consist of the following:

   a. Generally well appearance of infant

   b. No previous or underlying disease; no perinatal complications

   c. No treatment with antimicrobial agents

   d. No evidence of skin, soft tissue, bone, joint, or ear infection

   e. Peripheral WBC count: 5000-15,000; absolute band count: <1500

   f. U/A: <10 WBC/HPF

   g. Stool: <5 WBC/HPF (in infants with diarrhea)

NOTE: Among infants evaluated for suspected sepsis, approximately 40% meet the Rochester low-risk criteria.

7. Laboratory evaluation

   a. WBC count/differential/smear: Findings suggestive of SBI include a ratio of

$$\frac{\%\ \text{lymphocytes} + \%\ \text{monocytes}}{\%\ \text{PMNs} + \%\ \text{bands}}$$

that is <1, as well as the presence of vacuolization and toxic granulations on the peripheral blood smear.

   b. U/A and urine culture
     1) In febrile infants, the prevalence of UTI ranges from 4.0%-7.5%.
     2) U/A may not accurately predict urine culture results; 20%-50% of febrile infants with UTI do *not* have pyuria. A Gram's stain of urine sediment may be a better screen.
     3) Except when there is an unequivocal source of fever, a urine culture should be obtained regardless of the results of the U/A.
     4) Urine should be collected by catheterization or suprapubic aspiration.

   c. Chest x-ray study
     1) In the absence of respiratory signs and symptoms, a febrile infant is unlikely to have an abnormal CXR.
     2) Indications include cough, tachypnea, rales, retractions, or rhonchi.

   d. Blood culture
     1) In febrile infants there is a 20% probability that an initially positive blood culture is a contaminant.
     2) The length of time before positivity helps distinguish "true" pathogens from contaminants; 97% of "true" pathogens result in a positive blood culture within 24 hours.

   e. Stool exam and culture
     1) A stool exam is of value only in infants with diarrhea. In such cases, stool should be examined for blood (hemoccult) and PMNs (methylene blue stain), and a culture should be sent for enteric pathogens.
     2) The best predictor of bacterial enteritis is the presence of blood in the stool.

   f. Lumbar puncture
     1) An LP is indicated for any child in whom the diagnosis of sepsis or meningitis is being considered on the basis of the history, observational assessment, or PE.
     2) It is extremely rare for bacterial meningitis to be manifest solely as a febrile seizure in the absence of other findings (altered sensorium, toxic appearance, nuchal rigidity, abnormal neurologic exam) that would mandate an LP.
     3) The work-up of a child who has had a febrile seizure and recovered consists solely of the work-up of the fever. A *routine* LP in all children with a fever and seizures(s) is not warranted. However, an LP is indicated in infants <3 months of age.

    4) In young infants it is important to consider CSF VDRL to rule out congenital syphilis.

  g. Viral cultures

    1) The highest yield comes from the nasopharynx and stool.

    2) Among febrile infants <3 months of age, more than half have an identified viral etiology (RSV, enterovirus, influenza). In many cases the infection can be detected early enough to alter management.

G. MANAGEMENT OF THE FEBRILE INFANT <3 MONTHS OF AGE

1. Febrile neonates 0-28 days

  a. Under most circumstances, febrile neonates <28 days, including those that meet the Rochester low-risk criteria, should have a full sepsis work-up (including LP, U/A, urine culture). They should be hospitalized for parenteral antibiotic therapy pending culture results.

  b. An alternative strategy for low-risk infants is a complete sepsis work-up, hospitalization, and close observation pending culture results.

2. Febrile infants 28-90 days

  a. Infants who do not meet the low-risk criteria should have a full sepsis work-up and be hospitalized for parenteral antibiotics pending culture results.

  b. For infants who meet the low-risk criteria, the probability of an SBI is approximately 0.2%. Such patients can be managed in one of two ways, which are listed as follows:

    1) If the parents are reliable and prompt medical follow-up can be ensured, the infant can be managed as an outpatient with IM ceftriaxone (50 mg/kg) after blood, CSF, and urine cultures have been obtained. The infant should be rechecked in 18-24 hours, at which time a second dose of ceftriaxone can be administered. At the time of recheck, the following should occur:

      a) Infants whose CSF or blood culture is positive or who show clinical deterioration should be admitted for antibiotic therapy.

      b) Infants with occult bacteremia for *Streptococcus pneumoniae* who are afebrile and appear well can be managed as outpatients with oral amoxicillin or penicillin. In such patients it is important to test susceptibility to penicillin and cephalosporins because there is an increasing incidence of resistance to both.

c) Infants with otitis media should receive a 10-day course of an oral antibiotic (e.g., amoxicillin).

d) Infants with a positive urine culture who are afebrile and not toxic should be treated with a 10-day course of an appropriate oral antibiotic plus a follow-up radiologic evaluation.

2) An alternate strategy for low-risk infants is outpatient observation without antibiotic treatment. Infants managed in this manner should have a urine culture but do not necessarily need a blood culture or LP. The patient should be evaluated in 18-24 hours. Infants with positive cultures should be treated as described previously.

H. FEVER IN THE CHILD 3-36 MONTHS OF AGE

1. In this age group most children with fever turn out to have a viral illness, but treatable conditions such as otitis, pneumonia, osteomyelitis, meningitis, UTI, and bacteremia need to be ruled out.

2. Occult bacteremia is present in approximately 4% of febrile children in this age group: 85% *S. pneumoniae,* 10% *Haemophilus influenzae* (lower since the widespread immunization of infants with HIB vaccine), and 3% *Neisseria meningitidis.* Risk factors for bacteremia include the following:

   a. Temperature >39°C
   b. WBC >15,000; >20,000, 25% risk of bacteremia; >30,000, 40% risk of bacteremia
   c. ESR >30 mm/h
   d. Toxic appearance (most important)

3. Untreated bacteremia is associated with a 56% risk of persistent fever, a 21% risk of persistent bacteremia, and a 9% risk of meningitis. These rates vary by organism (for meningitis, *H. influenzae* 26%, *S. pneumoniae* 6%) and are significantly reduced by outpatient antibiotic therapy.

I. EVALUATION AND MANAGEMENT OF THE FEBRILE CHILD 3-36 MONTHS OF AGE

1. Clinical assessment by an experienced clinician is most important.
2. The WBC and differential count can be used to determine the risk of bacteremia.
3. An algorithm for the management of a previously healthy child who

has fever without source is shown in Fig. 7-1. If a patient is considered at high risk for bacteremia (temperature >39°C, WBC >15,000), obtain a blood culture and administer IM ceftriaxone 50 mg/kg.

NOTE: In a child fully immunized with HIB vaccine, treatment with PO amoxicillin and IM ceftriaxone should be equally effective in preventing the majority of serious complications associated with occult bacteremia. However, this situation may change as the prevalence of penicillin-resistant pneumococcal strains increases.

4. U/A and a urine culture should be obtained before antibiotic treatment.
5. Close follow-up of children treated as outpatients is essential.

J. PETECHIAE AND FEVER

1. Among patients who have fever and petechiae, 7%-10% have meningococcemia. The evaluation of such patients should include a CBC with differential, a TC and/or streptococcus antigen test, a blood culture, and an LP.
2. Hospital admission and treatment with IV antibiotics should be strongly considered, especially for an ill-appearing child with an abnormal WBC, an increased band count, or an abnormal CSF exam result. Less aggressive management may be appropriate in the patient >3 years of age with signs and symptoms of pharyngitis (especially with a positive streptococcus antigen test).
3. The differential diagnosis includes streptococcal infection and respiratory virus infections.

NOTE: Meningococcal disease is more likely in patients with generalized petechiae, including the trunk and lower extremities. The risk of serious disease is low if the petechiae are only above the nipple line.

K. HEAT STRESS

1. The clinical features of heat-related illness are compared in Table 7-1.
2. Complications of heat stroke
   a. Cardiovascular: ECG changes, hypotension, myocardial dysfunction
   b. Hematologic: DIC, fibrinolysis, thrombocytopenia
   c. Hepatic: Cholestasis, ↑ liver enzymes, jaundice (often delayed 1-3 days)
   d. Metabolic: Hypernatremia, hypoglycemia, hypocalcemia, hypokalemia, lactic acidosis
   e. Renal: Acute renal failure, myoglobinuria
   f. Neurologic: Coma, focal neurologic signs, seizures

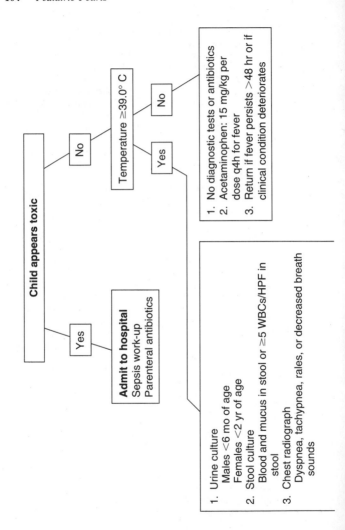

Child appears toxic

Yes

Admit to hospital
Sepsis work-up
Parenteral antibiotics

No

Temperature ≥39.0° C

No

1. No diagnostic tests or antibiotics
2. Acetaminophen: 15 mg/kg per dose q4h for fever
3. Return if fever persists >48 hr or if clinical condition deteriorates

Yes

1. Urine culture
   Males <6 mo of age
   Females <2 yr of age
2. Stool culture
   Blood and mucus in stool or ≥5 WBCs/HPF in stool
3. Chest radiograph
   Dyspnea, tachypnea, rales, or decreased breath sounds

4. Blood culture
   Option 1: All children with temperature ≥39.0° C
   Option 2: Temperature ≥39.0° C and WBC count ≥15,000
5. Empiric antibiotic therapy
   Option 1: All children with temperature ≥39.0° C
   Option 2: Temperature ≥39.0° C and WBC count ≥15,000
6. Acetaminophen
   15 mg/kg per dose q4h for temperature ≥39.0° C
7. Follow-up in 24-48 hr
   Blood culture positive
   Streptococcus pneumoniae
      Persistent fever: Admit for sepsis evaluation and parenteral antibiotics pending results.
   All others
      Admit for sepsis evaluation and parenteral antibiotics pending results.
   Urinalysis positive
   All organisms
      Admit if febrile or ill-appearing.
      Outpatient antibiotics if afebrile and well.

FIG 7-1. Algorithm for the management of a previously healthy child 91 days to 36 months of age with fever without source. (From Baraff LJ et al: *Pediatrics* 82(1):9, 1993.)

TABLE 7-1.
Heat Stress

	Heat exhaustion	Heat stroke
Onset	Often gradual	Usually acute, but may be prodrome
Temperature	Normal or mild elevation	40.6°C or above
Blood pressure	Normal or slightly hypotensive	Hypotensive
Skin	Pale, clammy, profuse sweating	Usually hot and dry but may be moist
CNS	Dizziness, headache, irritability, mild confusion but usually oriented	Agitation, disorientation, seizures, lethargy, coma
GI	Nausea, vomiting	Vomiting, diarrhea
Serum Na	Normal or elevated	Elevated
Mortality	Rare	Significant

3. Treatment
    a. Heat cramps
        1) Cessation of exercise
        2) Rest in cool environment
        3) Oral fluid and electrolyte replacement
    b. Heat exhaustion (heat collapse)
        1) Remove to a cool environment; remove constrictive clothing; cover the body with cold, wet towels.
        2) Replace fluid losses, orally if sensorium is clear and otherwise with IV fluids.
    c. Heat stroke
        1) Treat heat stroke as a true emergency; transport the patient to the nearest emergency medical facility.
        2) During transport, remove all clothing and cool the patient with cold, wet towels.
        3) In the ED, place the patient in an ice-water bath and rapidly cool to a core temperature of 38.3-38.8°C.
        4) Massage extremities to increase peripheral blood flow.
        5) Replace fluid and electrolyte losses with Ringer's lactate solution.
        6) Provide supplemental O_2.
        7) Monitor ECG and rectal temperature.
        8) Monitor and treat complications.
Do not use antipyretics or drugs to prevent shivering.

NOTE: Regardless of climate, a diagnosis of heat stroke should be considered when acute encephalopathy in infants is associated with fever.

BIBLIOGRAPHY

Fever

Baker MD et al: Failure of infant observation scales in detecting serious illness in febrile, 4- to 8-week-old infants, *Pediatrics* 85:1040, 1990.

Baker MD et al: Outpatient management without antibiotics of fever in selected infants, *N Engl J Med* 329:1437, 1993.

Baker RC et al: Fever and petechiae in children, *Pediatrics* 84:1051, 1989.

Banco L, Veltri D: Ability of mothers to subjectively assess the presence of fever in their children, *Am J Dis Child* 138:976, 1984.

Baraff LJ et al: Effect of antibiotic therapy and etiologic micro-organism on the risk of bacterial meningitis in children with occult bacteremia, *Pediatrics* 92:140, 1993.

Baraff LJ et al: Practice guideline for the management of infants and children 0-36 months of age with fever without source, *Pediatrics* 92:1, 1993.

Bass JW et al: Antimicrobial treatment of occult bacteremia: a multicenter cooperative study, *Pediatr Infect Dis J* 12:466, 1993.

Bramson RT et al: The futility of the chest radiograph in the febrile infant without respiratory symptoms, *Pediatrics* 92:524, 1993.

Crain EG, Gershel JC: Urinary tract infections in febrile infants younger than 8 weeks of age, *Pediatrics* 86:363, 1990.

Dagan R et al: Epidemiology and laboratory diagnosis of infection with viral and bacterial pathogens in infants hospitalized for suspected sepsis, *J Pediatr* 115:351, 1989.

Fleisher GR et al: Intramuscular versus oral antibiotic therapy for the prevention of meningitis and other bacterial sequelae in young febrile children at risk for occult bacteremia, *J Pediatr* 124:504, 1994.

Hoberman A et al: Prevalence of urinary tract infection in febrile infants, *J Pediatr* 123:17, 1993.

McCarthy CA et al: Outpatient management of selected infants younger than two months of age evaluated for possible sepsis, *Pediatr Infect Dis J* 9:385, 1990.

Muma BK et al: Comparison of rectal, axillary, and tympanic membrane temperatures in infants and young children, *Ann Emerg Med* 20:41, 1991.

Schmitt BD: Fever phobia: misconceptions of parents about fevers, *Am J Dis Child* 123:204, 1972.

Stephen M, Baraff LJ: Care of the febrile child: an annotated bibliography, *Am J Emerg Med* 9:281, 1991.

Heat stress

Bacon C et al: Heat stroke in well-wrapped infants, *Lancet* 1:422, 1979.

Robinson MD, Seward PN: Heat injury in children, *Pediatr Emerg Care* 3:114, 1987.

Rosenstein BJ: The twin perils of heat exhaustion and heat stroke, *Contemp Pediatr* 3:46, 1986.

GASTROINTESTINAL DISORDERS

8

A. ABDOMINAL PAIN

1. Abdominal pain may be acute or chronic/recurrent (at least three episodes in 3 months). It may represent surgical, medical, and emotional conditions. Chronic/recurrent abdominal pain occurs in approximately 10% of children between 5 and 10 years of age; however, less than 10% of these cases have an organic basis (often genitourinary) for the pain.
2. The history should be tailored to the circumstances of the pain (acute vs. chronic/recurrent).
   a. Where is the pain located? Does it radiate? Is it cramping, sharp, dull, constant, or intermittent?
   b. Does the pain make the child cry or abandon his or her usual activities? Does it occur at particular times of the day or certain days of the week? Does the pain awaken the child from sleep? Is it present on awakening? What is its relation to meals?
   c. How long does the pain last? Is the child totally well between episodes?
   d. What are the events, factors, or medications (including prescriptions, OTC preparations, home remedies) that relieve the pain?
   e. What is the child's diet? (Check especially for intake of lactose, fiber, fruit juices.)
   f. Does the child have any allergies or food intolerances? Which ones?
   g. Is the child taking any medications? Which ones?
   h. Does the child have a chronic medical condition? Which one?
   i. Has the child ever had a diagnosed GI medical problem or GI surgery? Elaborate.
   j. Is the pain accompanied by anorexia, nausea, reflux, vomiting, bloating, flatulence, diarrhea, or constipation?
   k. Are non-GI symptoms present (e.g., fever, oral ulcers, sore throat, rash, cough, headache, joint symptoms)?

l. Is there a history of trauma? Elaborate.

m. Do other family members have similar symptoms?

n. In the female adolescent, when did menses begin? Is there a history of vaginal discharge or bleeding?

o. Has there been a change in the child's environment (e.g., home, friends, school) or behavior (e.g., poor school performance, apathy, argumentativeness)?

3. A complete PE is essential, with special emphasis on the abdomen and rectal exam.

a. With the patient in the supine position, the abdomen should be inspected for evidence of trauma (e.g., bruises, lacerations), chronic medical conditions (café au lait spots, neurofibroma, ash-leaf spots, tuberous sclerosis), rashes, petechiae, asymmetries, or distension. Is there a scaphoid abdomen or is a hernia present? Is there reverse peristalsis?

b. Palpation of the abdomen should be performed to elicit evidence of tenderness (including rebound), masses, or organomegaly. Are fluid waves present?

c. Detection of tenderness may be difficult in a crying, frightened child; performing the exam with the child sitting on the parent's lap may sometimes lessen the child's fear. In addition, if a child reports that "everything hurts" but does not act accordingly, palpation with the stethoscope ("I'm going to listen to you now") may help sort out real areas (if any) of tenderness. The child in real pain will say, "Ow," flinch, jump, blink, dilate pupils, or tear if the stethoscope palpation is painful.

d. Percussion of the abdomen is performed to determine the liver span, areas of dullness (shifting?), and overall tympanicity.

e. Auscultation should be used to determine the presence and quality of bowel sounds in each quadrant (hypoactive, normal, hyperactive, tinkles, rushes).

f. Try to elicit the presence of peritoneal signs (obturator, psoas).

g. A rectal exam should be performed to detect masses, tenderness, hard stool, and other signs.

h. If the patient is a female adolescent, a pelvic exam should be considered.

i. To gain some insight into the degree of incapacitation or emotional overlay that may be present, patients with abdominal pain should be observed walking, climbing onto the exam table, getting down from the table, and interacting with both parents and staff.

4. Selected causes of abdominal pain
    a. Infectious: Viral GE, bacterial enteritis, food poisoning (especially *Stapylococcus aureus, Salmonella* organisms), *Clostridium difficile* infection, parasite infestation, hepatitis, pneumonia (basilar), urinary tract infection, group A streptococcal infection
    b. Surgical: Obstruction, stenosis, malrotation, intussusception, Meckel's diverticulum, appendicitis, cholelithiasis, tumor. The diagnosis of appendicitis in young children is difficult to make before rupture. Pain is often periumbilical early in the course and only later moves to the RLQ. Anorexia and vomiting are often associated symptoms, whereas diarrhea is not.
    c. Medical: Peptic gastritis, reflux, esophagitis, cholecystitis, pancreatitis, renal calculi, constipation, ulcerative colitis, regional enteritis, Hirschsprung's disease, abdominal migraine, indigestion, allergic reactions to foods, medication use (especially erythromycin), porphyria, lactase deficiency, sickle cell crisis
    d. Trauma: Blows to the abdomen or back, falls (remember duodenal hematoma and pancreatic pseudocyst)
    e. Emotional: Depression, anxiety, school phobia, irritable bowel (spastic colon), abuse
5. Laboratory tests are dictated by the history and physical findings.
    a. If an acute surgical condition is suspected, a CBC with differential, ESR, serum chemistry studies (electrolytes, BUN, creatinine, glucose), and type and crossmatch are indicated in conjunction with radiographic studies of the abdomen, a stool test for occult blood, and U/A.
    b. The same studies may be indicated with blunt abdominal trauma. An ultrasound study may be needed to locate the site and extent of hematomas and other conditions.
    c. If pancreatitis is suspected or if there is diffuse abdominal pain, a serum amylase should be obtained.
    d. If stones are suspected, U/A and radiologic (or ultrasound) studies of the abdomen may be diagnostic.
    e. When inflammatory bowel disease is being considered, a CBC with differential; ESR; stool for occult blood, culture, and *C. difficile* toxin; and flat and upright abdominal x-ray studies may be helpful initially. Sigmoidoscopy and biopsy confirm the diagnosis.
    f. When gastroesophageal reflux/esophagitis is suspected, a stool for occult blood is obtained; diagnosis of these entities is confirmed by endoscopy. Results of a barium swallow may be normal if reflux is only intermittent. A barium swallow often shows reflux in young

infants and should not be the only basis for a diagnosis of pathologic gastroesophageal reflux.

g. Lactase deficiency is diagnosed by an abnormal lactose breath hydrogen test.

h. When uncomplicated viral GE is suspected, no laboratory tests (except perhaps U/A) are mandatory. However, when a bacterial enteritis is suspected, a stool for occult blood, a methylene blue exam (to detect WBCs), and culture are indicated. A CBC with differential and blood culture should be performed if the child is ill.

i. If parasitic infestation is suspected, a fresh stool sample for *Giardia* antigen, ova, and parasites should be obtained.

j. The possibility of hepatitis necessitates U/A, stool exam, serum bilirubin, liver enzymes (ALT, AST, GGT), and serologic screen for hepatitis A, B, and C.

k. Group A streptococcus pharyngitis, urinary tract infection, and pelvic inflammatory disease require appropriate cultures.

l. The child with suspected emotion-related pain should undergo few studies: U/A (to R/O occult urinary tract infection); a stool for occult blood, culture, *Giardia* antigens and ova/parasites (to R/O occult infection); and *perhaps* a CBC with differential and ESR.

6. Treatment is directed at the underlying cause of the pain.

a. Surgical problems are treated accordingly.

b. Infections are treated with the appropriate antibiotic or antimicrobial.

c. Inflammatory bowel disease responds to proper diet, antiinflammatory medications, and aggressive nutrition intervention.

d. Individuals with a lactase deficiency benefit from a lactose-free diet or exogenous lactase replacement (available in tablets).

e. Patients with reflux esophagitis benefit from small, frequent meals rather than infrequent, large ones; sitting upright or sleeping at a 45-degree angle after eating; avoidance of late-evening meals; an H_2 blocker (see p. 131); and properistaltic medication (cisapride, metoclopramide, bethanechol).

f. Patients with ulcers benefit from eliminating foods that seem to exacerbate symptoms and from the use of antacids, H_2 blockers, and relaxation techniques (see p. 131). The exclusion of *Helicobacter pylori* is indicated if symptoms persist or recur.

g. Children with emotion-related abdominal pain, as well as their parents, require patience and reassurance. Psychotherapy may be indicated in children with handicapping pain (missing school) whether or not it is organic.

B. ANAL FISSURE
1. An anal fissure is a break in the anal skin or rectal mucosa.
    a. Such breaks are caused by passing (with straining) hard stools; external fissures suggest Crohn's disease or possible child abuse.
    b. Blood is either on the outside of a hard stool or is mixed in a linear pattern in a looser stool.
    c. Fissures are particularly common in infants.
    d. The child is otherwise well but may cry before or during stooling.
    e. A history of incomplete evacuation, constipation, or attempts to stimulate stooling may be obtained.
2. The PE is important. With the child in the supine position, the buttocks are spread to stretch the anus. The location of the fissure is compared to the position of the hands on a clock (e.g., "fissure at the 8-o'clock position"). A proctoscopic exam is performed to ascertain the presence of internal fissures. It is best to use a true proctoscope and not a test tube.
3. Treatment of anal fissures is simple; soften the stools (see Section D), keep the area as clean as possible, and apply petroleum jelly locally with each diaper change.

C. GASTROINTESTINAL BLEEDING
1. Bleeding can occur anywhere in the GI tract. Such bleeding may be acute or chronic, gross or microscopic, and manifested in vomitus (hematemesis) or stool or both. Hematemesis and melena (black stool resulting from blood) usually indicate a proximal GI site as the source of bleeding. Hematochezia (bright red blood in stool) usually indicates bleeding in the distal small intestine or colon. However, if there is rapid GI transit time, the patient can have hematochezia after a proximal GI bleed.
2. Important historical information includes the following:
    a. Onset and duration of the bleeding
    b. Color (bright red vs. dark red)
    c. Rate (brisk vs. gradual)
    d. Possible non-GI sources (e.g., epistaxis)
    e. Presence of clots
    f. Description of any vomiting or diarrhea
    g. Child's condition or mental status (normal vs. semiconsciousness or shock)
    h. Presence of pain (location, radiation)
    i. Presence of previous GI bleeding, trauma (e.g., lye ingestion), surgery, or medical condition

   j. Presence of a chronic medical condition (e.g., hemosiderosis) or medication use (which?)
   k. Hematologic problems
   l. The possibility of an ingestion (elaborate as to what, how much, and when)
   m. Remember, many episodes of "red" vomitus or diarrhea are not secondary to bleeding but instead are the result of the ingestion of red fluids or foods. Therefore a dietary history of the previous 24-48 hours is necessary for all patients.
3. The PE should be complete, and particular attention should be given to the following:
   a. Vital signs (look for evidence of shock, orthostatic changes, and other abnormal signs), capillary refill time
   b. Mental status (clues to pain, shock), spontaneous movements (clues to presence of peritonitis, surgical abdomen)
   c. Skin: Petechiae, purpura, trauma
   d. Mouth and nose: Evidence of previous bleeding
   e. Abdomen: Distension, areas of tenderness, organomegaly, presence of masses or bruits, quality and location of bowel sounds
   f. Rectal exam: Fissures, hemorrhoids, trauma
   g. Is active bleeding occurring? From what orifice?
4. A CBC with differential, ESR, a platelet count, and coagulation studies should be performed unless the source of the bleeding is clearly from the oropharynx, epistaxis, an anal fissure, or hemorrhoids.
   a. Urine should be examined for the presence of blood.
   b. If the stool is bloody, a methylene blue stain and a stool culture should be performed.
   c. A sepsis work-up may need to be considered for certain patients, especially neonates.
   d. A CXR may be indicated if the respiratory exam is abnormal.
   e. If the child is actively bleeding, in shock, or has an acute surgical abdomen, other laboratory tests may be necessary (e.g., clotting studies, serum electrolytes, BUN, creatinine, type and crossmatch, imaging studies).
5. Causes of GI bleeding include the following:
   a. Swallowed blood: Neonate postdelivery, infant nursing at cracked or bleeding nipple, epistaxis, oral or pharyngeal trauma or bleeding; amount of bleeding may vary
   b. Esophagitis/gastritis: Results from ingestion of a corrosive material, alcohol, iron or aspirin overdose; amount of bleeding may vary

c. Esophageal varices: Secondary to portal hypertension; massive or chronic low-grade bleeding

d. Esophageal tear: Results from trauma or foreign body ingestion; variable bleeding (usually large)

e. Esophagitis: Results from hiatal hernia or gastroesophageal reflux; variable bleeding

f. Gastritis: Results from intractable vomiting (viral infection, ipecac use, anorexia nervosa, pyloric stenosis); small amount of bleeding

g. Hemorrhagic gastritis of the neonate: Result of sepsis, CNS disease, overwhelming systemic illness; massive bleeding

h. Gastric ulcer/duodenal ulcer: Midepigastric pain, vomiting; variable bleeding (may be massive)

i. Stress ulcer: Result of sepsis, CNS disease; large amount of bleeding

j. Gastric outlet obstruction (especially pyloric stenosis); small amount of bleeding

k. Enteritis: Result of infection with certain viruses, especially rotavirus, *Salmonella* and *Shigella* organisms, invasive *Escherichia coli, Campylobacter* organisms, and *C. difficile* overgrowth after antibiotic therapy; variable bleeding

l. Intestinal surgical disorders: Volvulus, obstruction, intussusception (currant jelly stools), Meckel's diverticulum, polyps, masses, perforation resulting from foreign-body ingestion; variable bleeding (usually large)

m. Intestinal hemangiomas; variable bleeding

n. Infantile milk allergy; variable bleeding

o. Hemosiderosis; may be massive bleeding

p. Ingestions, especially iron or aspirin; may be massive bleeding

q. Henoch-Schönlein purpura: Hemorrhagic rash, melena, abdominal pain, arthritis, hematuria; variable bleeding, may be marked

r. Hemolytic-uremic syndrome: Bloody diarrhea, renal failure, anemia, thrombocytopenia, CNS disturbances; may be massive bleeding

s. Ulcerative colitis: Bloody diarrhea, weight loss, abdominal pain, awakening during the night, arthritis, uveitis; variable bleeding

t. Regional enteritis: Bloody diarrhea, weight loss, abdominal pain, growth failure, perirectal disease, anemia, arthritis, fever; variable bleeding, may be marked

u. Anal fissure: Small amount of bleeding

v. Hemorrhoids: Small-to-moderate bleeding

w. Proctitis resulting from gonorrhea: Usually a small amount of bleeding

x. Hematologic disorders: Vitamin K deficiency in the neonate, aplastic anemia, leukemia, thrombocytopenia, hemophilia; may be massive bleeding

y. Sepsis, especially as a result of *Neisseria meningitidis*

6. The child with moderate-to-massive upper GI bleeding should be given nothing by mouth.

   a. A nasogastric tube is inserted and gastric lavage is instituted using normal saline; lavage until the return is clear. Leave the tube in place (intermittent suction). If active bleeding continues, the child may need to go to the operating room. Diagnostic endoscopy often is indicated.

   b. Surgical conditions should be corrected. Intussusception is treated by hydrostatic reduction with contrast enema or by surgery (if nonsurgical correction is unsuccessful).

   c. Infections should be treated with the appropriate antibiotic.

   d. Iron ingestion is treated with fluids and electrolytes (and base if pH <7.10) and IV deferoxamine if the serum iron is >300 μ/dL 2-4 hours after ingestion (see p. 210).

   e. ASA ingestion is treated with lavage, activated charcoal, fluids, electrolytes, and base if pH <7.10; dialysis may be necessary (see p. 211).

   f. Uncomplicated Henoch-Schönlein purpura can be treated with steroids.

   g. Patients with a milk allergy and hemosiderosis require the elimination of milk from their diets.

   h. The management of ulcerative colitis, regional enteritis, anal fissure, hemolytic-uremic syndrome, and foreign-body ingestion is discussed elsewhere in this text.

   i. Hemorrhoids are treated by keeping the stools soft and applying topical anesthetics; recalcitrant cases may require proctoscopic evaluation.

D. CONSTIPATION

1. Constipation is the condition in which the child fails to completely empty the colon with bowel movements. Stools are often hard, difficult to pass, and infrequent.

   a. The usual cause of constipation is voluntary withholding and is commonly associated with a diet that is high in dairy products and complex carbohydrates or low in fiber and bulk.

   b. Starvation or intractable vomiting may lead to infrequent stooling.

   c. Resistance to toilet training and psychologic problems may lead to constipation (with or without encopresis) in the absence of an organic condition.

   d. Irritation of the anus (rashes, fissures) may cause avoidance of stooling.

   e. Miscellaneous causes of constipation include Hirschsprung's disease, hypothyroidism, and certain medications, especially antidepressants.

2. Important historical information includes the following:

   a. Onset, duration, and recurrences of the constipation. Most patients with Hirschsprung's disease have a history of abnormal stools beginning with the first month of life.

   b. Patient's usual stool pattern and daily diet

   c. Age of successful toilet training (if applicable)

   d. Presence of anorexia or vomiting

   e. Presence of diarrhea or fecal spotting that alternates with periods of constipation (Hirschsprung's disease, encopresis)

   f. Presence of anal lesions, fissures, rashes

   g. Psychologic difficulties

   h. Medication use (which ones?)

   i. Hypothyroidism (see p. 85).

3. The PE is usually normal except for the presence of hard stool palpable in the lower abdomen or in the rectum. The anus and surrounding area should be examined for rashes, lesions, and fissures.

4. Most children with constipation require no laboratory tests. If hypothyroidism is suspected, T_4 and TSH determinations are indicated. A rectal mucosal biopsy confirms the diagnosis of Hirschsprung's disease.

5. Treatment

   a. The child with constipation with impaction must be managed initially with an enema (Fleet or Pediatric Fleet, depending on the child's age) to achieve complete evacuation.

   b. The child with constipation without impaction does not require an initial enema.

   c. The diet should be improved, which specifically involves increasing fluid intake, decreasing the amount of complex carbohydrates (especially junk food) and cheese, increasing the amount of fiber and bulk (leafy vegetables work well), and encouraging daily ingestion of undiluted apple juice or pineapple juice.

   d. Stool softeners and stimulants should be reserved for children (not infants) in whom dietary measures are insufficient.

1) Softeners include mineral oil, docusate (Colace), and lactulose.

2) Stimulants must be free of phenolphthalein.

e. The child is encouraged to develop (with behavior modification) a habit of regular toilet use.

f. Anal fissures that can be associated with constipation are discussed on p. 113.

g. Battles over toilet training and emotional dysfunction require patience and counseling; emotional dysfunction may also require psychotherapy.

h. Hirschsprung's disease should be managed in consultation with a pediatric surgeon. Affected children also require emotional support.

E. DIARRHEA

1. Diarrhea is manifest by increased frequency and water content of stools.

2. The history should elicit the duration (chronic, acute, recurrent), frequency, amount, and consistency of the stools; compare with the patient's usual stooling pattern.

   a. What are the characteristics of the stool (e.g., blood, mucus, black, pale, greasy, foul-smelling)?

   b. Determine the diet history, which may give clues to lactose intolerance, celiac disease, and food poisoning; also determine medication (especially antibiotic) and travel history.

   c. Is there fever, vomiting, anorexia, cramps, headache, rash, lethargy, or a decrease in urination?

   d. Can the patient tolerate oral liquids?

   e. Has there been a recent exposure to others with diarrhea or previous *Salmonella* infection, or to food handlers?

   f. Is the child in day care? Are day-care contacts ill?

3. The PE should assess the child's vital signs, weight, appearance (toxic vs. well), degree of hydration, and perfusion.

   a. Other possible foci of infection (ear, throat, lungs, urinary tract) should be checked.

   b. Emphasize the abdominal exam, the skin exam (turgor, mucous membranes, purpura, exanthem), and the neuro exam (alertness, activity, tone, seizures).

   c. A rectal exam may be necessary if the diarrheal illness is more than mild.

4. Laboratory assessment of diarrhea includes the following:

    a. Stool exam: Evaluate for blood, mucus, appearance, and consistency. Obtain a methylene blue stain of stool smear to look for PMNs. Obtain a culture for bacteria if organisms such as *Salmonella, Shigella,* and *Campylobacter* are suspected or if the child is febrile or appears toxic. Test stool for parasites (if warranted by history) or *Clostridium* toxin, if indicated.

    b. Urine: Dipstick, specific gravity, microscopic; culture if indicated

    c. Blood: Obtain CBC, electrolytes, BUN; culture when indicated

5. Cause

    a. Acute diarrhea

        1) Viral

            a) Rotavirus

                (1) Common cause of acute diarrhea in infants; often preceded or accompanied by vomiting

                (2) Occurs year-round but usually in winter

                (3) Incubation 1-3 days; duration 5-8 days

                (4) May have fever and vomiting

                (5) May have $\downarrow$ HCO_3

                (6) Diagnosis by ELISA

            b) Enterovirus

                (1) Occurs usually in summer

                (2) Diagnosis by ELISA

            c) Adenovirus

                (1) Year-round occurrence

                (2) Causes GI/respiratory symptoms

                (3) Diagnosis by ELISA

            d) Norwalk virus

                (1) Epidemic

                (2) Self-limited (24-48 hours); prominent emesis

                (3) Diagnosis by electron microscopy of stool (research purposes only)

        2) Bacterial (accounts for 20% of acute GE)

            a) *Shigella* organisms

                (1) Seasonal; peak July to September

                (2) Peak incidence 1-5 years

                (3) Invades gut wall; bloody, mucoid stools

                (4) May be associated with febrile seizures

                (5) Vomiting not prominent

                (6) PMNs in stool

                (7) Bands in blood

(8) Treatment: Ampicillin (*not* amoxicillin) 75-100 mg/kg/d ÷ qid or TMP/SMZ 8 mg/kg/d (dose based on TMP) ÷ bid

b) *Salmonella* organisms

(1) Any age, but higher incidence under 1 year of age

(2) Invades gut wall; bloody, mucoid stools

(3) Temperature elevation possible

(4) Vomiting not prominent

(5) PMNs in stool

(6) Incubation 6-48 hours; 2-5–day course

(7) Organism may be shed in stool for months

(8) Transient bacteremia in 20%-40% of infants with salmonellal GE

(9) No treatment necessary for uncomplicated GE. Antibiotic indicated for infants <3 months of age (increased incidence of complications), highly febrile patients (enteric fever picture), debilitated patients, patients with sickle-cell disease or immune compromise, and day-care attendees.

c) *E. coli*

(1) Either invades mucosa (bloody stool) or produces an enterotoxin

(2) Patient (usually infant) may be very ill; requires IV antibiotics

d) *Campylobacter* organisms

(1) Invasive (blood and mucus); in neonates may cause bloody diarrhea without other clinical manifestations

(2) Severe abdominal cramps

(3) Vomiting/dehydration uncommon

(4) ↑ Incidence in summer

(5) Usually resolves spontaneously, but if treatment is needed, use erythromycin 40 mg/kg/d ÷ qid

e) *Yersinia enterocolitica*

(1) Mucoid stools

(2) PMNs often present in stools

(3) Severe abdominal pain possible

(4) Diarrhea × 1-2 weeks

(5) Often mimics appendicitis

(6) Treatment: Not usually indicated for infections confined to GI tract. If treatment is indicated, use TMP/SMZ 8 mg/kg/d ÷ bid × 5 days.

3) Noninfectious
   a) Acute poisoning: Fe, Hg, Pb, fluoride
   b) Antibiotic-induced: Ampicillin in particular; pseudomembranous enterocolitis caused by *C. difficile* overgrowth after antibiotic use
   c) Hemolytic-uremic syndrome: Hemolysis, thrombocytopenia, melena, hematuria, renal failure; CNS symptoms such as seizures, behavior changes, coma, and shock
   d) Toxic shock syndrome: Mediated by *S. aureus* toxin; has been associated with tampon use and with osteomyelitis, abscess, pneumonia, GU infection. Signs and symptoms include fever, diarrhea, hyperemic mucous membranes, generalized macular red rash, hypotension, and shock.
   e) Intussusception: Paroxysms of pain, bloody diarrhea, currant jelly stools, and irritability *or* pale apathetic state
b. Chronic diarrhea (infectious causes)
   1) Amebiasis
      a) Chronic diarrhea, lower abdominal pain, or perianal abscess
      b) May be asymptomatic
      c) Stool PMNs may be present
      d) Recurrent fever may be present
      e) Mucoid stool
      f) Treatment: Iodoquinol 30-40 mg/kg/d ÷ tid × 20 days (max = 2 g/d) or metronidazole 30-50 mg/kg/d ÷ tid × 10 days (max = 750 mg/d)
   2) Giardiasis
      a) Chronic diarrhea or lower abdominal pain
      b) May be asymptomatic or have frequent relapses
      c) Treatment: Furazolidone 6-9 mg/kg/d ÷ tid × 10 days or metronidazole 15-30 mg/kg/d ÷ tid × 10 days (max = 750 mg/d)
   3) *E. coli, Salmonella,* and *Yersinia* diarrhea may occasionally become persistent or recurrent.
c. Chronic diarrhea (noninfectious causes)
   1) Ulcerative colitis: Fever, abdominal pain, diarrhea (may be bloody), arthralgias, arthritis, growth failure
   2) Regional enteritis: Fever, abdominal pain, arthritis, diarrhea (may be bloody), growth failure
   3) Hirschsprung's disease: Constipation alternating with diarrhea or fecal spotting
   4) Lactase deficiency

5) Metabolic/malabsorption diseases: Cystic fibrosis, disacchari-
   dase deficiencies, celiac disease, and other conditions
6) Irritable colon
7) Encopresis
8) Food allergies
9) Excessive fructose intake

6. Treatment: There is controversy regarding the most appropriate way
   to manage outpatient acute diarrhea. Some authorities recommend
   stopping lactose-containing products; others do not. The following
   procedures are guidelines. The goal is to correct hydration and
   electrolyte imbalances and to maximize nutrition.

   a. Consider discontinuing lactose-containing formulas and milk.
      Older children may be able to tolerate a solid diet plus oral
      glucose-electrolyte solution. Breast-fed infants appear to tolerate a
      continuation of nursing. Children who continue regular formula or
      solids, as well as breast-fed infants who continue nursing, may
      have an initial slight increase in stooling but no prolongation of
      total duration of diarrhea. If the stool output is excessive, an infant
      may be managed with oral glucose-electrolyte solutions (see Point
      b) and advance to a lactose-free formula. If an infant is not or is
      only mildly dehydrated and is tolerating oral feedings, he or she
      may also be managed with a full-strength lactose-free formula (see
      the following discussion).

   b. Oral glucose-electrolyte solutions (OGESs)
      1) If an infant can take PO fluids and is mildly to moderately
         dehydrated (<8%), rehydration may proceed with OGESs.
         Rehydration with OGESs can be carried out even in patients
         with mild-to-moderate hyponatremia or hypernatremia. Some
         OGESs are low in Na concentration (30 mEq/L), which is
         usually not a problem with mild, self-limited diarrhea. Continue
         OGESs × 12-36 hours.
      2) The child with moderate-to-severe dehydration (>7%-8%) may
         need admission for appropriate replacement of fluids and
         electrolytes; replacement may be PO, if tolerated, or IV.

   c. Dehydration
      1) If a child is severely dehydrated (≥10%), provide rapid volume
         expansion by IV Ringer's lactate solution (20 ml/kg/h) × 1-2
         hours. Calculate estimated deficits of water and electrolytes.
         Replace deficits over 4-8 hours. Give patient his or her
         maintenance and cover ongoing losses for that same period.
      2) After this initial period, continue calculated maintenance and

TABLE 8-1.
Composition of Solutions Available for Oral Therapy

	Lytren	Ricelyte (rice syrup solids)	Pedia-lyte	WHO std.	Resol	Rehy-dralyte
Na (mEq/L)	50	50	45	90	50	75
K (mEq/L)	25	25	20	20	20	20
Cl (mEq/L)	45	45	35	80	50	65
HCO_3 or citrate (mEq/L)	30	34	30	30	34	30
Glucose (g/L)	20	30	25	20	20	25

ongoing loss therapy. Patient may be given OGESs (Table 8-1) after initial 4-8–hr therapy if tolerated. Continue × 12-36 hours.

3) Never treat diarrhea with half-strength Pedialyte or Lytren; those dilutions do not even supply *maintenance* electrolytes for someone *without* diarrhea.

4) Other commonly used "clear liquids" (e.g., apple juice, cola, ginger ale, Kool-Aid) are inadequate in electrolyte composition for rehydration or maintenance therapy; thus they should not be used as a mainstay of therapy except for very brief intervals or as "free-water" replacement.

5) Homemade solutions are fraught with all the hazards of errors in measuring and mixing, and their use should be discouraged.

d. Advance diet to nonlactose formula (e.g., LactoFree, ProSobee, Isomil) for infants who are not breast-feeding; advance to BRATS diet (*B*ananas, *R*ice, *A*pplesauce, *T*oast, *S*altines) for older children × 24 hours. Continue to normalize diet as tolerated.

e. Treat for underlying cause of diarrhea.

1) Treatment for bacterial and parasitic infections includes the use of the appropriate antimicrobial.

2) Pseudomembranous colitis resulting from *C. difficile* is treated by discontinuing the offending antimicrobial, restoring fluid and electrolyte balance, and metronidazole 30-50 mg/kg/d ÷ tid × 7-10 days or vancomycin 10-40 mg/kg/d ÷ q6h (max 2 g) × 7-10 days.

3) Other antibiotic-associated diarrheas are treated by discontinuing the drug.

4) Hemolytic-uremic syndrome is treated with appropriate IV fluid and electrolytes, blood transfusions (if necessary), seizure

control, and management of renal disease or increased intracranial pressure.
5) Toxic shock syndrome should be treated with IV nafcillin or
   oxacillin 100-200 mg/kg/d, IV fluids, vasopressors to maintain
   a normal BP, and ventilatory support, if necessary.
6) Intussusception is treated by hydrostatic reduction with contrast
   enema or surgery (unsuccessful hydrostatic reduction, symptoms ≥2 days, recurrent episodes, obstruction, or peritonitis).

F. ENCOPRESIS

1. Encopresis is recurrent fecal incontinence in the absence of organic
   disease. Approximately 1% of 7- to 8-year-olds (the peak age) are
   affected, with a male-to-female ratio of 3:1. Approximately half of the
   children have never been completely bowel trained. A single episode
   of fecal incontinence should not be regarded as encopresis.
   a. Hypotheses regarding possible causes include premature or
      coercive toilet training, fear of defecation because of previous
      "accidents" or pain (such as from an anal fissure), mental
      retardation, and isolated areas of neurodevelopmental delay.
   b. Organic lesions that can cause encopresis include those discussed
      under Section E, Point c, as well as several others such as central
      and peripheral nervous system disease, defects in rectal or anal
      musculature, chronic constipation with resultant overflow, and
      chronic laxative or enema use.
2. Important historical information includes the following:
   a. Onset and duration of the problem
   b. Current and previous stooling patterns
   c. Age of attainment of bowel control
   d. Appearance and consistency of stools
   e. Presence of constipation
   f. Chronic enema or laxative use
   g. Pattern of growth
   h. Psychosocial, emotional, familial, and scholastic assessments
3. The PE is usually normal. Emphasis should be placed on the
   neurologic exam and abdominal/rectal exams. The anal tone should
   be normal but may be patulous with chronic enema use, and the rectal
   vault should be of normal or enlarged size with feces present.
4. The possibility of organic disease should be obvious from the history
   and PE; if suspected, the work-up is as discussed for chronic diarrhea.
   a. A U/A and urine culture may demonstrate an occult urinary tract
      infection secondary to chronic constipation.

    b. Serum chemistry studies, ESR, CBC, and radiographic studies are usually normal in children with true encopresis.

5. Treatment of encopresis includes diet manipulation, colon evacuation with enemas or laxatives, establishment of (and reward for) a normal defecation pattern, reassurance, patience, counseling and, occasionally, psychotherapy.

G. GASTROESOPHAGEAL REFLUX

1. GER is the return of stomach contents into the esophagus as a result of increased relaxation of the lower esophageal sphincter. This incompetence may result from immaturity (as in infants), esophageal disease, obstructive lung disease, or overdistension of the stomach (because of overeating). A small degree of reflux is probably universal. GER may be accompanied by effortless vomiting (infants), aspiration pneumonia (infants), apnea (infants), belching, esophagitis (all ages), and midepigastric pain. Pain is worse after eating, especially if the patient is supine; in contrast, the pain of an ulcer is similarly located but is relieved by eating, especially in older children and adolescents.

2. In infants with suspected GER, the following questions are helpful:
    a. Is the infant vomiting (forceful projection) or "spitting up"?
    b. When does this occur (e.g., how long after a meal)?
    c. How is the infant fed (sitting up, laying down)? In what position is the infant placed after feeding? Does the position make a difference as to whether the infant is likely to spit up?
    d. Is the infant a rapid eater? Does he or she belch?
    e. How much (and what type of) formula does the infant take with each feeding? What other foods are ingested?
    f. Does the infant appear hungry?
    g. Is the infant gaining weight?
    h. What does the vomitus look like? Is it tinged with green or red?
    i. Does the infant wheeze, cough, or turn blue? When? Has the infant ever had pneumonia? When?
    j. Are there feeding difficulties? Elaborate.
    k. Does the infant have fever or diarrhea? Elaborate on the time and degree of fever and on the onset, duration, and appearance of diarrhea.
    l. Is the infant taking any medications? Which one(s)?

NOTE: Theophylline may worsen GER.

    m. Have any OTC preparations or home remedies been used to stop the vomiting? Which ones?

n. In the older patient, where is the pain (if any) located? Does it radiate? What is its relation to eating and lying down? What precipitates it? What causes relief?

o. Is the pain accompanied by fever, vomiting, diarrhea? If yes, elaborate.

p. Has the child ever vomited blood?

q. Does pain interfere with activities? Does it awaken the child from sleep?

3. The PE is usually normal. Young infants, however, may have failure to thrive or (rarely) torticollis (Sandifer's syndrome).

4. If significant vomiting, diarrhea, or failure to thrive is present, certain laboratory tests are useful to secure a diagnosis.

a. Except for those (especially infants) who have significant reflux and may be anemic, alkalotic, and hypochloremic, patients with GER (but without failure to thrive) usually have a normal CBC and serum chemistry profile.

b. If the chest exam is abnormal, a CXR (to R/O aspiration pneumonia) is indicated.

c. The diagnosis of mild reflux is made by the characteristic history. With moderate-to-severe reflux (especially if accompanied by failure to thrive or pulmonary symptoms), the diagnosis of GER may be confirmed by pH monitoring of the lower esophagus, measurement of lower esophageal sphincter pressure, a technetium "milk scan," or an endoscopy to look for evidence of esophagitis.

d. For any patient with moderate-to-severe GI symptoms or weight loss, a barium swallow should be performed to confirm normal anatomy and normal gastric emptying.

NOTE: Many normal infants show some reflux on barium swallow, and some infants with pathologic GER have a normal swallow because of the intermittent nature of the reflux.

5. Treatment of the infant with GER includes small, frequent feedings in the upright position; formula thickened with cereal (1 tsp/1 oz); and maintenance of a prone head-up position after feeding.

a. If these measures fail, a trial of bethanechol (0.1-0.3 mg/kg/dose tid-qid), metoclopramide (0.1 mg/kg/dose qid before meals), or cisapride (0.3 mg/kg/dose tid) may be efficacious in relieving symptoms.

b. If esophagitis is present, an H_2 blocker is indicated. The use of antacids is limited by concern regarding the side effects in infants and young children.

c. If medical management fails, fundoplication may be necessary.

d. Treatment of the older child with GER includes small, frequent meals; maintenance of an upright position after meals; eating slowly; and no meals after 7 PM. Bethanechol or metoclopramide should be considered if antireflux measures do not work. An H_2 blocker (cimetidine 5-10 mg/kg/dose before meals and hs or ranitidine 3-4 mg/kg/d ÷ bid) may be necessary for recalcitrant cases.

H. FOREIGN-BODY INGESTION

1. The most common foreign bodies ingested by children are metal objects (especially coins), buttons, small parts of toys, hair, tablets, and button batteries.
2. Foreign bodies that lodge in the esophagus may cause dysphagia, midsternal pain or fullness, gagging, choking, coughing, or respiratory embarrassment.
   a. Diagnosis is by posteroanterior and lateral x-ray studies of the chest and neck.
   b. The foreign body is usually located in the upper esophagus (C4 level).
   c. Removal may be accomplished in two ways: (1) during endoscopy in the OR, or (2) using a No. 8-14 Foley catheter. With the second method, a deflated catheter is passed into the sedated child's nose and into the esophagus; the balloon is inflated, and the foreign body is removed by traction on the catheter. The child should be taken to the OR if there is any concern about the safety of removing the foreign body in the office or ED. Because of their potential to leach chemicals, button batteries lodged in the esophagus must be removed as soon as possible.
3. Foreign bodies that pass into the stomach generally pass out of the body in 2-10 days. To localize the object's position, an x-ray study should be obtained when the child first arrives. If the object does not pass in 10 days or if GI symptoms occur, the child should return for evaluation (and possibly treatment). Emetics and cathartics should not be used.

I. JAUNDICE

1. Jaundice is clinically obvious yellowing of the skin, mucous membranes, and sclera as a result of an excess of bilirubin in the blood. Tears, saliva, secretions, and CSF may also be icteric. Jaundice is apparent when the bilirubin reaches 6-7 mg/dL in neonates and 2 mg/dL in older children and adolescents.

2. Important historical information to be elicited includes the following:
   a. Duration of symptoms? Worsening? Improvement?
   b. Associated GI or constitutional symptoms?
   c. Weight loss?
   d. Stool color change (e.g., clay color)?
   e. Darkening of urine?
   f. Pruritus?
   g. Exposure to the following:
      1) IV drug use?
      2) Sexual activity, especially anal sex?
      3) Persons with known hepatitis or jaundice?
3. A thorough PE is mandatory, with emphasis on the following:
   a. Skin color
   b. Scleral color
   c. Liver size (palpation and percussion)
   d. Abdominal (especially RUQ) tenderness
   e. Abnormal abdominal vascular pattern or distension
4. Laboratory work-up includes the following:
   a. CBC with differential, smear, and reticulocyte count (R/O hemolysis)
   b. Bilirubin (direct and indirect)
   c. SMA-7, SMA-12, amylase
   d. PT/PTT
   e. Hepatitis serology panel
   f. U/A; stool exam (acholic stools)
   g. Radiographic or imaging studies if a surgical cause seems likely
5. Differential diagnosis ($\uparrow$ indirect bilirubin)
   a. Hemolysis (e.g., ABO, Rh incompatibility, sickle-cell disease, α-thalassemia, drug reaction)
   b. Physiologic (neonate)
   c. Hypothyroidism (neonate)
   d. Hereditary/constitutional hepatic dysfunction
   e. Massive internal hemorrhage
   f. Pyloric stenosis, duodenal atresia, annular pancreas
6. Differential diagnosis ($\uparrow$ direct and indirect bilirubin)
   a. Infections
      1) Hepatitis A, B, C
      2) Epstein-Barr virus
      3) Cytomegalovirus
      4) Congenital rubella

     5) Herpes virus
     6) Syphilis
     7) Sepsis (bacterial)
     8) Toxoplasmosis (congenital)
     9) Amebiasis
     10) Leptospirosis
  b. Inborn errors of metabolism
     1) Wilson's disease
     2) Galactosemia
     3) Hereditary fructose intolerance
     4) Hereditary tyrosinemia
  c. Cirrhosis
  d. Chemicals, including cleaning fluids, heavy metals, certain drugs
  e. Congenital
     1) Biliary atresia
     2) Hypoplasia or atresia of hepatic ducts
     3) Cystic fibrosis
     4) α_1-antitrypsin deficiency
     5) Inspissated bile syndrome
     6) Dubin-Johnson syndrome
  f. Cholelithiasis
  g. Neoplasms
     1) Benign
     2) Primary malignant
     3) Metastasis
  h. Pancreatic disease
7. Treatment
  a. Treatment depends on the cause of the jaundice.
  b. Infectious viral hepatitis is treated by symptomatic and supportive measures; persistent viral hepatitis may respond to interferon-α.
  c. Bacterial infections require appropriate antibiotics.
  d. Hemolysis and internal hemorrhage require blood transfusions and control of any bleeding.
  e. Surgical disorders and oncologic disease are treated in consultation with those specialists, respectively.
  f. Pancreatitis is treated supportively unless complications develop. Such patients are generally given nothing by mouth and are given IV fluids with careful monitoring of vital signs, I&O, WBC, amylase, glucose, LFTs, BUN, Ca, albumin, and oxygen saturation. Pain relief is necessary.

J. PARASITES

1. Pinworms
   a. Diagnosis
      1) Intense pruritus ani, especially at night; vulvovaginitis; urinary tract infection; irritability; no eosinophilia
      2) Worms may be seen in the rectal area or stool; eggs are seen in anal skinfolds or the vaginal introitus.
      3) Scotch tape test; press tape to perianal area (best in evening before going to bed). Mount tape over a drop of toluene on a glass slide and look for ova with a microscope.
   b. Treatment
      1) It is often best to also treat other children at home. If recurrent, treat the entire family; make sure the mother is not pregnant.
      2) Launder bedclothes and undergarments; make sure children sleep in underwear to avoid contact of fingers with anus.
      3) Medication
         a) Mebendazole (Vermox); same dosage for all ages; 100 mg × 1; not much experience in children <2 years of age; contraindicated in pregnant women
         b) Pyrantel pamoate (Antiminth) 11 mg/kg to maximum of 1 g; given in a single dose
   c. Consider retreatment in 2 weeks. The chance for reinfestation is very high.
2. *Giardia* organisms (see p. 121)

K. PEPTIC ULCER DISEASE

1. PUD is the ulceration of the gastric or duodenal mucosa and results from an imbalance between the protective mechanisms of the mucosa and the effects of acid, pepsin, injury, and infection.
2. Most primary ulcers in children under 6 years of age are gastric and equally affect boys and girls. After age 10, most ulcers found in boys are duodenal. A primary duodenal ulcer is a chronic condition; at least two thirds of patients have recurrent disease after the completion of therapy.
3. Ulcers may occur because of the use of certain drugs (e.g., steroids and antiinflammatory agents), alcohol use, the stress of critical illness (e.g., Curling's ulcer associated with burns, Cushing's ulcer associated with trauma), a secondary manifestation of certain illnesses, and infection. Any condition that interferes with the protective mechanism of the mucosa or increases acid production contributes to the genesis and persistence of an ulcer.

4. *H. pylori* is an infection specific to gastric mucosa by a spirochete-like organism, which elaborates an enzyme (urease) that is capable of degrading gastric mucin. Epidemics have been related to contaminated water, travel, and raw milk. It seems to be a seasonal disease, peaking in June and November, and has been recognized as the most common cause of recurrent PUD in adults. In children, infection with *H. pylori* manifests primarily as antral gastritis.

5. Psychologic factors play a role in some patients. They have been described as bright overachievers, and they sometimes have anger or hostility (overt or covert). Peptic complaints are also common during times of divorce, an impending move, or child abuse.

6. Symptoms vary with age. In infants and young children, the symptoms are often feeding difficulties, vomiting, unexplained crying, or upper/lower GI bleeding. The pain may be periumbilical or poorly localized, may not be more prevalent at certain times of the day, and may not be affected by the types of foods or beverages ingested. On the other hand, older children and adolescents have adultlike symptoms, such as epigastric (or RUQ) pain approximately 1 hour after meals. When pain is related to esophagitis, it is relieved by eating or by antacids and is exacerbated by the ingestion of soda, juices, tomatoes, any acidic food or beverage, alcohol, and spices.

7. The PE often reveals epigastric tenderness to palpation. There may also be evidence of blood in the vomitus or stools. Therefore every child with suspected ulcer disease should have a stool test for occult blood. A baseline CBC is also useful to assess the degree and chronicity of bleeding.

8. If any significant or recurrent GI bleeding is noted, consultation with a pediatric gastroenterologist is advisable.

9. Treatment of uncomplicated PUD

   a. Antacids are no longer the mainstay of therapy because they are weak buffers of hydrochloric acid and cause diarrhea (magnesium) or acid-rebound (calcium). They may also interfere with the absorption (or excretion) of other medications.

   b. H_2 blockers inhibit gastric secretion. Cimetidine is used in a dosage of 20-40 mg/kg/d (use half of this amount for infants and young children) either tid or qid × 6-8 weeks; it might interfere with the hepatic processing of certain drugs, especially theophylline, warfarin, phenytoin, diazepam, propranolol, and lidocaine. Ranitidine is used in a dosage of 3-4 mg/kg/d ÷ bid; it has less effect on hepatic metabolism than does cimetidine.

c. The use of anticholinergics is limited to severe ulcer disease in combination with H_2 antagonists.

d. The therapy of *H. pylori* in childhood includes antibiotics (amoxicillin or clarithromycin [Biaxin] plus metronidazole) and bismuth given for 3-6 weeks.

e. Treatment must continue for several weeks to months; exacerbations and recurrences are common. Psychotherapy may be in order for patients with marked psychologic symptoms.

L. VOMITING

1. The history should differentiate between real vomiting and "spitting up."

   a. Important questions about vomiting relate to its frequency, severity, appearance (blood- or bile-tinged), amount, time of occurrence, projectile nature, and duration after meals.

   b. What has the child taken by mouth (foods, medicines, poison)?

   c. How has the parent treated the vomiting?

   d. Are there associated symptoms (e.g., fever, headache, earache, sore throat, cough, asthma, abdominal pain, diarrhea, rash, lethargy, seizures)?

   e. If the patient is a young infant (1-3 months of age) with projectile vomiting, suspect pyloric stenosis or other gastric outlet processes (malrotation, annular pancreas).

2. The PE should include an assessment of the patient's vital signs, weight, and hydration. Specific areas to highlight in the exam include the following:

   a. HEENT: Fundi (papilledema), ears (otitis media), throat (pharyngitis, cervical adenopathy), fontanelle (bulging vs. sunken)

   b. Respiratory tract: Coughing/wheezing

   c. Abdomen: Pain, distension, bowel sounds, hepatosplenomegaly, palpable "olive"

   d. Genitourinary: R/O infection, pregnancy, toxic shock syndrome

   e. Skin: Rash

   f. Neurologic: Lethargy, paresthesias, seizures, focal signs

3. Laboratory studies depend on the suspected cause.

   a. Blood: CBC, electrolytes, glucose, BUN, ammonia, medication, or toxicology levels

   b. Urine: ± Metabolic screen, urine specific gravity, glucosuria, ketonuria, microscopic, ± culture

4. Causes include infection (viral, rotavirus, Norwalk virus, bacterial

enterotoxins), metabolic (diabetic ketoacidosis, inborn error of
metabolism), ↑ ICP (meningitis, Reye's syndrome, tumor), GI
obstruction (pyloric stenosis).
5. Treatment: Outpatient therapy should be tried if the cause appears to
   be a self-limited infectious process (e.g., viral, enterotoxin) and if the
   patient is not significantly dehydrated and can retain sufficient liquids
   to maintain hydration.
   a. Discontinue solid foods and milk for 12-18 hours.
   b. Infants: Oral glucose-electrolyte solution, with frequent, small
      feedings × 12-24 hours. Advance to regular diet as tolerated over
      24-48 hours.
   c. Older children: Cola, Kool-Aid, Hawaiian Punch; popsicles;
      frequent, small feedings × 12-24 hours. Advance to BRATS diet as
      quickly as tolerated; finally, advance to a regular diet.

BIBLIOGRAPHY

Abdominal pain

Gartner JC: Recurrent abdominal pain: who needs a work-up?
  Contemp Pediatr 6:62, 1989.
Harberg F: The acute abdomen in childhood, *Pediatr Ann*
  18:169, 1989.
Oberlander T, Rappaport L: Recurrent abdominal pain during
  childhood, *Pediatr Rev* 14:313, 1993.
Olson A: Recurrent abdominal pain: an approach to diagnosis
  and management, *Pediatr Ann* 16:834, 1987.
Reynolds S, Jaffe D: Children with abdominal pain: evaluation in
  the pediatric emergency department, *Pediatr Emerg Care* 6:8,
  1990.
Silverberg M: Chronic abdominal pain in adolescents, *Pediatr
  Ann* 20:179, 1991.
Stevenson R, Ziegler M: Abdominal pain unrelated to trauma,
  Pediatr Rev 14:302, 1993.
Tunnessen W: *Signs and symptoms in pediatrics,* Philadelphia,
  1983, JB Lippincott.

Gastrointestinal bleeding

Ament M: Diagnosis and management of upper gastrointestinal
  tract bleeding in the pediatric patient, *Pediatr Rev* 12:107,
  1990.

Milov D, Andres J: Sorting out the causes of rectal bleeding, *Contemp Pediatr* 5:80, 1988.

Rudolph A, Hoffman J: *Pediatrics,* Norwalk, Conn, 1987, Appleton & Lange.

Silber G: Lower gastrointestinal bleeding, *Pediatr Rev* 12:85, 1990.

Tunnessen W: *Signs and symptoms in pediatrics,* Philadelphia, 1983, JB Lippincott.

Constipation

Fitzgerald J: Constipation in children, *Pediatr Rev* 8:299, 1987.

Pettei M: Chronic constipation, *Pediatr Ann* 16:796, 1987.

Schmitt B: Soiling with constipation in preschoolers, *Contemp Pediatr* 8:55, 1992.

Sondheimer J: Helping the child with chronic constipation, *Contemp Pediatr* 1:12, 1985.

Diarrhea

Avery ME, Snyder J: Oral therapy for acute diarrhea, *N Engl J Med* 323:891, 1990.

Barkin R: Treatment of the dehydrated child, *Pediatr Ann* 19:597, 1990.

DeWitt T: Acute diarrhea in children, *Pediatr Rev* 11:6, 1989.

Fitzgerald J: Management of acute diarrhea, *Pediatr Infect Dis J* 8:564, 1989.

Harrison H: Dehydration in infancy: hospital treatment, *Pediatr Rev* 11:139, 1989.

Levine J: Chronic nonspecific diarrhea, *Pediatr Ann* 16:821, 1987.

Lo C, Walker WA: Chronic protracted diarrhea of infancy: a nutritional disease, *Pediatrics* 72:786, 1983.

Merritt R et al: Treatment of protracted diarrhea of infancy, *Am J Dis Child* 138:770, 1984.

Northrup R, Flanigan T: Gastroenteritis, *Pediatr Rev* 15:461, 1994.

Encopresis

McClung HJ et al: Is combination therapy for encopresis nutritionally safe? *Pediatrics* 91:591, 1993.

Nolan T, Oberklaid F: New concepts in the management of encopresis, *Pediatr Rev* 14:447, 1993.

Partin J et al: Painful defecation and fecal soiling in children, *Pediatrics* 89:1007, 1992.

Schmitt B: Soiling with constipation in the school-age child, *Contemp Pediatr* 8:75, 1992.

Schmitt B, Mauror R: 20 common errors in treating encopresis, *Contemp Pediatr* 9:47, 1992.

Gastroesophageal reflux

Orenstein S: Effects on behavior state of prone vs seated positioning for infants with GER, *Pediatrics* 85:765, 1990.

Orenstein S: Gastroesophageal reflux, *Pediatr Rev* 13:174, 1992.

Rudolph A, Hoffman J: *Pediatrics,* Norwalk, Conn, 1987, Appleton & Lange.

Tunnel W: Gastroesophageal reflux in childhood, *Pediatr Ann* 18:192, 1989.

Foreign-body ingestion

Bonadio W: Coin ingestion, *Contemp Pediatr* 8:71, 1992.

Paul R et al: Foreign body ingestions in children, *Pediatrics* 91:121,1993.

Schunk J et al: Fluoroscopic Foley catheter removal of esophageal foreign bodies in children, *Pediatrics* 94:709, 1994.

Jaundice

Committee on Infectious Diseases: Universal hepatitis B immunization, *Pediatrics* 89:795, 1992.

Gartner L: Neonatal jaundice, *Pediatr Rev* 15:422, 1994.

Krugman S: Viral hepatitis A, B, C, D & E: infection, *Pediatr Rev* 13:203, 1992.

Krugman S: Viral hepatitis A, B, C, D & E: prevention, *Pediatr Rev* 13:245, 1992.

Pickering L: Management of the infant of a mother with viral hepatitis, *Pediatr Inf Dis J* 9:315, 1988.

Peptic ulcer disease

Gryboski J: Peptic ulcer disease in children, *Pediatr Rev* 12:15, 1990.

Mezoff A, Balistreri W: New GI therapies: any better than antacids? *Contemp Pediatr* 6:101, 1990.

Vomiting

Fuchs S, Jaffe D: Vomiting, *Pediatric Emerg Care* 6:164, 1990.
Ramos A, Tuchman D: Persistent vomiting, *Pediatr Rev* 15:24, 1994.

GENITOURINARY DISORDERS

9

A. DYSURIA, HESITANCY, URGENCY, DRIBBLING

1. Dysuria (painful urination), hesitancy (inability to start stream), urgency (heightened pressure to void), and dribbling (passing a few drops of urine after voiding is completed) may be signs of a UTI, genital infection, perineal irritation (trauma, tight clothing, harsh soaps, bubble baths, shampooing in the bath, masturbation), sexual abuse, or emotional disorders.
2. Obtain a pertinent history, physical, and laboratory work-up (see Section B).
3. Treatment is directed toward the underlying disorder.

B. FREQUENCY

1. *Frequency* denotes a pattern of increased urination compared with an individual's normal pattern. There may be more frequent voiding episodes, more urine produced with each episode, or both.
2. Important historical information includes the following:
   a. Age of attainment of bladder control
   b. Normal voiding pattern
   c. Duration of new pattern
   d. Amount and types of fluids ingested each day
   e. Ingestion of medications or caffeine-containing products
   f. Possibility of trauma or abuse
   g. Presence of other GU symptoms (dysuria, hesitancy, urgency, enuresis, change in urine color or odor)
3. The PE should be complete. Pay particular attention to the perineum (e.g., redness and swelling of urethral meatus and penile discharge; redness, bruises, swelling, or excoriations of the urethral meatus, labia, or clitoral areas; vaginal discharge or odor). The perianal area should be examined for excoriations and signs of trauma.
4. Urine should be microscopically examined for blood cells and bacteria. The pH and specific gravity of the urine should be assessed;

the presence of glucose, protein, ketones, blood, and bilirubin should be determined by dipstick. A culture and Gram's stain are indicated if there is penile or vaginal discharge.

5. Causes of frequency
   a. UTI (see p. 155)
   b. Diabetes mellitus: Dipstick positive for glucose (±ketones) necessitates a serum glucose determination (see Chapter 6).
   c. Diabetes insipidus: Failure to raise urine specific gravity above 1.010, even with 6-12 hours of fluid deprivation, necessitates a serum osmolality determination.
   d. Vaginitis/urethritis/labial adhesions (see Section P)
   e. Excessive fluid intake
   f. Diuretic, caffeine, or theophylline intake
   g. Irritation of urethra/vagina, especially trauma, tight clothing, harsh soaps, bubble baths or shampooing in the bath, masturbation
   h. Emotional problems
   i. Sexual abuse
6. Treatment of frequency is accomplished by correcting the underlying condition.

C. ENURESIS

1. Enuresis is involuntary urination that occurs after a child has reached the age when bladder control is usually attained (4 years of age).
   a. Children who have never attained bladder control have primary enuresis; those who have had such control but subsequently lose it have secondary enuresis.
   b. Before 5 years of age, primary enuresis is more common; secondary enuresis is more common after 5 years of age.
   c. Enuresis may be nocturnal, diurnal, or both. Diurnal enuresis in a child older than 5 years of age usually is associated with an organic disorder.
2. Important historical information includes the following:
   a. Age of attainment of bladder control
   b. Type of enuresis (nocturnal, diurnal); if nocturnal, the time in the night during which urination occurs
   c. Frequency of accidents
   d. How the child is treated after an accident
   e. Possible precipitating events (e.g., too busy playing to go the bathroom)
   f. Presence of other GU symptoms (dysuria, obvious hematuria, frequency, urgency, hesitancy, dribbling, itching)

    g. Presence of constipation

    h. Amount and types of fluids ingested in an average day

    i. Presence of psychologic problems or a change in the child's familial, social, or scholastic milieu

    j. Age of successful toilet training of siblings and parents

    k. Concomitant presence of encopresis

3. A complete PE, including a full neurologic assessment, should be performed; it is usually normal.

    a. The BP should be measured (initial screen for a renal pathologic condition).

    b. Give particular attention to the perineum to determine the presence of erythema, edema, signs of trauma, anatomic anomalies, or the presence of urethral/vaginal discharge. Give particular attention to the sacral area for dimpling or cutaneous anomalies that might indicate a spinal abnormality.

    c. The abdomen should be palpated for organomegaly (bladder and kidneys), stools, and masses.

    d. A rectal exam should be performed; especially note sphincter tone.

4. U/A and urine culture should be performed on all children with enuresis. Radiologic evaluation and/or ultrasound of the GU tract is necessary for children with diurnal enuresis, recalcitrant enuresis, constant dribbling, or external GU anatomic anomalies.

5. Some causes of enuresis are as follows:

    a. UTI (see p. 155)

    b. Ectopic ureter

    c. Other GU organic lesions

    d. Small bladder capacity (maturational delay in size)

    e. Ingestion of increased amounts of fluids

    f. Intake of caffeine, theophylline, chocolate, diuretics

    g. Inattention (too busy to void)

    h. Psychologic problems (e.g., fear, anger, resentment, especially in conjunction with a new sibling or a change in the child's social, familial, or scholastic milieu)

    i. Diabetes mellitus, diabetes insipidus

    j. Post-ictal states

    k. Child abuse, especially sexual abuse

    l. Perineal irritation (e.g., masturbation, trauma, infection, chemical irritation)

6. Treatment of primary enuresis includes the following:

    a. Reassurance (spontaneous cure rate of 10% per year after 5 years of age)

b. Bladder stretching exercises are recommended by some authorities. The family establishes the child's baseline I&O; the child is then encouraged to force fluids and hold urine for as long as possible each day—3-6 months required.

c. A reward system for a certain number of dry nights (goal should be attainable and dynamic)

d. Discouraging fluid intake after dinner

e. Encouraging voiding before bedtime

f. An enuresis alarm (alarm sensitizes sleeping child to sensation of a full bladder so that ultimately he or she awakens when his or her bladder is full but he or she has not yet voided)

g. Counseling, hypnotherapy, or psychotherapy (if indicated)

h. The use of imipramine had been widely advocated; it depresses both bladder contractions and REM sleep. However, recent studies have questioned the association of enuresis with a particular stage of sleep. Concerns regarding the myocardial effects of imipramine and its potential for overdosage have discouraged its use.

i. The use of intranasal DDAVP has been explored with mixed results in clinical trials. Relapse rates have been high, and better results are seen in older children than in younger ones. The initial dose is 10 μg in each nostril hs with a gradual increase to 40 μg nightly. Side effects are few; nasal irritation is associated with the use of nasal spray, and there is a slight risk of water intoxication.

j. Children with secondary enuresis should have the precipitating disorder addressed and managed.

D. GLOMERULONEPHRITIS (ACUTE)

1. AGN refers to a disorder characterized by smoke-colored, tea-colored, or grossly bloody urine with proteinuria, RBC casts, hyaline casts, and granular casts.

2. Many etiologies are implicated in the genesis of AGN; the best described is poststreptococcal AGN. In this entity, immune complexes are deposited along the glomerular basement membrane and activate the complement system, which leads to a release of more inflammatory agents and recruitment of inflammatory cells to the area.

3. Clinically, a child can have brown, smoky, or red urine 1-3 weeks after a sore throat. Urine output may be decreased, and edema (especially periorbital) may be present. The child may (rarely) have florid CHF or acute hypertensive encephalopathy. Regardless of the etiology, any of the nephritides can appear in this manner.

4. On PE, the child may be entirely asymptomatic or severely ill depending on the amount of renal involvement at the time of presentation.
5. Laboratory tests include the following:
   a. Urine for culture and for U/A; U/A shows hematuria and ≥2+ proteinuria. Microscopic exam of the urine reveals RBC casts and leukocyturia.
   b. Electrolytes may be normal or markedly abnormal ($\downarrow$ Na, $\uparrow$ K, $\uparrow$ BUN, $\uparrow$ creatinine). Total proteins may be normal or $\downarrow$ (especially albumin).
   c. CBC is usually normal but may show anemia depending on the amount and duration of blood loss. The ESR is elevated during the acute phase.
   d. Streptococcus serologic tests (ASO, antihyaluronidase, antideoxyribonuclease), as well as ANA and C3 ($\downarrow$), should be obtained. A TC and a culture of any area of pyoderma should be obtained.
   e. If the patient is hypertensive, a CXR should be obtained to assess the presence/degree of CHF.
6. Therapy
   a. Admit any child with AGN who has oliguria or hypertension. If oliguria and edema are present, fluids are restricted to 300-400 ml/m^2 and Na intake is limited to 1-2 mEq/kg/d. If severe edema does not respond to furosemide, metolazone (Zaroxolyn) 0.07-0.14 mg/kg/d might be useful.
   b. If the patient is in CHF, administer O_2, place the head up, and give 0.5-1.0 mg/kg furosemide IV.

NOTE: The daily dosage of furosemide varies between 1 and 5 mg/kg/d, depending on the degree of renal impairment.

   c. If the patient is hypertensive, give nifedipine 0.25-0.5 mg/kg sublingually *or* diazoxide 2.5-5.0 mg/kg IV push *or* hydralazine 0.5 mg/kg IV over several minutes.
   d. If the patient is severely hypoalbuminemic, infuse albumin (0.3-1 g/kg/dose) followed by furosemide (1-2 mg/kg/dose) q6-12h IV.
   e. If a child is only mildly affected, he or she may be discharged home. The parent should place the child on a low-sodium diet, weigh him or her each day, and measure the urine output. The parent should also be aware of signs of increasing BP and fluid retention. Follow-up is mandatory in 2-3 days, sooner if there are problems. Consultation with a pediatric nephrologist is advisable.

E. HEMATURIA
1. The presence of microscopic hematuria may be noted by dipstick in asymptomatic children during health assessment visits. Remember, a dipstick is very sensitive and may be positive in the presence of only 2-5 RBCs/HPF. When macroscopic hematuria is present, it is usually the reason for the child's visit.
2. Causes of macroscopic hematuria
   a. Trauma, masturbation
   b. Tumors
   c. Sickle cell trait
   d. Renal stones
   e. Hypercalciuria without stones
   f. Hyperuricosuria
   g. GU disorders
   h. Thin basement membrane (benign recurrent hematuria)
   i. Alport's syndrome (hereditary nephritis with nerve deafness)
   j. Glomerulonephritis (smoke-colored urine, hypertension, oliguria, edema)
   k. Hemorrhagic cystitis
   l. UTI
   m. Hematospermia (in adolescent males)
   n. IgA nephropathy (Berger's disease)
3. Microscopic (or variable) hematuria may be present in the conditions listed previously and also in the following:
   a. Connective tissue disease–induced nephritis
   b. HUS
   c. HSP
   d. Leukemia
   e. Certain malignancies
   f. Thrombocytopenia or clotting disorders
   g. Renal vein thrombosis
   h. Subacute bacterial endocarditis
   i. Hemangiomas of the GU tract
   j. Polycystic renal disease
   k. Urinary tract anomalies
   l. Renal tuberculosis
   m. Hydronephrosis
   n. Mumps
   o. Rubeola
   p. Varicella
   q. Malaria

r. Schistosomiasis

s. Exercise, running, boxing, wrestling

t. Drugs or toxins (e.g., aspirin, anticoagulants, amitriptyline [Elavil], lead, methicillin, phenol, sulfa drugs, and turpentine)

4. History should elicit the following:

a. Onset and duration of the hematuria

b. Urine color (or color change) and intensity

c. Any other GU symptoms; previous GU disease, surgery, or instrumentation

d. History of edema, rash, joint symptoms

e. History of trauma, chronic medical conditions, medication use or ingestions

f. Antecedent sore throat and date of its occurrence (AGN)

g. Colicky pain, back pain (stones)

h. Allergies

i. Diet history, including ingestion of red/orange/purple substances

j. Easy bleeding or bruising (hematologic disorders); history of sickle-cell disease

k. Bloody diarrhea (HUS, HSP)

l. Dyspnea, fatigue, or change in a known murmur (SBE); other history of heart disease

m. Other illnesses present concomitantly (e.g., mumps, varicella, rubeola)

n. Travel history (malaria, schistosomiasis)

o. Exertion

p. History of connective tissue disease

q. Deafness in patient or other family members (Alport's syndrome)

r. Other family members with hematuria (familial hematuria) or other renal disease, connective tissue disease, or sickle-cell disease

5. A complete PE must be performed. It may be normal or markedly abnormal depending on the cause of the bleeding. The child's vital signs should be assessed and stabilized if unstable. The presence or absence of the following should be noted:

a. HEENT: Periorbital edema, malformed ears, pharyngeal erythema/exudate

b. Chest: Rales or rubs, precordial activity, cardiac murmurs or gallops

c. Abdomen: Masses, ascites, bruits, trauma

d. Back: Flank tenderness

e. GU: Meatal stenosis, discharge, trauma

   f. Extremities: Edema, arthritis
   g. Skin: Rash, petechiae, purpura
6. Laboratory tests are dictated by the clinical findings
   a. Macroscopic hematuria should be evaluated with a CBC, differential, and platelet count. Obtain serum BUN and creatinine, electrolytes, and sickle cell preparation (if the child is African-American and his or her sickle status is unknown).
   b. If AGN is suspected, an ESR, ANA, IgA, serum complement (C3) level, ASO titer, and TC should be obtained.
   c. If SBE is suspected, a cardiac ECHO and multiple blood cultures should be obtained.
   d. When stones are suspected, an ultrasound or a flat plate of the abdomen should be obtained.
   e. If trauma has occurred, an IVP may localize the lesion.
7. Treatment is directed toward the underlying condition.
   a. Some conditions require no specific therapy but only reassurance (sickle trait, benign hematuria, Alport's syndrome).
   b. Other conditions have recurrent hematuria as part of their constellation (e.g., connective tissue diseases). Patients should be alerted with instructions regarding which symptoms require attention.
   c. Surgical problems and significant trauma should be addressed.
   d. Infections should be treated with the appropriate antimicrobials.
   e. Malignancies and tumors are treated surgically or with chemotherapy.
   f. Hematologic disorders are treated with replacement therapy, when appropriate (e.g., fresh-frozen plasma, whole blood).
   g. HSP and HUS are discussed elsewhere (see Sections F and G, respectively).
   h. AGN is discussed in Section D.
   i. Hypercalciuria may be treated with sodium citrate/citric acid (Bicitra) or a chlorothiazide diuretic.
   j. Hyperuricosuria is treated with allopurinol.

F. HEMOLYTIC-UREMIC SYNDROME

1. HUS is characterized by microangiopathic hemolytic anemia (in association with glomerular endothelial injury), thrombocytopenia, and azotemia.
2. HUS is reported worldwide and in all races; it seems to be more common during the summer and fall.
3. HUS is associated with a number of infectious agents, including

cytotoxic *Escherichia coli* strains (especially *E. coli* 0157:H7), *Shigella dysenteriae,* and *Streptococcus pneumoniae.*

4. Important historical information includes diarrhea (watery or bloody) 3-12 days before the onset of HUS symptoms with or without vomiting or abdominal pain. Symptoms of HUS include irritability, restlessness, pallor, oliguria/anuria, edema, and signs of fluid overload (↑ BP, pulmonary congestion, and edema).

5. The PE should be complete with careful attention to the neurologic exam (irritability, lethargy, ataxia, hemiparesis, focal signs, seizures, coma), the GI exam (hyperactive bowel sounds, ascites, enlarged liver), the extremities (edema), the chest exam (rales, rubs, cardiac gallop, new or worsening murmur), and the skin (petechiae, purpura, oozing from orifices or venipuncture sites).

6. Laboratory evaluation includes a CBC (↑ WBC with shift to the left, ↓ Hct), peripheral smear (evidence of fragmented RBCs), platelet count (commonly <40,000), fibrin degradation products (↑), PT/PTT (usually normal), electrolytes (↑ K, ↓ Na), BUN and creatinine (↑), uric acid (↑), P (↑), triglycerides (↑), bilirubin (sometimes ↑), and LFTs (↑).

7. Differential diagnosis
   a. Other renal diseases
      1) AGN
      2) SLE with nephropathy
      3) Overwhelming sepsis
      4) Vasculitis
   b. Other causes of microangiopathic hemolytic anemia
      1) Acute liver failure
      2) Nephrotic syndrome with intravascular thrombosis
      3) Malignant hypertension
      4) SBE
      5) Valvular heart disease
      6) Coarctation of the aorta
      7) DIC
      8) Sepsis (especially with meningococcus or herpes)

8. Therapy
   a. Renal manifestations
      1) Follow weights carefully.
      2) Restrict fluids to insensible losses plus measured losses.
      3) Consider IV furosemide (1-2 mg/kg/dose q6-12h) with replacement of urine losses.
      4) Monitor electrolytes frequently; correct as needed.

    5) Consider dialysis if there is severe fluid overload, severe hyperkalemia, severe acidosis, hyponatremia, or oliguria/anuria unresponsive to diuretics.

    6) Control hypertension by maintaining normovolemia, avoiding overtransfusion, and using antihypertensive agents (hydralazine 0.15-0.5 mg/kg/dose IV q4-6h, *or* captopril 0.15-2 mg/kg/dose PO q8h, *or* nifedipine 0.15-0.5 mg/kg/dose PO q6h).

  b. Hematologic abnormalities
    1) Maintain Hgb over 6-8 g/dL with infusions of washed RBCs.
    2) Use platelet transfusion for symptomatic bleeding.
    3) Consider plasma transfusion for hereditary HUS or prolonged or recurrent HUS.
    4) Avoid plasma transfusion in pneumococcal-neuraminidase HUS.

  c. Maintain caloric intake parenterally or enterally.

G. HENOCH-SCHÖENLEIN PURPURA

1. HSP is also referred to as anaphylactoid, allergic, or rheumatoid purpura; leukocytoclastic vasculitis; or allergic vasculitis.

2. The etiology of HSP is unresolved. Seventy-five percent of the cases occur in children between 2 and 11 years of age; the disease is rare in adults. The male-to-female ratio is 1.5-2.0:1. More cases occur during the spring and fall.

3. HSP is thought to be an IgA-mediated vasculitis involving the small vessels of involved organs. The renal lesions of HSP are indistinguishable from those of IgA nephropathy (Berger's disease).

4. Seventy-five percent of patients give a history of preceding upper respiratory infection.

5. The hallmarks of HSP are nonthrombocytopenic purpuric rash, abdominal pain, arthritis, and nephritis.

  a. The rash may consist of urticarial wheals, erythematous maculopapules, petechiae, or purpura; there is no associated thrombocytopenia. Lesions usually occur on the lower extremities and buttocks. They may initially blanch on pressure. Purpuric lesions evolve from red to purple and become rust-colored with a brownish hue; eventually they fade. Angioedema (nonpitting) of the scalp and extremities occurs.

  b. Arthralgias and arthritis occur commonly in HSP. Joint involvement (most commonly ankles and knees) tends to be periarticular; involved joints are swollen, tender, and painful on motion.

  c. Most patients with HSP have colicky abdominal pain, which usually follows the skin changes in timing. Vomitus and stools may contain blood, either grossly or microscopically. The pain is a result of submucosal and intramural extravasation of fluid and blood into the intestinal wall. Intussusception (usually ileoileal) may occur and is best diagnosed by ultrasound.

   d. Patients who develop renal disease do so within 3 months of the onset of rash; persistence of the rash for 2-3 months is associated with nephropathy. Renal disease ranges from transient microscopic hematuria to rapidly progressive glomerulonephritis. Patients may develop a nephritic syndrome (hematuria, hypertension, azotemia, oliguria) or a nephritic-nephrotic syndrome (24-hour protein excretion >50 mg/kg/d and serum albumin <2.5 mg/dL). A syndrome with components of both nephritis and nephrosis is more predictive of renal failure and chronic renal disease than is nephritis alone, and the presence of nephrotic-range proteinuria is the most accurate predictor of long-term renal failure.

   e. Patients with HSP can have thrombocytosis, $\uparrow$ ESR, factor VIII deficiency, vitamin K deficiency, and hypoprothrombinemia.

   f. CNS involvement in HSP is rare and usually manifests as headache and mood or mental status changes. However, nearly every type of central and peripheral nervous system dysfunction has been reported anecdotally.

   g. Testicular swelling or pain may result from vasculitis of the scrotal vessels.

6. Differential diagnosis

   a. Abdominal symptoms: R/O acute abdomen, intussusception

   b. Joint symptoms: R/O acute rheumatic fever, rheumatoid arthritis, SLE, periarteritis nodosa

   c. Rash: R/O sepsis, drug reaction, hemorrhagic diathesis (e.g., immune thrombocytopenic purpura), abuse

   d. Renal symptoms: R/O AGN

   e. Testicular symptoms: R/O hernia, testicular torsion, orchitis

7. Laboratory tests include CBC (normal-low Hct, $\uparrow$ WBC with shift to the left), ESR ($\uparrow$), electrolytes (normal), BUN and creatinine ($\uparrow$ according to degree of renal disease), serum proteins (occasionally $\downarrow$ albumin), factors VIII and XIII ($\downarrow$), C3 (occasionally low), serum IgA (may be $\uparrow$). Many children with HSP present with the majority of their laboratory studies in the normal range.

8. Therapy

   a. No specific therapy is available.

b. Prednisone 1-2 mg/kg/d × 5-7 days is useful for abdominal colic, marked joint symptoms, and testicular swelling.
c. In the acute presentation monitor hydration, Hct, blood in stools; D/C all unnecessary drugs.
d. For any child with HSP and a nephritic-nephrotic picture, involve a pediatric nephrologist *early* in the illness.

H. HERNIA

1. An inguinal hernia is the protrusion of abdominal structures into the scrotum or inguinal region. This protrusion is a result of the persistence of a peritoneal sac, the processus vaginalis, which normally becomes fibrotic late in gestation after testicular descent.
   a. Hernias may occur in both males and females because the processus vaginalis precedes both the testis in its descent into the inguinal canal and scrotum and the round ligament in its descent into the canal and labia.
   b. The male-to-female ratio of hernias is 5-6:1. In a female patient, bilateral inguinal hernias with palpable contents (gonads?) should prompt suspicion of an endocrine or intergender problem.
   c. Most (85%-90%) hernias are unilateral; the right side predominates, and the size is variable.
2. Important historical information includes duration and location of the mass, whether it changes in size (especially if it becomes larger on exertion or crying), and the events that precipitate size changes. If incarceration of the hernia is suspected, a history of vomiting, scant stooling, melena, irritability, and abdominal distension should be sought.
3. On PE, a mass may be palpated in the scrotum or labia. This mass may be more easily appreciated if the child is crying or straining (increased intraabdominal pressure).
   a. The hernia usually does not transilluminate, and bowel sounds are usually heard on auscultation over the hernia sac.
   b. Most hernias are manually reducible by the examiner because the contents of the processus ordinarily slide in and out of the abdominal cavity. However, the hernia may not be reducible if the neck of the sac closes over the herniated abdominal contents (incarcerated hernia).
   c. If the hernia is tender, swollen, and warm, it is strangulated. Vascular compromise may lead to bowel ischemia and perforation.
4. Treatment is surgical.
   a. The hernia sac (patent processus vaginalis) is closed at the inguinal

ring. Because there is a significant incidence of contralateral hernia sacs, bilateral exploration may be performed. Surgical repair should be performed as soon as possible after the hernia is discovered.

b. An incarcerated hernia may be manually reduced under sedation. If successful, a herniorrhaphy should be performed within 1-2 days; if unsuccessful, immediate surgery is necessary.

I. HYDROCELE

1. A hydrocele is a collection of peritoneal fluid in the scrotum. An accompanying hernia may or may not be present. If the size of the hydrocele varies over time, suspect a somewhat open tunica vaginalis (communicating hydrocele). If the size of the hydrocele is constant, the tunica vaginalis is closed.

2. Important historical information includes the duration of scrotal swelling and whether the size of the swelling varies both during rest and during times of emotional unrest (crying, fear).

3. On PE, the hydrocele feels ovoid or round, smooth, and nontender. Scrotal skin is normal. A hydrocele may be differentiated from a hernia in several ways. A hydrocele cannot be reduced; a hernia usually can. A hydrocele is translucent when transilluminated, whereas a hernia is not. Auscultation of the scrotum reveals bowel sounds when a hernia is present but not when there is a hydrocele.

4. A hydrocele that is constant in size usually indicates that a hernia is not present; no treatment is necessary because the fluid gradually reabsorbs. If the hydrocele is accompanied by a hernia, treatment is as discussed for hernia (see p. 148).

J. PENILE PROBLEMS (ACQUIRED)

1. Phimosis/paraphimosis
   a. Phimosis exists when a tight foreskin precludes its ability to be retracted so that the glans can be exposed. Paraphimosis is an inability to replace the foreskin over the glans after retracting it.
   b. The foreskin should never be forcibly retracted to "clean the penis" because doing so may lead to paraphimosis.
   c. Paraphimosis is a medical emergency because venous and lymphatic congestion results.
   d. On PE, phimosis presents as a tight foreskin incapable of any retraction; paraphimosis presents as markedly edematous foreskin in a retracted position.
   e. A child with phimosis should be referred to a urologist, especially

if hygiene is a problem or if the patient has had a UTI.

    f. A child with paraphimosis should be referred to a urologist emergently. Steps must be taken to decompress the edema so that there is no vascular compromise to the penis. Various techniques have been suggested: applying ice or a compression dressing followed by manual pressure on the glans (similar to turning a sock inside out) to return the foreskin to its usual position **(Note:** This procedure is performed after a local anesthetic is administered); a dorsal slit; or a "puncture" in the edematous foreskin (with subsequent manual reduction), which obviates the need for a dorsal slit.

    g. Counseling must be given to parents to prevent recurrence of the problem.

2. Balanitis

    a. Balanitis is an infection or inflammation of the foreskin as a result of trauma, poor hygiene, or an STD that may extend onto the glans.

    b. History reveals a painful penis; PE reveals a swollen, tender, erythematous penis.

    c. If there is a penile discharge, it should receive a Gram's stain and be sent for culture. Urine should be examined microscopically and sent for culture, if appropriate.

    d. Therapy includes sitz baths (warm soaks) and ampicillin 50-100 mg/kg/d ÷ q6h.

3. Penile trauma

    a. Bruising or minor lacerations of the penis usually result from straddle injuries, falls, blunt trauma (e.g., hit with a ball or bat, toilet seat entrapment), and zipper entrapment. The possibility of abuse must always be considered.

    b. The history should ascertain how the injury occurred; be careful to ascertain whether the story fits the injury. The penis can appear swollen and bruised with or without a laceration. Be sure to check for other signs of trauma, anal tears, and penile discharge. Make sure the child can void. Check urine for the presence of blood.

    c. Obtain a GU consult if blood is seen at the meatus, if a large amount of blood is in the urine, or if there is significant penile laceration or swelling. A VCUG and exploration with the patient under anesthesia may be needed to verify urethral integrity.

    d. If zipper entrapment is the problem, consider applying mineral oil to the foreskin and zipper, which eases the skin's release from the zipper; unfastening the zipper one tooth at a time; cutting the median bar of the zipper with a wire cutter; or cutting the cloth strips that are holding the zipper. If in doubt, call a urologist.

  e. Therapy is directed toward decreasing the swelling. Sitz baths (warm soaks) are useful.

4. Strangulation

  a. Strangulation of the penis may occur as a result of an encircling hair, thread, or fiber and produces venous engorgement and edema.

  b. Obtain a GU consult even if the hair/thread can be cut. Sometimes it is difficult to locate the hair/thread because of the degree of edema.

  c. Keep in mind the possibility of abuse.

5. Priapism

  a. Priapism is prolonged, painful (because of ischemia) penile erection.

  b. Common causes of priapism are trauma, sickle-cell disease, and leukemic infiltration.

  c. Treatment of sickle-cell disease–associated priapism includes hydration and hypertransfusion or exchange transfusion.

  d. Other therapies suggested are ice baths or, alternatively, warm soaks.

K. PROTEINURIA

1. When protein is present in the urine, its concentration may be estimated by a dipstick impregnated with tetrabromophenolphthalein:

$$
\begin{aligned}
\text{Trace} &= 10 \text{ mg/100 ml} \\
1+ &= 30 \text{ mg/100 ml} \\
2+ &= 100 \text{ mg/100 ml} \\
3+ &= 300 \text{ mg/100 ml} \\
4+ &= 1000 \text{ mg/100 ml}
\end{aligned}
$$

  a. Some degree of proteinuria is found in 5%-15% of routine U/As. A falsely positive dipstick test for proteinuria may occur if the urine pH is basic.

  b. Total daily protein excretion should be <100 mg.

2. Transient proteinuria

  a. Transient proteinuria may result from fever, epinephrine, cold exposure, blood transfusions, burns, or exercise.

  b. Orthostatic proteinuria is present in the upright position but absent in the supine position. It is diagnosed by obtaining one urine sample *before* the child gets out of bed and another *after* he or she has been up for several hours, or his or her last void before going to bed. Orthostatic proteinuria is benign; rarely is more than 1 g of protein spilled per day.

3. Other causes of proteinuria include analgesic abuse, nephritis, and nephrosis.

4. When proteinuria is discovered as an incidental finding during a health-assessment visit, the history and physical usually do not reveal its cause.

   a. Questions should be asked regarding GU symptoms, edema and its location, exercise, weight gain, antecedent sore throat (especially if hematuria is also present), and family members with proteinuria.

   b. The PE should determine if the kidneys can be palpated (i.e., enlargement), if there is edema, or if the perineum is abnormal in any way.

   c. The urine, which is usually foamy, should be examined microscopically for evidence of infection and sent for culture as appropriate.

5. If the child has proteinuria of at least 1+, a second urine sample (on another day) should be obtained. If this sample is also positive, orthostatic and exercise-induced proteinuria should be ruled out. A urine culture should also be obtained.

   a. If the evaluation is unrevealing and proteinuria (2+ or greater) continues, a 24-hour urine collection for protein should be obtained.

   b. Also indicated are serum proteins (including albumin), creatinine, BUN, cholesterol, complement (C3 and C4), and ASO titer, *especially* if hematuria is present because the proteinuria may be secondary to poststreptococcal nephritis.

   c. A renal biopsy may eventually be needed to secure a diagnosis.

   d. Nephrotic syndrome is manifest by hypoproteinemia (serum albumin <3 g/dL), large proteinuria (>40 mg/m^2/h in a 24-hour urine), edema, and hyperlipidemia.

      1) There is a worldwide distribution, with males affected more commonly than females. The typical age of presentation of primary nephrotic syndrome is between 18 months and 5-6 years.

      2) The chief presenting sign is localized or diffuse edema. The amount of edema reflects both the lack of urine output and decreased serum albumin concentration.

      3) Laboratory tests include serum albumin and globulin (both $\downarrow$), serum cholesterol ($\uparrow$), urine protein ($\uparrow$), urine specific gravity

($\uparrow$), U/A (check for the presence of blood), serum immuno-globulins, C3, ANA, HBsAg, CBC ($\uparrow$ Hct), electrolytes (Na$\downarrow$), Ca ($\downarrow$), BUN, and creatinine (normal or $\uparrow$). A CXR is also indicated.

4) Therapy
   a) If the patient is shocky, infuse normal saline at 20 ml/kg/h.
   b) If the patient is severely dehydrated with $\uparrow$ Hct but is not shocky, give Na-deficient fluids PO at twice maintenance. Give 1-4 oz q1-4h to avoid vomiting.
   c) If the patient is well-hydrated but severely edematous, management should be carried out in conjunction with a pediatric nephrologist.
   d) Begin prednisone at 2 mg/kg/d (max 80 mg/d) ÷ q8-12h after a PPD has been placed and the need for a renal biopsy has been considered. If the patient has been on prednisone, return to full-dose therapy.
   e) Any patient with nephrotic syndrome and fever, especially if receiving prednisone, cyclophosphamide (Cytoxan), or chlorambucil, should be considered to have a bacterial infection and be cultured and started on antibiotics to cover both gram-positive and gram-negative organisms.

5) Admit any child who has severe dehydration, fever, refractory edema, peritonitis, or renal insufficiency. Consider admission for newly diagnosed cases.

6) Acute and long-term management should be in concert with a pediatric nephrologist, who can advise on the need for a renal biopsy, prednisone dosing (and tapering), and alkylating drugs.

L. TESTICULAR SWELLING/PAIN

1. The normal prepubertal testis is 1×2 cm in diameter; by adulthood, the testis measures $2.5\text{-}3.0 \times 4.0\text{-}4.5$ cm. Several diagnoses must be considered when there is testicular enlargement or pain.

2. Testicular torsion (torsion of the spermatic core): This condition is an emergency because continued torsion results in gangrene of the testis. The child has sudden, unilateral testicular pain; his testis is swollen and tender, and the overlying scrotal skin is red and warm. Gently lifting the testis does not relieve the pain (Prehn's sign). The child may have fever and vomiting. A lack of urinary symptoms is the rule, and the U/A is normal. If the diagnosis is in doubt, a technetium-99m pertechnetate scan can confirm it. However, because the risk of gangrene is high, there should be no delay in definitive treatment,

which is surgery. Orchiectomy is usually necessary if the torsion has been present for a prolonged period.

3. Epididymitis (inflammation of the epididymis): The child has unilateral testicular pain; the epididymis is swollen and tender, and the testis may also be involved (see Point 4). Scrotal skin is red on the affected side. Unlike with testicular torsion, lifting the scrotum diminishes the pain. The child may have fever, chills, dysuria, or frequency. A microscopic urine exam may demonstrate bacteria and pyuria; *E. coli* is the common infecting agent in prepubertal boys. In postpubertal, sexually active boys (especially those with a penile discharge), a gonorrhea or chlamydia infection must be considered; obtain a Gram's stain and culture of the discharge. Treatment consists of immediate antibiotic use (initially ampicillin; the final choice is based on the culture and sensitivity results of urine or urethral discharge), sitz baths tid-qid, and scrotal support. If an STD is diagnosed, sexual partners must be treated.

4. Orchitis (inflammation of the testis): The prepubertal child has fever, chills, scrotal swelling, and pain; the postpubertal boy has similar symptoms and may also have urinary symptoms and a penile discharge (usually gonorrhea). In both age groups, elevating the scrotum diminishes the pain. Urine and penile discharge should be appropriately stained, examined microscopically, and cultured. The usual cause of orchitis in a prepubertal child is mumps (with or without parotid swelling); the serum amylase level will be elevated. Treatment for self-limited (7-14–day) mumps orchitis consists of sitz baths and scrotal support. Treatment for orchitis resulting from gonorrhea includes sitz baths, scrotal support, and antibiotic therapy (see Chapter 20).

5. Testicular trauma: Usually results from a direct blow to the scrotum, which then is tender, bruised, and swollen. A PE may be extremely painful for the child. A urine sample should be examined for the presence of blood (urethral, renal trauma). Treatment consists of ice packs to the area (24-48 hours followed by sitz baths), elevation of the scrotum, or scrotal support.

6. Tumor

M. UNDESCENDED TESTIS

1. A testis may be considered "undescended" if it rides high in the scrotum or is not palpable (testicular agenesis or ectopic testis).
   a. A retractile testis is normally descended but is intermittently retracted because of the action of the cremasteric muscle.

b. Undescended testes may be unilateral or bilateral. In the neonate with bilateral undescended testes, serum FSH and LH levels should be obtained to rule out anorchism.

c. An undescended testis is common in neonates, especially premature infants. If spontaneous descent is going to occur, it does so by 9-12 months of age.

2. A retractile testis may be brought back into the scrotum manually or may descend spontaneously when the child is relaxed, squats, or bathes in warm water. Retractile testes require no therapy.

3. The administration of human chorionic gonadotropin over several weeks may medically reposition bilaterally undescended testes. However, to preserve fertility, most children require surgery (orchiopexy with concomitant inguinal herniorrhaphy) before 2 years of age.

N. URETHRITIS

1. Urethritis is characterized by erythema of the urethra and dysuria; there may or may not be purulent discharge.

2. Etiology includes the following:

   a. Purulent urethritis: Gonococcus (most common pathogen); also *Staphylococcus aureus,* streptococci, and enteric organisms

   b. Nonpurulent urethritis: Gonorrhea, *Chlamydia trachomatis, Ureaplasma urealyticum,* and *Trichomonas* and *Mycoplasma* organisms

   c. Noninfectious causes: Chemicals (soaps, bubble baths, powders), trauma, physical irritation to urethra (masturbation), Reiter's syndrome (urethritis, arthritis, and conjunctivitis; cause unknown)

3. Evaluation

   a. Obtain a Gram's stain. Obtain a culture for gonococci and other pathogens. *Trichomonas* and *Chlamydia* organisms require special media.

   b. Obtain a wet saline preparation (look for *Trichomonas* organisms).

   c. Treatment

      1) Gonococcal: See Chapter 20

      2) Nongonococcal (e.g., *Chlamydia* organisms most common): Tetracycline 500 mg qid × 14 days (erythromycin is alternate treatment during pregnancy) (see Chapter 20)

      3) Noninfectious: Removal of irritating factor

O. URINARY TRACT INFECTIONS

1. Symptoms vary and can be nonspecific (especially in younger children).

    a. Associated symptoms include dysuria, frequency, urgency, and enuresis.

    b. Nonspecific symptoms include vomiting, diarrhea, fever, lethargy, irritability, failure to thrive, and abdominal pain.

    c. Dysuria and frequency also may be associated with urethritis (check for vaginal infection, history of tight underwear, bubble baths, trauma). Consider gonococci, *Chlamydia* organisms, or other STDs.

    d. Some UTIs are asymptomatic; both symptomatic and asymptomatic UTIs can lead to renal compromise.

    e. Pyelonephritis is usually but not always associated with high fever, an elevated ESR, and the presence of leukocytosis.

2. The PE is often normal, but emphasis should be placed on the abdominal exam (masses, suprapubic tenderness), CVA area (tenderness), and perineum (redness, excoriations, discharge). The BP should be checked.

3. Diagnosis varies with the method of obtaining the specimen.

    a. Urine culture

        1) Clean-catch urine: >100,000 colonies/ml of single organism × 2 consecutive specimens

        2) Catheterized urine: >100 colonies/ml of single organism × 1 specimen

        3) Suprapubic urine: Growth of any organism

NOTE: The traditional standard of >100,000 colonies of any organism per ml of midstream urine as diagnostic of a UTI is based on studies of adult women. This standard is probably not valid for pediatric patients; therefore strict adherence to it may result in missed diagnoses of UTIs in symptomatic patients. Make certain the patient or parent really knows how to obtain a clean-catch specimen. To obtain this type of specimen, the child's urethral meatus and surrounding area are cleaned, and the child begins to void. After the stream has started, the midstream specimen is collected.

    b. U/A: Examination of the urine is valuable but is *not* sufficient to diagnose UTI. A negative analysis does not rule out a UTI. A patient may or may not have any of the following on analysis:

        1) Pyuria: If >10 WBCs/HPF spun specimen, then positive culture rate is >40%

        2) Hematuria

        3) Bacteriuria: >1 organism/HPF on unstained, unspun urine associated with 10^5 colonies/ml (100,000 colonies/ml)

    4) Granular casts: Associated with pyelonephritis

    5) Also check for protein, sugar, pH, concentration

4. Causes: *E. coli* is the most common organism. Other common pathogens include enterococci and *Enterobacter, Klebsiella,* and *Proteus* organisms. *S. aureus* and *Pseudomonas* organisms are more likely to be recovered after antimicrobial therapy or instrumentation.

5. Treatment

    a. Sulfisoxazole (Gantrisin) 120-150 mg/kg/d ÷ qid (max 6 g/d) × 14 days *or* amoxicillin (Augmentin) 50 mg/kg/d ÷ tid *or* TMP/SMZ 6-12 mg TMP, 30-60 mg SMZ per day ÷ bid *or* cephalexin 50 mg/kg/d ÷ q6-8h *or* nitrofurantoin 5-7 mg/kg/d ÷ q6h

    b. If upper tract disease is suspected, use IV ampicillin 100 mg/kg/d ÷ qid or tid *and* (1) gentamicin 7.5 mg/kg/d ÷ tid *or* (2) cefotaxime 100 mg/kg/d ÷ tid. IV therapy should be continued until fever has resolved and repeat cultures are negative. At that point, the patient can be treated with oral antibiotics to complete a 4-6–week course.

    c. To avoid problems with equivocal urine culture results, do not start treatment until at least two clean-catch urine samples or one suprapubic or catheter specimen has been obtained.

    d. Sepsis is often associated with a UTI in infants <8 weeks of age (some authorities would be more conservative and state 6 months of age). Work up appropriately. Treatment involves IV ampicillin (100 mg/kg/d) and gentamicin (5-7.5 mg/kg/d) or IV cefotaxime (100 mg/kg/d) for 5 days; then complete a 10-15–day course of therapy with oral ampicillin or a cephalosporin. The infant should receive prophylactic antibiotic coverage (one third to half of the treatment dosage) hs until a VCUG and ultrasound or cortical scintigraphy are performed. Do not use sulfonamides or nitro-furantoins during the first 8 weeks of life.

    e. Eliminate the use of bubble bath and treat constipation, if present; both are risk factors.

6. Suggested follow-up

    a. Return in 48 hours for a repeat U/A and culture to document sterile urine and clinical improvement and to help identify resistant organisms.

    b. Return 1-3 weeks after antibiotics have been discontinued for U/A and culture.

    c. Obtain subsequent follow-up cultures every 1-3 months until patient has remained free of infection for 1 year, then yearly.

7. Recurrences
    a. Recurrence in 25% of males and 30%-80% of females within the first year; the recurrence is often asymptomatic.
    b. If necessary, consider prophylaxis with TMP/SMZ or nitrofurantoin for 6 months to 1 year.
    c. Avoid urologic procedures such as cystoscopy and urethral dilation.
8. Further evaluation
    a. The official recommendation of the American Academy of Pediatrics is that a radiologic work-up should be performed on all children (boys and girls) after one documented UTI.
    b. Children <4 years of age and boys are more likely to have structural problems (e.g., vesicoureteral reflux or ureteral obstruction). Renal scarring (usually secondary to reflux or obstruction) is most likely to occur in preschool-age children.
    c. The ideal work-up for a child with a first UTI is under debate.
        1) Some authorities favor a renal ultrasound and VCUG 2-4 weeks following adequate therapy of the UTI.
        2) To detect renal scarring, others favor cortical scintigraphy with technetium-99m dimercaptosuccinic acid (DMSA) or ^{99m}Tc-glucoheptonate because of its greater sensitivity compared with ultrasound or VCUG. This is a real issue because renal scarring can occur in the absence of reflux. Cortical scintigraphy is also recommended for an infant with a UTI.
        3) The following types of children are likely to benefit from scintigraphy:
            a) Children with marked reflux for whom surgery is contemplated
            b) Children 6-12 years of age with moderate reflux who have been treated with antibiotic prophylaxis for several years
            c) Children with a history of multiple UTIs or previous pyelonephritis
            d) Children with breakthrough UTIs while on prophylaxis
            e) Children with suspected pyelonephritis
        4) Cortical scintigraphy is expensive but entails less radiation than a VCUG.
    d. Radionuclide cystography is used to follow patients with reflux and in children whose first UTI is diagnosed at 6 years of age or older. Some authorities would also advocate its use in siblings of children with reflux and in children whose parents have reflux.

P. VAGINAL PROBLEMS

1. Vulvovaginitis and vaginitis: May occur at any age

   a. Symptoms include itching, discharge, dysuria (if urethritis also present), and erythema/edema of vulva or vagina.

   b. Etiology may be noninfectious or infectious.

   1) Noninfectious

      a) Trauma, foreign body (malodorous, often bloody discharge), labial adhesions, chemical irritant or allergen (OTC douches, powders, bubble bath), masturbation, tumor

      b) Nylon panties prevent evaporation of normal moisture, and therefore their use may promote vaginitis.

   2) Infectious

      a) Nonspecific: Bacterial overgrowth of enteric organisms secondary to poor perineal hygiene; *Gardnerella vaginalis*

      b) Specific: Gonorrhea, *Monilia* or *Trichomonas* organisms, β-hemolytic streptococcus, *Chlamydia* organisms, pinworms, herpes simplex virus

   c. Evaluation

   1) Examine external genitalia for scratches, tears, redness, ulcers, discharge, or swelling. Use toluidine blue dye if necessary. Vaginoscopy may be performed in a prepubertal female using a veterinary otoscope speculum. A gynecologic consult may be needed.

   2) A culture is indicated if clinical symptoms are present with or without discharge or ulcerations. In young girls, may need to obtain a culture using a medicine dropper filled with nonbacteriostatic saline solution; inject saline solution and aspirate for vaginal culture. Evaluate the vaginal specimen by a wet saline mount (*Trichomonas* organisms), KOH preparation (*Monilia* organisms), and Gram's stain (intracellular gram-negative diplococci). Perform both a gonococcal and a routine culture.

   3) Foreign bodies are characteristically associated with foul-smelling discharge. Foreign bodies may be palpable by digital rectal exam in a prepubertal girl; however, toilet paper is the most common foreign body and usually is not palpable. A vaginal flush can be performed using normal saline solution introduced into the vagina via an infant feeding tube that is connected to a 30-ml syringe. Do not exert excess force to the plunger of the syringe; by doing so there is the possibility of retrograde flow up the cervix. Examination under sedation might be necessary.

d. Agent-specific treatment

   1) Nonspecific vaginitis

      a) Remove the irritating factor (e.g., foreign body, douche, bubble bath).

      b) Parents should instruct the child on the proper wiping technique (front to back, not back to front).

      c) Prescribe warm sitz baths tid.

      d) Instruct the patient to wear loose-fitting white cotton panties.

      e) Reassure parents about the normalcy of masturbation. If the patient is old enough to understand, she might also be counseled.

      f) Reassess cases that are resistant to such therapies. Make sure that adequate cultures have been performed and that abuse, foreign bodies, anatomic defects, and other such conditions have been ruled out. If reassessment still does not elicit a cause, a 10-day course of oral antibiotics (e.g., amoxicillin) may be helpful.

   2) *Monilia* organisms

      a) Intense pruritus, thick curdy discharge, dysuria

      b) Predisposing factors: Oral contraceptives, antibiotics, diabetes; very common in postpubertal females

      c) Diagnosis is made with a KOH preparation. Darkly stained hyphae sometimes can be seen on Gram's stain. KOH may miss 50% of culture-positive specimens.

      d) Treatment

         (1) Miconazole (Monistat) cream intravaginally qhs × 1-2 weeks; minipad to keep cream from coming out during the day

         (2) Clotrimazole 100-mg intravaginal tablets, 1 hs × 1-2 weeks

   3) *Trichomonas* organisms

      a) Greenish yellow discharge, foul odor, pruritus, dyspareunia

      b) Diagnosis by saline wet mount

      c) Treatment

         (1) Metronidazole (Flagyl) if not pregnant, 2 g PO in a single dose (preferred) or 125 mg (15 mg/kg/d) tid × 7-10 days

         (2) Clotrimazole 100 mg intravaginally hs × 7 days if pregnant; partner treated to prevent reinfection

   4) *G. vaginalis* (formerly *Haemophilus vaginalis*)

      a) Gray frothy discharge, fishy odor; pruritus not prominent

      b) Diagnosis is made by the presence of "clue cells" (epithelial cells covered with bacteria) and the absence of *Trichomonas* and *Monilia* organisms.

   c) Treatment

      (1) Ampicillin 500 mg qid × 10 days or tetracycline 500 mg qid × 10 days (if patient is not pregnant and is older than 8 years of age). Not all cases respond to this regimen. It is often a good idea to treat concomitantly with nystatin cream to avoid superinfection with *Monilia* organisms.

      (2) Metronidazole (Flagyl) 500 mg bid × 7 days. This therapy is effective, but uncertainty about carcinogenicity remains.

      (3) Treat the sexual partner if antibiotics are used.

  5) Group A β-hemolytic streptococcus: Oral penicillin in same dosage as for streptococcus pharyngitis (i.e., 125-250 mg PO qid × 10 days)

  6) Gonococcal and herpes simplex virus: See Chapter 20

2. Vaginal bleeding

  a. Vaginal bleeding may result from trauma (straddle injury, inanimate object penetration, sexual abuse), menstruation, spotting during early pregnancy, abortion, ingestion or improper use of birth control pills, maternal estrogen effect (neonates who may also have breast enlargement), vaginal infections, foreign bodies, and tumors.

  b. Obtain a history of the duration and amount of vaginal bleeding, precipitating events, whether bleeding waxes and wanes, history of trauma, abuse, foreign body, ingestion of birth control pills, other GU symptoms.

  c. Examine the perineum carefully.

    1) Look for contusions and lacerations of the labia, vagina, and urethra; use toluidine blue dye if necessary.

    2) Check hymenal integrity (virginal prepubertal hymen <1 cm).

    3) Is bleeding brisk, or is it slow and sporadic?

    4) Are there any masses present?

    5) If the patient is sexually active or has had previous pelvic exams, perform a pelvic exam to determine if blood is coming from the cervical os (if os is open), if the cervix is eroded, or if a foreign body is present. Perform a bimanual and rectal exam to check for masses and foreign bodies.

    6) If the child is prepubertal, she may require sedation for an adequate inspection of the vagina and cervix. Vaginoscopy may

be performed using a veterinary otoscope speculum. A rectal exam should be performed to check for masses or foreign bodies.

d. If vaginal bleeding is profuse, Hct should be checked.

   1) Clotting studies may be indicated if there are petechiae, purpura, or other bleeding sites.

   2) If there is evidence of an infection, appropriate cultures and a Gram's stain of the discharge or exudate should be obtained.

   3) If the girl is sexually active, a urine or serum pregnancy test should be obtained.

e. Treatment is directed toward the underlying condition.

   1) The trauma victim may require surgical repair under sedation or anesthesia.

   2) Foreign bodies should be removed and the vagina flushed with normal saline.

   3) Vaginal/cervical infections should be appropriately treated (see Chapter 20).

   4) The proper strength of oral contraceptives should be chosen, and their proper administration should be encouraged and monitored closely.

   5) Mothers of neonates with vaginal bleeding should be reassured. Such bleeding should cease by 10 days of age.

3. Labial adhesions

   a. Labial adhesions are epithelial agglutinations that cover the hymen and sometimes the urethral meatus. They are caused by superficial inflammation of the labia minora and usually occur in prepubertal girls. Adhesions may be complete or partial. Girls with adhesions should be observed while voiding to ensure an adequate stream.

   b. Adhesions disappear by puberty when estrogen levels rise.

   c. If the girl has dysuria, a UTI, or chronically poor hygiene, an estrogen cream may be applied bid for 7-10 days to simulate the estrogen effect that occurs at puberty. Estrogen cream should not be used for more than 14 days; doing so may promote signs of precocious puberty. After separation, petroleum jelly (Vaseline) should be applied to the area tid × 4 weeks to prevent readherence.

   d. Adhesions should never be cut or manually broken because they will recur.

BIBLIOGRAPHY

Enuresis

Foxman B et al: Childhood enuresis: prevalence, perceived impact and prescribed treatments, *Pediatrics* 77:482, 1986.

Hurley RM: Enuresis: the difference between night and day, *Pediatr Rev* 12:167, 1990.

Marshall F: Urinary incontinence in children, *Pediatr Rev* 5:209, 1984.

Miller K: Concomitant nonpharmacologic therapy in the treatment of primary nocturnal enuresis, *Clin Pediatr* (special edition), 32:32, July 1993.

Moffatt M et al: Desmopressin acetate and nocturnal enuresis: how much do we know? *Pediatrics* 92:420, 1993.

Schmitt B: Nocturnal enuresis, *Contemp Pediatr* 7:70, 1990.

Stenberg A, Lackgren G: Desmopressin tablets in the treatment of severe nocturnal enuresis in adolescents, *Pediatrics* 94:841, 1994.

Tunnessen W: *Signs and symptoms in pediatrics,* Philadelphia, 1983, JB Lippincott.

Warady B et al: Primary nocturnal enuresis, *Pediatr Ann* 20:246, 1991.

Glomerulonephritis

Burg F et al: *Gellis and Kagan's current pediatric therapy,* ed 14, Philadelphia, 1993, WB Saunders.

Fleisher G, Ludwig S: *Textbook of pediatric emergency medicine,* ed 3, Baltimore, 1993, Williams & Wilkins.

Hematuria

Boineau F, Levy J: Evaluation of hematuria in children and adolescents, *Pediatr Rev* 11:101, 1989.

Fitzwater D, Wyatt R: Hematuria, *Pediatr Rev* 15:102, 1994.

Hogg R: Recent advances in the diagnosis of hematuria in children, *Pediatr Ann* 17:560, 1988.

Kallen R: What's causing hematuria? *Contemp Pediatr* 2:55, 1986.

Tunnessen W: *Signs and symptoms in pediatrics,* Philadelphia, 1983, JB Lippincott.

Hemolytic-uremic syndrome

Burg F et al: *Gellis and Kagan's current pediatric therapy,* ed
  14, Philadelphia, 1993, WB Saunders.
Cimolai N et al: Risk factors for CNS manifestations of
  gastroenteritis-associated HUS, *Pediatrics* 90:616, 1992.
Fleisher G, Ludwig S: *Textbook of pediatric emergency medicine,*
  ed 3, Baltimore, 1993, Williams & Wilkins.
Havens P et al: Laboratory and clinical variables to predict outcome in HUS, *Am J Dis Child* 142:961, 1988.
Neill M et al: *E. coli* 0157:H7 as the predominant pathogen associated with HUS, *Pediatrics* 80:37, 1987.
Pickering L et al: Hemolytic-uremic syndrome and enterohemor-
  rhagic *E. coli, Pediatr Infect Dis J* 13:459, 1994.
Stewart C, Tina L: Hemolytic-uremic syndrome, *Pediatric Rev*
  14:218, 1993.

Henoch-Schöenlein purpura

Fleisher G, Ludwig S: *Textbook of pediatric emergency medicine,*
  ed 3, Baltimore, 1993, Williams & Wilkins.
Furley T et al: Epidemiology of a cluster of HSP, *Am J Dis
  Child* 143:798, 1989.
Lanzkowsky S et al: Henoch Schöenlein purpura, *Pediatr Rev*
  13:130, 1992.

Hernia/hydrocele

Nakayama D, Rowe M: Inguinal hernia and the acute scrotum in
  infants and children, *Pediatr Rev* 11:87, 1989.
Ziegler M: Diagnosis of inguinal hernia and hydrocele, *Pediatr
  Rev* 15:286, 1994.

Penile problems

Gorman R, Oderda G: Penile trauma: small slam revisited,
  Pediatr Emerg Care 5:108, 1989.
Kanegaye J, Schonfeld N: Penile zipper entrapment: a simple
  and less threatening approach using mineral oil, *Pediatr Emerg
  Care* 9:90, 1993.

Proteinuria

Burg F et al: *Gellis and Kagan's current pediatric therapy,* ed
  14, Philadelphia, 1993, WB Saunders.
Feld L et al: Evaluation of the child with asymptomatic

proteinuria, *Pediatr Rev* 5:248, 1984.

Fleisher G, Ludwig S: *Textbook of pediatric emergency medicine,* ed 3, Baltimore, 1993, Williams & Wilkins.

Kelsch R, Sedman A: Nephrotic syndrome, *Pediatr Rev* 14:30, 1993.

Vehaskari VM, Rapola J: Isolated proteinuria: analysis of a school-age population, *J Pediatr* 101:661, 1982.

Warshaw B, Hymes L: Daily single-dose and daily reduced-dose prednisone therapy for children with the nephrotic syndrome, *Pediatrics* 83:694, 1989.

Testicular swelling/pain

Fleisher G, Ludwig S: *Textbook of pediatric emergency medicine,* ed 3, Baltimore, 1993, Williams & Wilkins.

Hermann D: The pediatric acute scrotum, *Pediatr Ann* 18:198, 1989.

Klein B, Ochsenschlager D: Scrotal masses in children and adolescents, *Pediatr Emerg Care* 9:351, 1993.

Likitnukul S et al: Epididymitis in children and adolescents, *Am J Dis Child* 141:41, 1987.

Nakayama D, Rowe M: Inguinal hernia and the acute scrotum in infants and children, *Pediatr Rev* 11:87, 1989.

Petrack E, Hafeez W: Testicular torsion vs epididymitis: a diagnostic challenge, *Pediatr Emerg Care* 8:347, 1992.

Stillwell T, Kramer S: Intermittent testicular torsion, *Pediatrics* 77:908, 1986.

Undescended testis

Berkowitz G et al: Prevalence and natural history of cryptorchidism, *Pediatrics* 92:44, 1993.

Hawtney C: Undescended testis and orchiopexy: recent observations, *Pediatr Rev* 11:305, 1990.

Koyle M et al: The undescended testis, *Pediatr Ann* 17:39, 1988.

Neely E, Rosenfeld R: The undescended testicle: when and how to intervene, *Contemp Pediatr* 7:21, 1990.

Rabinowitz R, Hulbert W: Cryptorchidism, *Pediatr Rev* 15:272, 1994.

Urethritis

Rosenfeld W, Litman N: Urogenital tract infections in male adolescents, *Pediatr Rev* 4:257, 1983.

Urinary tract infections

Andrich M, Majid M: Diagnostic imaging in the evaluation of the first urinary tract infection in infants and young children, *Pediatrics* 90:436, 1992.

Belman AB: Urinary imaging in children, *Pediatr Infect Dis J* 8:548, 1989.

Benador D et al: Cortical scintigraphy in the evaluation of renal parenchymal changes in children with pyelonephritis, *J Pediatr* 124:17, 1994.

Burg F et al: *Gellis and Kagan's current pediatric therapy,* ed 14, Philadelphia, 1993, WB Saunders.

Conway J, Cohn R: Evolving role of nuclear medicine for the diagnosis and management of UTI, *J Pediatr* 124:87, 1994.

Feld L et al: Urinary tract infections in infants and children, *Pediatr Rev* 11:71, 1989.

Hellerstein S: Evolving concepts in the evaluation of the child with UTI, *J Pediatr* 124:589, 1994.

Hoberman A et al: Pyuria and bacteruria in urine specimens obtained by catheter from young children with fever, *J Pediatr* 124:513, 1994.

McCracken G: Diagnosis and management of acute urinary tract infections in infants and children, *Pediatr Infect Dis J* 6:107, 1987.

McCracken G: Options in antimicrobial management of urinary tract infections in infants and children, *Pediatr Infect Dis J* 8:552, 1989.

Rosenfeld D et al: Current recommendations for children with UTI, *Clin Pediatr,* 34:261, 1995.

Todd J: Management of urinary tract infections, *Pediatr Rev* 16:190, 1995.

Vaginitis

Altchek A: Recognizing and controlling vulvovaginitis in children, *Contemp Pediatr* 2:59, 1985.

Arsenault P, Oerbie A: Vulvovaginitis in the preadolescent girl, *Pediatr Ann* 15:557, 1986.

Emans S: Vulvovaginitis in the child and adolescent, *Pediatr Rev* 8:12, 1986.

Paradise J, Willis E: Probability of vaginal foreign body in girls with genital complaints, *Am J Dis Child* 139:472, 1985.

Sanfilippo J: Adolescent girls with vaginal discharge, *Pediatr Ann* 15:509, 1986.

Tunnessen W: *Signs and symptoms in pediatrics,* Philadelphia, 1983, JB Lippincott.

Vandeven A, Emans S: Vulvovaginitis in the child and adolescent, *Pediatr Rev* 14:141, 1993.

Vaginal bleeding

Anderson M et al: Abnormal vaginal bleeding in adolescents, *Pediatr Ann* 15:697, 1986.

Labial adhesions

Burg F et al: *Gellis and Kagan's current pediatric therapy,* ed 14, Philadelphia, 1993, WB Saunders.

Williams T et al: Vulvar disorders in the prepubertal female, *Pediatr Ann* 15:588, 1986.

HEMATOLOGY 10

A. ANEMIA (TABLE 10-1)

1. Anemia is only a sign of a disease or blood loss; the cause must be determined.
2. For normal values and indices, see *The Harriet Lane Handbook,* ed. 14; in blacks, Hgb may run 0.5 g% lower.
3. Nadir: "Physiologic anemia" of a term infant at 8-12 weeks of age. Hct should not be <30%; after this nadir, Hct should be >32% and MCV >77 μm^3.
4. History
   a. Any known blood loss (e.g., stool, urine, nosebleeds), perinatal problems
   b. Source of dietary iron (formula, meats, cereals, vitamins with iron)
   c. History of excess whole-milk intake (>32 oz/d)
   d. History of pica (R/O lead poisoning)
   e. History of prior anemia
   f. Family history: Ethnic/racial background, hemoglobinopathy/ gallstones/anemia/splenectomy
   g. Is the patient taking any medications that may depress bone marrow or cause hemolysis?
   h. History of malaise, fatigue, palpitations
5. PE: Look for pallor, tachycardia, petechiae, purpura, icterus, lymphadenopathy, hepatosplenomegaly, positive stool test for blood, hematuria, maxillary prominence, cheilosis, spooning of nails.
6. Hematology laboratory: CBC with indices, reticulocyte count, peripheral blood smear (most important). Perform a more extensive work-up (e.g., lead level/hemoglobin-electrophoresis, G-6-PD, Coombs' test, haptoglobin) as indicated in selected patients.
7. Iron deficiency anemia
   a. Think of blood loss; the incidence of nutritionally based iron deficiency anemia has decreased dramatically.
   b. Smear: Hypochromic, microcytic RBCs; low MCV and/or MCHC; elevated RDW; low reticulocyte count; low serum ferritin; moderately elevated FEP

TABLE 10-1.
Hematologic Parameters in Common Causes of Anemia

	Mean corpuscular volume	RBC distribution width	Anemia	Morphologic abnormalities	Free erythrocyte protoporphyrin (µg/100 ml)	Hgb A_2
Iron deficiency	↓	>13.5	+	1+	30-200	Normal or decreased
Lead poisoning*	↓†	>13.5†	±	1-2+	>200	Normal
α-Thalassemia trait‡	↓	<11.5	±	2+	<90	Normal or decreased
β-Thalassemia trait§	↓	<11.5	±	2+	<90	Elevated

*Pb poisoning; peak age 6 mo-4 yr.
†Usually a result of concomitant iron deficiency.
‡α-Thalassemia trait predominant in Asians, blacks, and Mediterraneans.
§β-Thalassemia trait mainly in blacks and Mediterraneans.

c. Treatment of iron deficiency anemia
  1) Correct the basic problem (e.g., dietary, bleeding sources, and similar problems).
  2) Elemental iron (3-6 mg/kg/d ÷ tid with meals (e.g., Fer-in-Sol drops = 25 mg Fe/ml × 2-3 months adequately repletes iron stores). Check *The Harriet Lane Handbook,* ed. 14 for other preparations.
  3) Check 7-10 days after initiation of iron therapy; should see elevated reticulocyte count and RDW. By 4 weeks, Hct should be normal. Smear has two populations of RBCs (normal and iron deficient). The maximum rate of increase in Hgb is usually 1-2 g/wk.
d. Failure to correct presumed iron deficiency anemia
  1) Poor compliance: Did patient get iron? Teeth staining, dark stools indicate that iron was given. Ask parents to bring medication with them, or inquire how much iron is left in the bottle.
  2) Improper administration: Iron may not be well absorbed if administered with milk or other products high in P content.
  3) Malabsorption: Malabsorption of iron may be present in as many as 20% of patients with iron deficiency anemia who do not respond to iron.
  4) Ongoing blood losses; check stool for blood.
  5) Incorrect diagnosis
    a) Lead poisoning, thalassemia, and chronic infection are also associated with hypochromic anemia.
    b) Check blood-lead level.
    c) Check parent's indices and smears for thalassemia.
  6) Inability to use iron: In the presence of concomitant lead poisoning or certain chronic disease states, especially those associated with inflammation, iron may be absorbed but not incorporated into Hgb.

B. HEMOPHILIA
1. General
  a. Clinically, hemophilia A and B are indistinguishable; hemophilia A is much more common. The diagnosis is based on factor VIII and factor IX assays; in neonates a diagnosis of factor VIII or factor IX deficiency can be made on a cord blood assay.
  b. In neonates with hemophilia, there may be intracranial bleeding secondary to traumatic delivery or bleeding at the circumcision

site; otherwise bleeding complications (other than bruising) are uncommon during the first year. With a positive family history, circumcision should be avoided. The highest incidence of bleeding episodes occurs from age 4 through adolescence. Clinical severity correlates with the patient's levels of factor VIII and IX: <2% = severe, 2%-5% = moderate, >5% = mild. Patients who have mild hemophilia usually bleed only after surgery, dental procedures, or severe trauma.

c. Bleeding into joints is the hallmark of hemophilia. Acute hemarthroses require prompt therapy; when in doubt, treat (often by self-infusion at home). For frequent episodes of rebleeding into a joint, prophylaxis with factor VIII or IX qod over a 12-week period may be indicated. If this treatment fails, arthroscopic synovectomy may be helpful.

d. Bruises are seldom large enough to require treatment, but intramuscular bleeding should be treated with a clotting factor; such treatment may be needed over several days. Extensive soft-tissue bleeding into the forearm or leg may result in a "compartment syndrome." Treatment includes ice, elevation, factor replacement; fasciotomy may be required to preserve function.

e. Episodes of CNS bleeding occur most often at an early age. Symptoms include headache, paralysis, behavioral changes, and aphasia. Any suspected intracranial bleeding demands immediate, aggressive therapy before diagnostic studies are initiated. After an initial bolus to achieve 100% replacement, a clotting factor should be given by continuous infusion to maintain a blood level >0.50 U/ml (>50%) and continued for as long as 3 weeks. Prophylaxis (bolus dose qod) is sometimes given for as much as 6 months following an initial episode of bleeding.

f. Spontaneous hematuria usually stops without specific treatment, but GU bleeding secondary to trauma should be treated with a clotting factor.

g. Tongue and mouth lacerations require clotting-factor replacement, an antifibrinolytic agent and, occasionally, sedation, NPO status, and IV fluids.

2. Treatment

a. Recommended dosages of factor VIII and IX concentrates for various clinical situations are shown in Tables 10-2 and 10-3. Recombinant human factor VIII products (Recombinate, Kogenate) are also now available. They are as effective as plasma-derived preparations and should reduce the possibility of viral

TABLE 10-2.

Hemophilia A: Recommended Dosages of Factor VIII*

Type of bleeding	Initial dose (factor VIII, U/kg)	Repeated doses (factor VIII, U/kg)	Other treatment
Acute hemarthrosis			Ice packs, non-weight-bearing sling or lightweight splint; rarely joint aspiration
Early	10	Seldom necessary	
Late	20	20 q12h	
Intramuscular hemorrhage†	20-30	20 q12h (often several days of treatment)	Non-weight-bearing support; complete bed rest for iliopsoas hemorrhage
Life-threatening situations‡	50	25-30 q8-12h or (preferably) as a continuous infusion (3-4 U/kg/h)	
Intracranial hemorrhage			
Major surgery			
Major trauma			
Tongue or neck bleeding with potential airway obstruction			
Painless spontaneous gross hematuria	None		Increased fluids by mouth; corticosteroids and factor VIII sometimes used
Severe abdominal pain‡	20-40	20-45 q12h	An antifibrinolytic agent (tranexamic acid or ε-aminocaproic acid), sedation; nothing by mouth in small child; local application of oral adhesive gauze may be beneficial for gum bleeding
Tongue and mouth lacerations‡	20	20 q12h	
Tooth extraction (permanent teeth)†	20	20 q12h (often not necessary in cases of uncomplicated extractions)	Antifibrinolytic agent beginning 1 d preoperatively; continue 7-10 d

From Lusher JM, Warrier I: Pediatr Rev 12:277, 1991.

*Refers to viral-attenuated factor VIII.

†In individuals who have mild hemophilia A, DDAVP (desmopressin) is the treatment of choice rather than factor VIII concentrates.

‡These situations should be treated in a comprehensive hemophilia center. If first seen in another hospital, the hemophilia center should be contacted and the patient transferred after emergency treatment is given at the local hospital.

TABLE 10-3.
Hemophilia B: Recommended Dosage Schedule*

Type of bleeding	Initial dose (factor IX, U/kg; and source of factor IX†)	Repeat dose (factor IX, U/kg; and source of factor IX†)	Other treatment
Acute hemarthrosis‡			Seldom necessary
In association with mild hemophilia B	10-15 (FIXCC)	None	Ice packs; non-weight-bearing support, sling; rarely, joint aspiration
Early, in association with severe hemophilia B	20 (FIXCC)	None	
Late (pain, swelling, limitation of motion) in association with severe hemophilia B	30 (FIXCC)	20-25 (FIXCC) q12h	
Intramuscular hemorrhage‡			Non-weight-bearing support; complete bed rest for iliopsoas hemorrhage
In association with mild hemophilia B	15 (FIXCC)	10-15 (FIXCC) q12h	
In associaton with severe hemophilia B	30-40 (FIXCC)	30 (FIXCC) q12h	
Life-threatening situations§ Intracranial hemorrhage Major trauma Tongue or neck bleeding with potential airway obstruction	50 (FIXCC)	20-25 (FIXCC) q12h or as a continuous infusion	AT-III concentrate as source of AT-III; add heparin to reconstituted prothrombin complex concentrate
Painless spontaneous gross hematuria	None		Increased fluids by mouth; corticosteroids and factor IX are used by some
Severe abdominal pain‡ In mild hemophilia B	15 (FIXCC)	10 (FIXCC) q12h	

In association with severe hemophilia B	40 (FIXCC)	20 (FIXCC) q12h	An antifibrinolytic agent (tranexamic acid or ε-aminocaproic acid), sedation; nothing by mouth in small children
Tongue and mouth lacerations	30	30 (FIXCC) q12h	Antifibrinolytic agent beginning 1 d preoperatively; continue 7-10 d
Tooth extraction (permanent teeth)	30	30 (FIXCC) q12h (often not necessary in cases of uncomplicated extractions)	

Modified from Lusher JM, Warrier I: *Pediatr Rev* 12:278, 1991.

*FFP = fresh-frozen plasma; FIXCC = Factor IX complex concentrate; AT-III = antithrombin III. If FIXCC is not available in an emergency situation, FFP can be used (not virus inactivated). One unit of FIXCC is equivalent to 1 ml FFP.

†FIXCC refers to heat-treated or otherwise virus-attenuated FIXCC. As soon as a nonthrombogenic factor IX concentrate (coagulant FIX) is licensed and available, it will become the preferred product for most of the above situations.

‡In infants and children younger than 4 yr of age, some physicians still prefer to use FFP rather than FIXCC, even in those with moderate or severe hemophilia B. However, FFP cannot be virus attenuated.

§These situations should be treated in a comprehensive hemophilia center. If first seen in another hospital, the hemophilia center should be contacted and the patient transferred after emergency treatment is given at the local hospital.

contaminants. The development of antibodies appears to be similar
to that seen with plasma-derived preparations.

b. Because of the risks of DIC and thromboembolism, the repetitive
use of large doses of factor IX concentrate has been avoided. The
incidence of such complications is much lower with newer, highly
purified products.

c. DDAVP is the treatment of choice for patients with mild-to-
moderate hemophilia A or type I von Willebrand's disease. An IV
dose of 0.3 μg/kg diluted in 50 ml normal saline results in a twofold
to fivefold (average is threefold) increase in factor VIII activity.
Need to monitor for hyponatremia, water intoxication, and
vasospasm. Tachyphylaxis may also develop with frequent dosing.
Testing is required to ensure an adequate response for each patient
before it can be prescribed routinely. A potent intranasal DDAVP
preparation is also being used but has not yet been approved for
pediatric patients.

d. Patients are best managed in collaboration with a regional
hemophilia center. With proper training and support, most patients
can carry out much of their infusion therapy at home.

3. Prophylaxis

a. With venipuncture, apply pressure to the site for at least 5 minutes.
Never use the femoral or jugular vein.

b. Immunizations should be given SQ with a 25-gauge needle or after
factor replacement; apply pressure for 5 minutes.

c. A clotting factor sufficient to raise the level to 30% of normal
should be given 30-45 minutes before an LP.

d. For surgical procedures, give an initial bolus of clotting factor to
100% 30-40 minutes preoperatively followed by a continuous
infusion to >50% levels. Maintain levels >50% for 5-7 days and
then >30% for an additional 5-7 days. Check for "inhibitors."

e. For dental procedures give an antifibrinolytic agent (α-
aminocaproic acid or tranexamic acid) before and 7-10 days after
the procedure. A dose of factor VIII or IX is generally given before
the procedure. Mandibular anesthetic blocks should be avoided.

f. Some patients with a severe clotting factor deficiency seem to
benefit from long-term qod prophylaxis beginning at 1-2 years
of age.

4. Complications

a. High-titer "inhibitor" antibodies develop in 10%-15% of patients
with hemophilia A and in 1% of those with hemophilia B. Such
cases can be treated with factor IX complex concentrates (standard

or activated), porcine factor VIII (Hyate:C), a human recombinant factor VIIa preparation, or immune tolerance regimens.

b. Ninety percent of patients who received plasma-derived products between 1979 and 1984 have become HIV seropositive. AIDS progression in these patients is somewhat delayed compared with other risk groups. Current products are safe with respect to HIV and hepatitis, but there is a risk of parvovirus transmission. Patients who are HBsAg seronegative should be immunized with hepatitis B vaccine.

5. Carrier detection and prenatal diagnosis: In families with a history of hemophilia, carrier testing and accurate prenatal diagnosis can be carried out using DNA analysis.

C. SICKLE-CELL DISEASE

The incidence of sickle-cell disease is 1 in 500 blacks; the course is very variable. In most cases, diagnosis is made as a result of neonate screening. Because of the presence of fetal Hgb, clinical manifestations are minimal before 4 months of age.

1. Clinical manifestations
   a. Anemia: Patients are usually not very symptomatic at their chronic Hgb level; however, there may be an acute drop in Hgb secondary to the following:
      1) Aplastic crisis: Usually secondary to viral infections, especially parvovirus. Treatment consists of transfusion therapy.
      2) Sequestration syndrome: Results from trapping sickled RBCs within an enlarging spleen; peak age 6 months to 2 years
         a) Manifestations: Pallor, splenomegaly, respiratory distress, ± thrombocytopenia, hypovolemia
         b) Treatment: Transfusion. Because of risk of recurrence, elective splenectomy may be indicated after 2 years of age.
   b. Infection: Because of functional asplenia, patients are at a significantly increased risk of overwhelming infection (sepsis, meningitis, pneumonia, osteomyelitis) with encapsulated organisms *(Haemophilus influenzae, Streptococcus pneumoniae)* and *Salmonella* organisms. It may be difficult to distinguish between a bacterial infection, self-limited viral disorder, and vasoocclusive crisis in a patient who has fever without an obvious source.
      1) Work-up: Consider CBC, blood culture, CXR, LP.
      2) Management: The treatment of a child with sickle-cell disease who is <4 yr of age and has a temperature >38.6°C should include the following at a minimum:

a) Evaluation by a primary care provider who is knowledgeable in the care of children with sickle-cell disease
b) IM or IV administration of an antibiotic (e.g., ceftriaxone) effective against *S. pneumoniae* and *H. influenzae*
c) Observation for at least 4 hours after parenteral administration of an antibiotic
d) Reevaluation 24 hours after antibiotic administration
e) Continuation of antibiotic for at least 3 days
f) Hospital admission if there is no reliable source of primary care follow-up

NOTE: The treatment strategy previously described is recommended whether or not the child has a focal source for the fever.

g) Other indications for hospitalization include the following:
   (1) Temperature >39.4°C
   (2) Age <12 months
   (3) Toxic appearance
   (4) Shock
   (5) Dehydration
   (6) Positive CXR findings
   (7) Respiratory distress
   (8) Neurologic abnormalities (e.g., meningeal signs: stiff neck, altered mental status, focal signs)
   (9) Rapidly enlarging spleen
   (10) Falling Hgb (drop of at least 2 g)
   (11) WBC count <5000 or >40,000
   (12) Severe abdominal pain
   (13) A significantly swollen extremity
   (14) Previous sepsis
   (15) Concurrent pain crisis

NOTE: The choice of antibiotics in treating a presumptive bacterial infection should take into consideration the high rate of *S. pneumoniae* strains resistant to penicillin and other antimicrobial agents among patients who have sickle-cell disease and are receiving penicillin prophylaxis.

c. Vasoocclusive crises: Results from areas of ischemic infarction. It may be precipitated by infection, dehydration, or cold exposure; however, in most cases no trigger is identified.
   1) Extremities are the most common site.
      a) Clinical features: Pain, ± erythema, ± localized soft-tissue swelling, ± localized tenderness of one or more bones or joints, ± fever. The possibility of osteomyelitis or septic

arthritis needs to be considered. However, infarction is much more common than infection; clues to infection include temperature >39°C, WBC >30,000, and systemic toxicity.

NOTE: Young infants may have painful swelling of the hands and feet because of dactylitis.

  b) Treatment: Hydration and analgesia; may start with bolus of normal saline (20 ml/kg) followed by fluids at 1.5 × maintenance. The drug of choice for analgesia is morphine, which may be given on a fixed IM schedule, by continuous IV infusion, or by a PCA pump. The risk of opiate addiction is low. Codeine and NSAIDs such as ketorolac may also be useful.

NOTE: The use of meperidine (Demerol) may be complicated by dysphoria and seizures.

 2) Abdominal crisis: Patient may have ileus and rebound tenderness, which mimicks an acute abdomen (e.g., appendicitis). The pain may be familiar to the patient and readily recognized as "crisis pain." Because painful crises are much more common than an acute surgical abdomen, a period of careful observation of clinical response to hydration and analgesia is warranted in most cases.

 3) Chest syndrome

  a) Clinical: Chest pain, fever, respiratory distress, rales, decreased breath sounds, infiltrates; difficult to distinguish infarction vs. infection

  b) Treatment: Antibiotics, IV hydration, oxygen

  c) Transfusion or *exchange* transfusion is indicated if Pao$_2$ is <75 mm Hg with mask O$_2$.

 4) Stroke: Most devastating form of vasoocclusive crisis, with a high risk of recurrence. Treatment consists of exchange transfusion followed by a chronic transfusion program to maintain Hgb S <30%. The duration of the chronic transfusion program is somewhat controversial. There may be a high stroke recurrence rate after transfusions are discontinued. Patients undergoing chronic transfusion therapy should receive chelation therapy with desferrioxamine to maintain a serum ferritin level <2000 ng/dL.

 5) Miscellaneous: Gallstones, cholecystitis, priapism, avascular hip necrosis, hepatomegaly, retinopathy, papillary necrosis, chronic renal failure, stunted growth, progressive CNS ischemia with neuropsychologic deficits

2. General management
  a. Comprehensive well-child care, including the following:
      1) Immunization against *H. influenzae* type B and hepatitis B
      2) Pneumococcal vaccine at 2 years of age and repeated between 4 and 6 years of age
      3) Family education and counseling
      4) Folic acid supplementation
  b. Penicillin prophylaxis starts at age 4 months and continues until at least 4-6 years of age. Prophylaxis probably can be stopped safely in children who have not had a prior severe pneumococcal infection or splenectomy and are receiving comprehensive care. However, the optimal timing of discontinuation has not been established. Parents must be counseled to seek immediate medical attention for all febrile events.
      1) <3 yr, 125 mg bid PO
      2) >3 yr, 250 mg bid PO
      3) If compliance is poor, consider IM penicillin G benzathine q21d.
  c. Refer to a comprehensive hemoglobinopathy treatment center. Operative procedures should be carried out by a surgeon who is experienced in treating patients with sickle-cell disease and in conjunction with an experienced anesthesiologist and hematologist.
  d. New therapies such as hydroxyurea and bone marrow transplantation are being used in selected patients.

D. THROMBOCYTOPENIA
1. Etiology
  a. Decreased production
      1) Acquired bone marrow hypoplasia: Idiopathic, drug-induced, viral infection, measles vaccine
      2) Congenital bone marrow hypoplasia: Fanconi's syndrome, TAR syndrome, Wiskott-Aldrich syndrome, amegakaryocytic thrombocytopenia
      3) Malignancy
  b. Increased destruction
      1) Drug-induced: Valproic acid, propylthiouracil, phenytoin, TMP/SMZ, penicillin, cephalothin, rifampin, acetaminophen
      2) Immune-mediated: Infection (torch), lupus erythematosus, post-transfusion, drug-induced, HIV infection, immune (idiopathic) thrombocytopenic purpura
      3) Vascular abnormalities: Catheters, prosthetic heart valves, giant

cavernous hemangioma (Kasabach-Merritt syndrome), congenital heart disease, hypersplenism (sequestration), portal hypertension, venous malformations
  4) Vasculitis with endothelial injury, hemolytic-uremic syndrome, thrombotic thrombocytopenic purpura, DIC
2. Neonatal thrombocytopenia
  a. Most commonly on immune basis
    1) Autoimmune (maternal SLE or chronic ITP)
    2) Alloimmune/isoimmune (platelet equivalent of Rh disease): Confirmed by platelet antigen typing of parents, antibody detection, genotyping (if necessary). This type of immunity is the most common cause of severe thrombocytopenia at birth.
  b. Other causes include TAR syndrome, trisomies 13 and 18, Wiskott-Aldrich syndrome, viral infection (TORCH), bacterial sepsis, cavernous hemangioma, cyanotic heart disease, and renal vein thrombosis.
3. Acute immune thrombocytopenic purpura
  a. Acute ITP usually occurs in a previously well child between 2 and 6 years of age who has easy bruising, hemorrhagic bullae of oral mucosa, and petechiae. The PE is otherwise normal. Intracranial and GI bleeding is uncommon.
  b. Often triggered by infection: Viral upper respiratory infection, varicella, Epstein-Barr virus, HIV, cat-scratch, measles, mumps, CMV, viral hepatitis, rubella. Look for recent medication use, immunizations, HIV risk factors, family history, or symptoms of autoimmune disease.
  c. Platelet count is usually <20,000; always confirm by exam of peripheral smear. Hgb concentration, WBC, and differential counts are characteristically normal. There is a risk of CNS bleeding when the count is <10,000 and there is evidence of oral/mucosal bleeding.
  d. A bone marrow exam is not generally indicated but is mandatory with other abnormalities of CBC or smear (nucleated RBCs, blasts) or with hepatosplenomegaly. The presence of at least a few large platelets on a smear is reassuring.
  e. Platelet antibodies are rarely positive and not diagnostically helpful.

NOTE: With *rare* exception, leukemia does not present as isolated thrombocytopenia. Rarely, aplastic anemia can present this way.

  f. Course
    1) The majority of children with ITP recover spontaneously

without recurrence. The time until the return of normal platelet counts ranges from a few days to 6 months (average 3 weeks).
2) In 4% of patients, resolution of the initial process is followed by recurrent episodes of thrombocytopenia. Chronic ITP (>6 months) develops in approximately 10% of children with acute ITP, and it is more common in older children and females.
3) The initial clinical and laboratory features may not distinguish between acute and chronic ITP or predict which acute patient will develop chronic ITP. However, older age, female gender, and a family history of autoimmune disease are seen more commonly with chronic ITP.
g. Treatment
1) Indications: Platelet count <20,000, active mucosal bleeding, or suspected internal bleeding
2) Prednisone 2 mg/kg/d (max 60 mg) × 3 weeks, with taper (response is often slow); for faster response, IV methylprednisolone 30 mg/kg (max dose 1 g) over 30 minutes q24h for 3 doses *and/or*
3) IV immune globulin
a) Single dose of 1 g/kg IV over 4-6 hours
b) A significant increase in platelet count is usually seen within 48 hours; it may be effective in children with steroid-resistant acute ITP.
c) Side effects include severe headache, fever, vomiting, vertigo, and myalgias and often appear 12-24 hours postinfusion. Side effects can be prevented in many cases by giving acetaminophen and diphenhydramine during and for 48 hours after infusion.
4) Recently, IV anti-D (WinRho) 25 μg qd × 2 or 50 μg × 1 has been recommended for the treatment of acute ITP.
5) Follow platelet counts until normal; a secondary drop with intercurrent viral illness may be seen.
6) Treatment of ITP with IV immune globulin or steroids does *not* decrease the likelihood of chronic ITP.
4. Chronic thrombocytopenic purpura
a. Platelet count is <50,000 for >6 months.
b. This condition is often seen in adolescents with other evidence of autoimmune disease or a positive family history for autoimmune disease.
c. Treatment options include intermittent doses of IV immune globulin, steroids, splenectomy, danazol, vitamin C, vincristine,

Rh$_o$ (D) immune globulin (RhoGam), plasmapheresis, and aza-thioprine.

E. NEUTROPENIA

1. Manifestations

Severity	Absolute neutrophil count	Symptoms
Mild	1000-1500	Asymptomatic
Moderate	500-1000	Superficial infections
Severe	<500	Deep tissue infections; sepsis

   a. WBC/neutrophil counts are higher in whites compared with blacks.
   b. Acute occurrence of bacterial infection in chronic neutropenia is significantly lower than in chemotherapy or HIV-infected patients.

2. Etiology
   a. Primary bone marrow disorder
      1) Fanconi's aplastic anemia
      2) Shwachman-Diamond syndrome
      3) Cyclic neutropenia
      4) Cartilage-hair hypoplasia
      5) Kostmann's syndrome (severe congenital neutropenia)
   b. Impaired neutrophil production secondary to metabolic or systemic disease
      1) Familial (associated with amino-acidopathy)
      2) Marrow replacement (leukemia, lymphoma, solid tumor); rare cause of isolated neutropenia
      3) Deficiency of vitamin B$_{12}$/folic acid, copper, protein
      4) Infection
   c. Infection
      1) Most common cause of neutropenia in childhood
      2) May be viral, bacterial, rickettsial, fungal, protozoal
      3) Often develops during first 24-48 hours of viral infection (Epstein-Barr virus, CMV, influenza); persists 3-6 days
   d. Alloimmune
      1) May follow leukocyte transfusion or fetomaternal sensitization
      2) Occasionally associated with infections, especially cutaneous
      3) Median recovery period of 7 weeks
   e. Autoimmune
      1) Peak age 3-30 months

      2) May be associated with autoimmune disease (antineutrophil antibodies may be detected)

      3) Generally benign outcome without therapy (median recovery, 20 months)

      4) Responds to steroids, IV immune globulin, anti-D, and G-CSF

NOTE: Chronic benign neutropenia of childhood may be autoimmune neutropenia with undetected antibody.

    f. Drug-induced

      1) Direct marrow suppression (TMP/SMZ, beta lactams)

      2) Suppression by drug metabolites

      3) Immune neutrophil destruction

3. Evaluation

   a. History

     1) Type, location, severity, frequency of infection

     2) Recent illnesses, drug exposure, family history

   b. PE

     1) Careful attention to skin, dental, and perineal areas

     2) Hepatosplenomegaly, congenital defects

   c. Laboratory studies

     1) Neutrophil counts, recent and past

     2) Other hematologic values, including MCV

     3) Special testing (e.g., antibodies) as indicated by H&P

4. Management

ANC count	Evaluation	Treatment
>1000	Exam, labs, ±x-rays	None, unless bacterial infection strongly suspected
500-1000	Exam, labs, cultures, ±x-rays	Same as above
0-500	Exam, labs, cultures, x-rays	Broad-spectrum antibiotic coverage

BIBLIOGRAPHY

Anemia

Dallman PR, Simes MA: Percentile curves for hemoglobin and red cell volume in infancy and childhood, *J Pediatr* 94:26, 1979.

Differential diagnosis of hypochromic microcytic anemia, *Pediatric Oncology/Hematology Newsletter,* Boston, vol 2, Spring 1979, Sidney Farber Cancer Institute.

Oski FA: Anemia in children, *Hosp Pract* 11:63, 1976.

Oski FA: The non-hematologic manifestations of iron deficiency, *Am J Dis Child* 133:315, 1979.

Oski FA: Iron deficiency: facts and fallacies, *Pediatr Clin North Am* 32:493, 1985.

Stockman JA III: Office hematology: how valid are the results, *Contemp Pediatr* 3:21, 1986.

Hemophilia

Bell B et al: Hemophilia: an updated review, *Pediatr Rev* 16:290, 1995.

Lusher JM, Warrier I: Hemophilia, *Pediatr Rev* 12:275, 1991.

Mannucci PMP: Desmopressin (DDAVP) for treatment of disorders of hemostasis, *Prog Hemost Thromb* 8:19, 1986.

Schwartz RS et al: Human recombinant DNA-derived antihemophilic factor (factor VIII) in the treatment of hemophilia A, *N Engl J Med* 323:1800, 1990.

Sickle-cell disease

Dover GJ: Management of sickle cell anemia in children, *Md Med J* 39:371, 1990.

Evans JPM: Practical management of sickle cell disease, *Arch Dis Child* 64:1748, 1989.

Falletta JM et al: Discontinuing penicillin prophylaxis in children with sickle cell anemia, *J Pediatr* 127:685, 1995.

Pearson HA: Sickle cell diseases: diagnosis and management in infancy and childhood, *Pediatr Rev* 9:121, 1987.

Pegelow CH: Survey of pain management therapy provided for children with sickle cell disease, *Clin Pediatr* 31:211, 1992.

Steele, RW et al: Colonization with antibiotic-resistant *Streptococcus pneumoniae* in children with sickle cell disease, *J Pediatr* 128:531, 1996.

Vichinsky EP: Comprehensive care in sickle cell disease: its impact on morbidity and mortality, *Semin Hematol* 28:220, 1991.

Wong W-Y et al: Infection caused by *Streptococcus pneumoniae* in children with sickle cell disease: epidemiology, immunologic mechanisms, prophylaxis and vaccination, *Clin Infect Dis* 14:1124, 1992.

Thrombocytopenia

Blanchette VS et al: Randomized trial of intravenous immunoglobulin G, intravenous anti-D and oral prednisone in childhood acute immune thrombocytopenia purpura, *Lancet* 344:703, 1994.

Bussel JB: Thrombocytopenia in newborns, infants, and children, *Pediatr Ann* 19:181, 1990.

Dunn HL, Maurer HM: Prednisone treatment of acute idiopathic thrombocytopenic purpura of childhood, *Am J Pediatr Hematol Oncol* 6:159, 1984.

Halperin DS, Doyle JJ: Is bone marrow examination justified in idiopathic thrombocytopenic purpura? *Am J Dis Child* 142:508, 1988.

Sartorius JA: Steroid treatment of idiopathic thrombocytopenic purpura in children, *Am J Pediatr Hematol Oncol* 6:165, 1984.

Souid AK, Sadowitz PD: Acute childhood immune thrombocytopenic purpura, *Clin Pediatr,* 34:487, 1995.

Walker RW, Walker W: Idiopathic thrombocytopenia, initial illness and long-term follow-up, *Arch Dis Child* 59:316, 1984.

IMMUNIZATIONS   *11*

A. RECOMMENDED SCHEDULE FOR IMMUNIZATIONS OF HEALTHY INFANTS AND CHILDREN (Table 11-1)

1. Recommended vaccines can be safely and effectively administered simultaneously, including Tetramune (DTP and Hib), DTaP/ActHib, and Comvax (Hib/hepatitis B vaccine).
2. DTP should be administered in the usual dose to preterm infants when they reach a chronologic age of 2 months, regardless of their size.
3. Recommended vaccine doses should never be reduced or divided in an effort to reduce adverse events.
4. A mild acute illness with a low-grade fever, mild diarrheal illness in an otherwise well child, pregnancy of mother or other household contact, current antimicrobial therapy, or recent exposure to an infectious disease are *not* contraindications to vaccination. Contraindications and precautions to immunizations are shown in Table 11-2.

B. RECOMMENDED IMMUNIZATION SCHEDULES FOR CHILDREN NOT IMMUNIZED DURING THE FIRST YEAR OF LIFE (Table 11-3)

1. A lapse in the immunization schedules does not require reinstitution of the entire series. If a dose of DTP or OPV is missed, immunization should occur on the next visit as if the usual interval had elapsed.
2. A patient whose immunization status is unknown should be considered susceptible, and appropriate immunizations should be administered. The administration of vaccines to already immune recipients is not harmful.

C. HEPATITIS B VACCINE

1. Universal immunization of all infants with the HBV vaccine is now recommended. The dose and schedule of the vaccine, as well as the use of HBIG, are based on the HBsAg status of the mother.
   a. Infants of HBsAg-negative mothers should be given the first dose of vaccine before hospital discharge, the second dose at 2 months

Text continued on p. 192.

187

TABLE 11-1.
Recommended Childhood Immunization Schedule: United States, January-June, 1996

Vaccines are listed under the routinely recommended ages. Bars indicate range of acceptable ages for vaccination. Shaded bars indicate *catch-up vaccination*: at 11-12 years of age, hepatitis B vaccine should be administered to children not previously vaccinated, and varicella-zoster virus vaccine should be administered to children not previously vaccinated who lack a reliable history of chickenpox.

Vaccine	Birth	1 mo	2 mo	4 mo	6 mo	12 mo	15 mo	18 mo	4-6 yr	11-12 yr	14-16 yr
Hepatitis B [a,b]	Hep B-1		Hep B-2		Hep B-3					Hep B [b]	
Diphtheria, Tetanus, Pertussis [c]			DTP	DTP	DTP	DTP [c] (DTaP at 15+ mo)			DTP or DTaP	Td	Td
H. influenzae type b [d]			Hib	Hib	Hib [d]	Hib [d]					
Polio [e]			OPV [e]	OPV	OPV				OPV		
Measles, Mumps, Rubella [f]						MMR			MMR [f] or MMR [f]	MMR [f]	
Varicella Zoster Virus Vaccine [g]						Var				Var [g]	

From Committee on Infectious Diseases: American Academy of Pediatrics, *Pediatrics* 97:143,1996.

Approved by the Advisory Committee on Immunization Practices (ACIP), the American Academy of Pediatrics (AAP), and the American Academy of Family Physicians (AAFP).

[a]*Infants born to HBsAg-negative mothers* should receive 2.5 μg of Merck vaccine (Recombivax HB) or 10 μg of SmithKline Beecham (SB) vaccine (Engerix-B). The 2nd dose should be administered ≥1 mo after the 1st dose.

Infants born to HBsAg-positive mothers should receive 0.5 ml Hepatitis B Immune Globulin (HBIG) within 12 hr of birth, and either 5 μg of Merck vaccine (Recombivax HB) or 10 μg of SB vaccine (Engerix-B) at a separate site. The 2nd dose is recommended at 1-2 mo of age and the 3rd dose at 6 mo of age.

Infants born to mothers whose HBsAg status is unknown should receive either 5 μg of Merck vaccine (Recombivax HB) or 10 μg of SB vaccine (Engerix-B) within 12 hr of birth. The 2nd dose of vaccine is recommended at 1 mo of age and the 3rd dose at 6 mo of age.

[b]Adolescents who have not previously received 3 doses of hepatitis B vaccine should initiate or complete the series at the 11-12-year-old visit. The 2nd dose should be administered at least 1 mo after the 1st dose, and the 3rd dose should be administered at least 4 mo after the 1st dose and at least 2 mo after the 2nd dose.

[c]DTP4 may be administered at 12 mo of age, if at least 6 mo have elapsed since DTP3. DTaP (diphtheria and tetanus toxoids and acellular pertussis vaccine) is licensed for the 4th and/or 5th vaccine dose(s) for children age ≥15 mo and may be preferred for these doses in this age group. Td (tetanus and diphtheria toxoids, adsorbed, for adult use) is recommended at 11-12 years of age if at least 5 years have elapsed since the last dose of DTP, DTaP, or DT.

[d]Three *H. influenzae* type b (Hib) conjugate vaccines are licensed for infant use. If PRO-OMP (Pedvaxhib [Merck]) is administered at 2 and 4 mo of age, a dose at 6 mo of age, is not required. After completing the primary series, any Hib conjugate vaccine may be used as a booster.

[e]Oral poliovirus vaccine (OPV) is recommended for routine infant vaccination. Inactivated poliovirus vaccine (IPV) is recommended for persons with a congenital or acquired immunodeficiency disease or an altered immune status as a result of disease or immunosuppressive therapy, as well as their household contacts, and is an acceptable alternative for other persons. The primary 3-dose series for IPV should be given with a minimum interval of 4 wk between the 1st and 2nd doses and 6 mo between the 2nd and 3rd doses.

[f]The 2nd dose of MMR is routinely recommended at 4-6 yr of age or at 11-12 yr of age but may be administered at any visit provided at least 1 mo has elapsed since receipt of the 1st dose.

[g]Varicella-zoster virus vaccine (Var) can be administered to susceptible children any time after 12 mo of age. Unvaccinated children who lack a reliable history of chickenpox should be vaccinated at the 11-12-year-old visit.

TABLE 11-2.
Guide to Contraindications and Precautions to Immunizations[a]

True contraindications and precautions	Not true (vaccines may be given)
General for all vaccines (DTP/DTaP, OPV, IPV, MMR, Hib, HBV)[b]	
Anaphylactic reaction to a vaccine contraindicates further doses of that vaccine	Mild-to-moderate local reaction (soreness, redness, swelling) following a dose of an injectable antigen
Anaphylactic reaction to a vaccine constituent contraindicates the use of vaccines containing that substance	Mild acute illness with or without low-grade fever
Moderate or severe illnesses with or without a fever	Current antimicrobial therapy
	Convalescent phase of illnesses
	Prematurity (same dosage and indications as for normal, full-term infants)
	Recent exposure to an infectious disease
	History of penicillin or other nonspecific allergies or relatives with such allergies
DTP/DTaP	
Encephalopathy within 7 d of administration of dose of DTP	Temperature of <40.5° C (105° F) following a previous dose of DTP
Precaution: Fever of ≥40.5° C (105° F) within 48 hr after vaccination with a dose of DTP[c]	Family history of convulsions[d]
Precaution: Collapse or shocklike state (hypotonic-hyperresponsive episode) within 48 hr of receiving a prior dose of DTP[c]	Family history of an adverse event following DTP administration
Precaution: Seizures within 3 d of receiving a prior dose of DTP[c] (see footnote d regarding management of children with a personal history of seizures at any time)	Family history of sudden infant death syndrome
Precaution: Persistent, inconsolable crying lasting ≥3 hr, within 48 hr of receiving a dose of DTP[c]	
OPV	
Infection with HIV or a household contact with HIV	Breastfeeding
	Current antimicrobial therapy
	Diarrhea

TABLE 11-2. (cont.)

True contraindications and precautions	Not true (vaccines may be given)
Known altered immunodeficiency (hematologic and solid tumors; congenital immunodeficiency; and long-term immuno-suppressive therapy) Immunodeficient household contact **Precaution:** Pregnancy[c]	
IPV	
Anaphylactic reaction to neomycin or streptomycin **Precaution:** Pregnancy[c]	None identified
MMR[e]	
Anaphylactic reactions to egg ingestion and to neomycin[f] Pregnancy Known altered immunodeficiency (hematologic and solid tumors, congenital immunodeficiency, and long-term immunosup-pressive therapy) **Precaution:** Recent (within 3 mo) immunoglobulin administration[c]	Tuberculosis or positive for purified protein derivative (PPD) of tuberculin Simultaneous tuberculosis skin testing[g] Breastfeeding Pregnancy of mother of recipient Immunodeficient family member or household contact Infection with HIV Nonanaphylactic reactions to eggs or neomycin
Hib	
None identified	None identified
HBV	
None identified	Pregnancy

National Vaccine Advisory Committee to the United States Public Health Service: *JAMA* 269:1817, 1993.
[a]This information is based on the recommendations of the Advisory Committee on Immunization Practices (ACIP) and those of the Committee on Infectious Diseases (Red Book Committee) of the American Academy of Pediatrics (AAP). Sometimes these recommendations vary from those contained in the manufacturers' package inserts. For more detailed information, providers should consult the published recommendations of the ACIP, the AAP, the American Academy of Family Physicians, and the manufacturers' package inserts.
[b]DTP, Diphtheria and tetanus toxoids and pertussis vaccine; DTaP, diphtheria, tetanus, and acellular pertussis vaccine; OPV, oral poliovirus vaccine; IPV, inactivated poliomyelitis vaccine; MMR, measles, mumps, rubella vaccine; Hib, *H. influenzae* b vaccine; HBV, hepatitis B vaccine; HIV, human immunodeficiency virus.

Continued.

TABLE 11-2. (cont.)

cAlthough not a contraindication, this should be carefully reviewed. The benefits and risks of administering a specific vaccine to an individual under the circumstances should be considered. If the risks are believed to outweigh the benefits, the immunization should be withheld; if the benefits are believed to outweigh the risks (e.g., during an outbreak or foreign travel), the immunization should be given. Whether and when to administer DTP to children with proven or suspected underlying neurologic disorders should be decided on an individual basis. It is prudent on theoretical grounds to avoid vaccinating pregnant women. However, if immediate protection against poliomyelitis is needed, OPV, not IPV, is recommended.

dAcetaminophen given before administering DTP and thereafter every 4 hr for 24 hr should be considered for children with a personal or family history of convulsions in siblings or parents.

eThere is a theoretical risk that the administration of multiple live virus vaccines (OPV and MMR) within 30 d of one another if not given on the same day will result in a suboptimal immune response. There are no data to substantiate this.

fPersons with a history of anaphylactic reactions following egg ingestion should be vaccinated only with extreme caution. Protocols have been developed for vaccinating such persons and should be consulted (*J Pediatr* 102:196-199, 1983; and *J Pediatr* 113:504-506, 1988.)

gMeasles vaccination may temporarily suppress tuberculin reactivity. If testing cannot be done the day of MMR vaccination, the test should be postponed for 4-6 wk.

of age, and the third dose at 6-18 months of age. There is some evidence of augmented response when the third dose is administered after 12 months of age.

  b. Infants of HBsAG-positive mothers should receive the first dose of vaccine at birth (along with HBIG), the second dose at 1 month of age, and the third dose at 6 months of age.

NOTE: Infants of HBsAg-positive mothers and patients with HIV infection should be tested for antibody response from 3-9 months after completion of the vaccination series. Revaccination with one or more additional doses should be considered for patients who do not respond to the initial series.

2. Vaccination is also recommended for the following groups:

  a. Unvaccinated children <11 years of age who are Pacific Islanders or who reside in households of first-generation immigrants from countries in which HBV is of high or intermediate endemicity

  b. All 11-12–year-old children who have not previously received HBV vaccine

  c. High-risk groups who should receive HBV vaccine regardless of age include the following:

TABLE 11-3.
Recommended Immunization Schedules for Children Not Immunized in the First Year of Life

Recommended time/age	Immunization(s)[a,b]	Comments
Younger Than 7 Years		
First visit	DTP, Hib, HBV, MMR, OPV	If indicated, tuberculin testing may be done at same visit. If child is 5 yr of age or older, Hib is not indicated.
Interval after first visit		
1 mo	DTP, HBV	OPV may be given if accelerated poliomyelitis vaccination is necessary, such as for travelers to areas where polio is endemic.
2 mo	DTP, Hib, OPV	Second dose of Hib is indicated only in children whose first dose was received when younger than 15 mo.
≥8mo	DTP or DTaP,[c] HBV, OPV	OPV is not given if the third dose was given earlier.
4-6 yr (at or before school entry)	DTP or DTaP,[c] OPV	DTP or DTaP is not necessary if the fourth dose was given after the fourth birthday; OPV is not necessary if the third dose was given after the fourth birthday.
11-12 yr	MMR	Given at entry to middle school or junior high school.
10 yr later	Td	Repeat every 10 yr throughout life.

From American Academy of Pediatrics: *Redbook Report of the Committee on Infectious Diseases,* ed 23, Elk Grove Village, Ill, 1994, American Academy of Pediatrics.
[a]DTP, diphtheria and tetanus toxoids and pertussis vaccine; DTaP, diphtheria, tetanus, and acellular pertussis vaccine; Hib, *H. influenzae* b vaccine; HBV, hepatitis B vaccine; MMR, measles, mumps, rubella vaccine; OPV, oral poliovirus vaccine; Td, tetanus and diphtheria toxoids. If all needed vaccines cannot be administered simultaneously, priority should be given to protecting the child against those diseases that pose the greatest immediate risk. In the United States, these diseases for children younger than 2 yr usually are measles and *H. influenzae* type b infection; for children older than 7 yr, they are measles, mumps, and rubella.
[b]DTP or DTaP, HBV, Hib, MMR and OPV can be given simultaneously at separate sites if failure of the patient to return for future immunizations is a concern.

Continued.

TABLE 11-3. (cont.)

Recommended time/age	Immunization(s)	Comments
7 years and older[d,e]		
First visit	HBV,[f] OPV, MMR, Td	
Interval after first visit		
2 mo	HBV,[f] OPV, Td	OPV may also be given 1 mo after the first visit if accelerated poliomyelitis vaccination is necessary.
8-14 mo	HBV,[f] OPV, Td	OPV is not given if the third dose was given earlier.
11-12 yr	MMR	Given at entry to middle school or junior high.
10 yr later	Td	Repeat every 10 yr throughout life.

[c]DTaP is not currently licensed for use in children younger than 15 mo of age and is not recommended for primary immunization (e.g., first 3 doses) at any age.
[d]If person is 18 yr or older, routine poliovirus vaccination is not indicated in the United States.
[e]Minimal interval between doses of MMR is 1 mo.
[f]Priority should be given to hepatitis B immunization of adolescents.

   1) Residents of long-term correctional facilities
   2) Clients in institutions for the developmentally disabled
   3) Hemodialysis patients
   4) Adoptees from countries in which HBV infection is endemic
   5) Recipients of clotting factor concentrates
   6) IV drug abusers
   7) Household and sexual contacts of HBV carriers
   8) International travelers who plan to spend more than 6 months in areas with high rates of HBV infection
   9) Sexually active homosexual and bisexual men
   10) Heterosexuals with multiple sex partners and/or a recent STD
3. The dose of licensed HBV vaccines is shown in Table 11-4.

D. NONROUTINE IMMUNIZATIONS
1. Pneumococcal vaccine
   a. Pneumococcal vaccine is recommended for children >2 years of age who have sickle-cell disease, functional or anatomic asplenia, nephrotic syndrome or chronic renal failure, conditions associated

TABLE 11-4.
Recommended Doses of Currently Licensed Hepatitis B Vaccines

Group	Recombivax HB* Dose (µg)	ml	Engerix-B* Dose (µg)	ml
Infants of HBsAg†-negative mothers and children <11 yr	2.5	0.25	10	0.5
Infants of HBsAg-positive mothers; prevention of perinatal infection	5	0.5	10	0.5
Children and adolescents 11-19 yr	5	0.5	20	1.0
Adults ≥ 20 yr	10	1.0	20	1.0
Dialysis patients and other immunocompromised persons	40	1.0‡	40	2.0§

From US Department of Health and Human Services: *MMWR* 40(RR-13):1, 1991.
*Both vaccines are routinely administered in a three-dose series. Engerix-B has also been licensed for a four-dose series administered at 0, 1, 2, and 12 mo.
†HBsAg, Hepatitis B surface antigen.
‡Special formulation.
§Two 1.0-ml doses administered at one site, in a four-dose schedule at 0, 1, 2, and 6 mo.

with immunosuppression (e.g., organ transplantation or cytoreduction therapy), CSF leaks, and HIV infection.
  b. It is given as a single dose (0.5 ml) SQ or IM.
  c. It should be given at least 2 weeks before elective splenectomy or initiation of chemotherapy or immunosuppression.
  d. Revaccination should be considered after 3-5 years for children younger than 10 years of age, patients with asplenia, and those with rapid antibody decline after the initial vaccination.
  e. Vaccination is *not* recommended for healthy children, during chemotherapy or radiation therapy, during pregnancy, or for prevention of otitis media.
2. Influenza vaccine (Table 11-5)
  a. Influenza vaccine is recommended for children >6 months of age with the following:
    1) Chronic pulmonary diseases, including moderate-to-severe asthma, bronchopulmonary dysplasia, and cystic fibrosis
    2) Hemodynamically significant cardiac disease
    3) Immunosuppression, including immunosuppression caused by medications
    4) Sickle-cell disease and other hemoglobinopathies
    5) Diabetes, chronic renal and metabolic diseases

TABLE 11-5.
Schedules for Influenza Vaccine

Age	Recommended vaccine	Dose (ml)	No. of doses*
6-35 mo	Split virus only	0.25	1-2
3-8 yr	Split virus only	0.5	1-2
9-12 yr	Split virus only	0.5	1
≥12 yr	Whole or split virus	0.5	1

*Two doses are recommended if the child is receiving influenza vaccine for the first time. If the hemagglutinin and neuraminidase of vaccine strains have not changed, subsequent immunizations may be achieved with 1 dose yearly.

   6) Symptomatic HIV infection

   7) Long-term aspirin therapy (increased risk of Reye's syndrome)
NOTE: Household contacts, including siblings and primary caretakers of high-risk children, should be immunized. Children in households with high-risk adults, including those with symptomatic HIV infection, should be immunized.

   b. Only the subvirion (split-virus) vaccine should be used for children <13 years of age. The IM route of administration is recommended; deltoid for adults and older children, and the anterolateral thigh for infants and young children.

   c. The vaccine should be administered in the autumn, before the start of the flu season; annual vaccination is recommended.

   d. The vaccine should *not* be given to individuals with a history of anaphylaxis to chicken or eggs.

   e. Children can receive the influenza vaccine at the same time they receive other routine vaccinations, including DTP or DTaP.

E. IMMUNIZATION OF IMMUNODEFICIENT AND IMMUNO-SUPPRESSED CHILDREN

1. Congenital disorders of immune function

   a. Live bacterial and viral vaccines are contraindicated in patients with congenital disorders of immune function; an inactivated vaccine (e.g., IPV) should be administered, if available.

   b. Inactivated vaccines are safe, but efficacy may be reduced; the postvaccination antibody response should be monitored. Normal immunologic response usually returns between 3 months and 1 year after discontinuing immunosuppressive therapy.

   c. Children with a deficiency of antibody synthesis may be protected by regular doses of immune globulin.

    d. Live virus vaccines are generally contraindicated; they may be administered at least 3 months after all immunosuppressive therapy has been discontinued. An exception is the use of live varicella vaccine in children with acute lymphocytic leukemia in remission.

    e. Immunologically normal siblings and other household contacts of persons with an immunologic deficiency should not receive OPV but can receive live MMR vaccines.

2. Corticosteroids

    a. Previously healthy children can become immunosuppressed because of corticosteroid therapy. However, there are no studies to determine with assurance the effect of such therapy on the immunity or side effects engendered by live vaccine or the exact amount and duration of administration needed to suppress the immune response.

    b. Previously healthy children treated with large amounts of systemic corticosteroids (≥ 2 mg/kg or ≥ 20 mg/d) should not be given live virus vaccines.

    c. Most experts agree that an interval of at least 1 month after discontinuation of steroid use is probably sufficient to safely administer the varicella vaccine (and probably other virus vaccines).

    d. Children who have a disease that suppresses the immune response and are being treated with systemic or locally administered steroids should not be given live virus vaccines, except under special circumstances.

    e. Otherwise healthy children who are receiving maintenance physiologic doses of corticosteroids and have no underlying immune defects can receive live virus vaccines.

3. HIV infection

    a. MMR vaccine is recommended, regardless of clinical status. The recommended age of administration is 12-15 months but may be given earlier if the risk of exposure is high.

    b. Children with symptomatic HIV infection should receive DTP, influenza, HBV, and *Haemophilus influenzae* conjugate vaccines; those 2 years of age or older should receive pneumococcal vaccine.

    c. IPV should be given in place of OPV.

    d. Household contacts of an adult or child with a proven or suspected HIV infection should *not* receive OPV.

4. Asplenia

    a. Polyvalent pneumococcal vaccine is recommended for all asplenic children who are at least 2 years of age.

b. Quadrivalent meningococcal polysaccharide vaccine should be administered to asplenic children who are at least 2 years of age.

c. Immunization against *H. influenzae* type B should be instituted in infancy as recommended for otherwise healthy children.

F. PASSIVE IMMUNIZATION

1. Immune globulin (human)
   a. For close personal exposure to a hepatitis A case (including day care and institutions for custodial care) as soon as possible after exposure but not >2 weeks after the last exposure. The dose is 0.02 ml/kg (max 2 ml) given IM.
   b. For measles prophylaxis (especially indicated for susceptible household or hospital contacts younger than 6 months). A single dose of 0.25 ml/kg (max 15 ml) is given as soon after exposure as possible. Immunosuppressed patients should be given 0.5 ml/kg.
   c. For travel to developing countries, the dose is 0.02 ml/kg for stays <3 months and 0.06 ml/kg for stays >3 months (repeated every 5 months).

2. Hepatitis B immune globulin
   a. Neonates born to patients with (or chronic carriers of) HBV should receive 0.5 ml IM as soon as possible after birth; the efficacy at 12-48 hours is presumed but unproven.
   b. Use for household contacts (<12 months of age) of persons with acute HBV infection.
   c. Use for percutaneous or permucosal exposure to HBsAg-positive blood; give HBIG 0.06 ml/kg (max 5 ml). If not previously vaccinated, initiate HBV vaccination.
   d. Use for sexual contacts of persons with HBV infection (0.06 ml/kg); susceptible sex partners should begin the HBV vaccine series.

3. Varicella-zoster immune globulin
   a. VZIG should be given to exposed, susceptible individuals at high risk of developing progressive varicella.
      1) Immunocompromised children
      2) Pregnant women
      3) Neonate of a mother who had an onset of varicella within 5 days before and 48 hours after delivery
      4) Hospitalized premature infant (>28 weeks' gestation) whose mother has no history of varicella
      5) Hospitalized premature infant (<28 weeks' gestation or ≤1000 g) regardless of maternal history

b. The dose is 1.25 ml (125 U, 1 vial) per 10 kg of body weight (minimum dose is 1 vial, maximum dose is 5 vials) given by IM injection. Never give IV.
c. VZIG should be given within 48 hours of and preferably not more than 96 hours after exposure.
d. VZIG is obtained by calling the local office of the American Red Cross Blood Services.

BIBLIOGRAPHY

American Academy of Pediatrics: Recommended childhood immunization schedule, *Pediatrics* 97:143, 1996.
Centers for Disease Control and Prevention: Prevention and control of influenza, *MMWR* 44:1, 1995.
Redbook Report of the Committee on Infectious Diseases, ed 23, Elk Grove Village, Ill, 1994, American Academy of Pediatrics.
Standards for pediatric immunization practices, *JAMA* 269:1817, 1993.

INGESTIONS 12

A. TELEPHONE TRIAGE

1. Many cases of ingestion come to attention by telephone call. Note time of call. Most parents will be frantic. *You* should remain calm.
2. Take a brief history. What was ingested? How much? (How many pills or how much liquid is missing?) The dose of ingested toxin should be calculated using a "worst case scenario." When? Where? Any vomiting? Was the event witnessed? Any treatment given? What is the child's present mental and physical status?
3. Assess urgency. Should parents come to the ED as soon as possible, or should an emergency vehicle be dispatched? If in doubt as to disposition, keep caller on hold and call local poison control center. Be sure to have parents bring ingested material with them plus the container, whether filled or empty.
4. Obtain name of caller, phone number, and address.
5. Advise emesis if the substance is not a caustic or hydrocarbon and if the patient is not obtunded, comatose, seizing, or at risk of rapid deterioration (tricyclics) or worsening by vagal stimulation of the cardiac conduction system. If there is any doubt about inducing emesis, the child should be sent straight to the ED.
   a. If emesis is indicated and the parent has syrup of ipecac at home, the recommended dose for children >6 months of age is as follows:

   > 6-9 months: 5 ml
   > 9-12 months: 10 ml
   > 1-12 years: 15 ml
   > >12 years: 30 ml

   b. The dose should be followed by 4-8 oz of clear tepid fluids. Ipecac also works best if the patient is kept active.
   c. If there is no emesis in 15-20 minutes and if the child is >1 year of age, repeat the dose × 1 (no more than once).

   NOTE: Ipecac may not be effective after the ingestion of an antiemetic.
6. Instruct the parents to bring the child to the ED if any potentially

dangerous substance has been ingested or if the child is <6 months of age.

B. EMERGENCY DEPARTMENT MANAGEMENT

1. Obtain a brief history as previously stated. If the nature of the ingestion is unknown, ask what medications or other toxic substances (e.g., household products, kerosene) are in the house.
2. PE: Note weight, vital signs, mental status, perfusion, respiratory status, cardiac status, pupils, unusual odors, and any spills on clothes.
3. Management of the highly symptomatic patient (see *The Harriet Lane Handbook,* ed. 14)
   a. Establish and maintain vital functions; establish and secure an airway.
   b. Insert an ETT for patients with impaired airway protection.
   c. Control hypotension, hypertension, pulmonary edema, arrhythmias, cerebral edema, renal failure, metabolic acidosis, and hypothermia as indicated.
   d. For the comatose patient, administer IV glucose; if no response, give naloxone.
   e. For seizures, give IV diazepam, lorazepam, or phenytoin (see p. 238).
4. Laboratory
   a. Urine 25-50 ml (essential for toxicology screen); urine ferric chloride as appropriate
   b. Blood (5-10 ml) for quantitation of substances picked up on urine screen and for detection of volatiles (alcohol, methanol, acetone); Dextrostix; measurement of osmolar or anion gap
   c. Talk to laboratory; be sure their testing is set up to detect the specific agent you have in mind.
   d. Testing gastric aspirate does *not* identify what is in the child's blood; hold, pending results of the urine screen.
   e. Consider blood-lead level on all children <5 years of age with ingestion.
5. GI decontamination: Absorbent, lavage, emesis
   a. Activated charcoal
      1) Most effective GI decontamination procedure for most acute ingestions in which it is known that charcoal is an effective absorbent; no significant side effects (rarely vomiting, aspiration, constipation, or intestinal obstruction); effective in preventing absorption of a toxin and also in promoting its excretion from the body (GI dialysis); in most cases may be given without prior gastric emptying

2) Very effective for phenobarbital, theophylline, tricyclics, dextropropoxyphene, digoxin, and salicylates

3) *Not* effective for iron, strong acids and alkalis, and simple alcohols

4) Contraindications include the absence of bowel sounds, intestinal obstruction, GI bleeding, and a lack of adequate airway protection, in which case a cuffed endotracheal tube should be placed before charcoal is given.

5) Usually given as a slurry in water; fruit juice may be added without a loss of efficacy. It is best tolerated if the liquid is cold and placed in an opaque container (e.g., cardboard orange juice container) to hide the ugly appearance. If refused, it can be given via a nasogastric or orogastric tube. Metoclopramide (Reglan) can also improve tolerance.

6) The usual dose is 1 g/kg (minimum 15 g). If the amount of toxin ingested is known, give 10 times as much charcoal. If this amount cannot be achieved with a single dose, serial dosing may be required.

7) In cases that involve enterohepatic circulation (e.g., theophylline overdose), repeat doses (0.5 g/kg q2-4h) may provide effective GI dialysis.

8) A cathartic such as sorbitol, magnesium sulfate, or magnesium citrate should be given along with or following charcoal to decrease intestinal transit time. There are preparations available that combine charcoal and sorbitol.

9) Suggested protocol

   a) Administer charcoal and cathartic.

   b) Repeat half of the initial dose (without cathartic) q4h until the blood level is nontoxic or there is an absence of clinical toxicity.

   c) Administer a cathartic q12h if the patient has not had a stool.

b. Gastric lavage

   1) Indicated for the ingestion of drugs with a low affinity for activated charcoal, including alcohols, aliphatic hydrocarbons, cyanide, glycols, metals (iron, lead, lithium, mercury), and drugs that are insoluble in aqueous solutions

   2) Use a large-bore orogastric or nasogastric tube (children, 22-28 Fr; adolescents, 36 Fr). Cutting large holes in the tube facilitates removal of tablet or capsule fragments. The patient should be in the Trendelenburg and left lateral decubitus position.

   3) Lavage with copious amounts (15-20 ml/kg/cycle) of warm normal saline solution until the return is clear; may need 2-5 L.

Save the first gastric sample for possible later analysis.

4) After lavage is clear, activated charcoal can be inserted via a nasogastric tube.

5) Contraindications to lavage include the following:

   a) Ingestion of caustics

   b) Coma, seizures, or other impairment of airway protective mechanisms. If lavage is mandatory in such cases, it can be carried out after intubation with a cuffed endotracheal tube.

   c) Presence of cardiac arrhythmia

c. Ipecac

   1) Ineffective if given >60 minutes after an ingestion

   2) In general, not very useful in ED; delays the administration of activated charcoal and may hinder its retention

   3) No added efficacy in using gastric emptying procedures before the administration of activated charcoal, except in patients who are obtunded and come to the ED within 1 hour of ingestion

   4) Note the appearance, odor, and color of any vomited material; save it for possible analysis.

6. Cathartics

   a. The efficacy of cathartics is questioned, but they are often used. Sorbitol produces the most rapid catharsis.

   b. Dose

   1) Sorbitol (50% solution): 2 g/kg; can be administered as a slurry with 1 g/kg of activated charcoal

   2) Magnesium citrate: 3-4 ml/kg to maximum of 8 oz

   3) Magnesium sulfate: 250 mg/kg of 10% solution to 15-20 g maximum

   4) Repeat q4-6h until there is passage of liquid stool or any administered charcoal.

   c. Magnesium-containing cathartic should be avoided in patients with potential nephrotoxicity.

   d. Cathartics should not be given following the ingestion of caustics or if there is GI irritation (such as occurs with iron poisoning), if bowel sounds are absent, or if the patient has a history of recent bowel surgery.

   e. Do not use sorbitol multiple-dose therapy; doing so may induce significant fluid and electrolyte losses, especially in children <12 months of age.

7. Whole-bowel irrigation

   a. Whole-bowel irrigation may be useful for specific ingestions (e.g.,

iron with radiographic evidence of retained material) and the
ingestion of sustained-release preparations.
  b. Use a colonic irrigation solution (GoLYTELY) at a rate of 0.5 L/h
  in children and 2 L/h in adolescents until there is clear effluent
  (usually 2-4 hours).

C. SYSTEMIC ANTIDOTES (Table 12-1)

D. SPECIFIC INGESTIONS
There are too many toxins ingested by children to list in this section.
Because management changes from year to year, it would be pointless
to list specific information. The best resource is the local poison control
center, which can provide up-to-date information regarding management.
The Poisondex data base is also useful. Some of the more common
ingestions are outlined as follows:
1. Acetaminophen
  a. Rapid intestinal absorption; peak plasma level in 70-120 minutes;
  may be earlier (30 minutes) with liquid preparations in children. GI
  symptoms such as abdominal pain, nausea, vomiting, and lethargy
  occur within hours. There may be a latent period of 1-5 days
  between ingestion and the onset of hepatic symptoms.
  b. Assessment of risk
    1) Amount ingested 70-140 mg/kg: No treatment. Hepatotoxicity
    is rare; give ipecac at home.
    2) Amount ingested >140 mg/kg: Toxic dose in children. Give
    ipecac at home and send to ED.
  c. A single plasma level is not reliable before 4 hours. If the 4-hour
  level is >300 µg/ml, there is a 90% chance of severe toxicity. If the
  level is <150 µg/ml, toxicity is unlikely (Fig. 12-1).
  d. Treatment consists of gastric lavage followed by oral administration of NAC. NAC is effective within 14-16 hours of ingestion
  (Fig. 12-2) but should never be given before 4 hours postingestion.
  The oral protocol takes 72 hours. Do not discontinue NAC
  treatment prematurely if the subsequent plasma acetaminophen
  level falls below the toxic line on the nomogram.
    1) Activated charcoal should be administered but separated from
    NAC by 1-2 hours.
    2) The administration of NAC may be associated with vomiting;
    the dose can be repeated one time if vomited with 1 hour of
    administration. NAC can be made more palatable by putting it
    in juice, on ice, and in a covered glass with a straw. If it is

TABLE 12-1.
Specific Antidotes

Indication	Antidote	Dose	Comments
Acetaminophen	N-acetylcysteine (5% solution)	Loading dose 140 mg/kg PO followed by 17 doses of 70 mg/kg q4h	Give cold and in soda
Anticholinergic agents Phenothiazines Antihistamines	Physostigmine	0.02 mg/kg by slow IV infusion (2 mg max); may repeat q30-60min	Atropine should be available; monitor cardiac status
Benzodiazepines	Flumazenil (Mazicon)	0.2 mg IV bolus; then 0.2 mg/min up to max of 3 mg	May precipitate convulsions; may not reverse respiratory depression; do not use if possibility of TCA ingestion
Digitalis	Fab fragments	80 mg Fab fragments/mg glycoside IV over ½ hr	For A-V conduction disturbances, arrhythmias, and hyperkalemia
Iron	Deferoxamine	For shock or coma, 15 mg/kg/h IV × 8 hr (max 6 g/d)	If no shock or coma, 90 mg/kg/dose IM q8h (max 6 g/d)
Methemoglobin	Methylene blue	1-2 mg/kg IV or (0.1-0.2 ml/kg/dose) over 5-10 min	May repeat after 1 hr
Opiates	Naloxone (Narcan)	0.1 mg/kg IV	If no response, give 2 mg IV
Organic phosphates Carbamate	Atropine sulfate	0.015-0.05 mg/kg/dose IV	May give q4-6h if needed; titrate dose to clinical effect
Phenothiazines	Diphenhydramine (Benadryl)	1-2 mg/kg/dose q6h IV or PO (max 50 mg/dose)	For oculogyric crisis; may cause sedation or paradoxical agitation

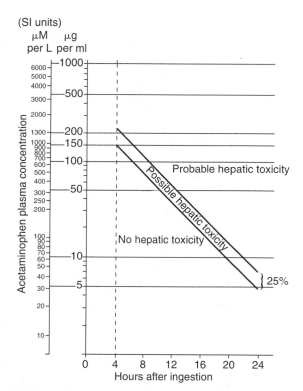

FIG 12-1. Rumack-Matthew nomogram for acetaminophen poisoning. Semilogarithmic plot of plasma acetaminophen levels vs. time. The following are cautions for the use of this chart: (1) time coordinates refer to time after *ingestion,* (2) serum levels drawn before 4 hours may not represent peak levels, (3) the graph should be used only in relation to a single acute ingestion, and (4) *lower solid line* 25% below the standard nomogram is included to allow for possible errors in acetaminophen plasma assays and estimated time from ingestion of an overdose. (From Rumack BH: *Poisondex: a computerized poison information system,* ed 47, Denver, 1986, Micromedex.)

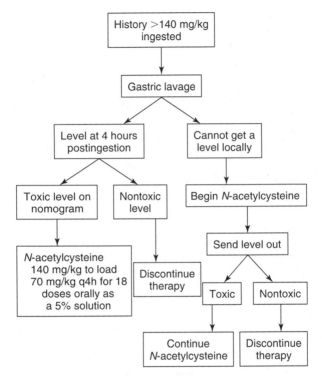

FIG 12-2. Acetaminophen poisoning treatment protocol. (From Peterson RG, Rumack BH: *Topics Emerg Med* 1:48, 1979.)

vomited, it may need to be administered by a slow drip via a tube in the duodenum; IV administration of metoclopramide may decrease vomiting.

3) The IV route of administration of NAC is faster and preferable but is not available for use in the United States.

e. In all patients with acetaminophen levels in the toxic range, AST,

ALT, bilirubin, and PT should be followed daily beginning 18 hours after the first NAC dose.

   f. Prognosis

      1) Significant toxicity is rare in children <6 years of age.

      2) Adolescents have a higher incidence of toxic plasma levels following ingestion, and one third of those with toxic levels are likely to develop ALT >1000 IU/L. Even with serious hepatotoxicity, the mortality rate is <0.5%. Patients who recover have no sequelae.

2. Hydrocarbons

   a. Hydrocarbons include gasoline, kerosene, lamp oil, lighter fluid, turpentine, paint thinner and remover, furniture polish, paraffin wax, and lubricating oil.

   b. Because of their bad taste, large volumes of hydrocarbons are rarely ingested (usually <1 oz).

   c. Pulmonary injury results from aspiration, *not* GI absorption. Aspiration can occur in the absence of vomiting. Evacuation of gastric contents is not indicated unless an aromatic (xylene, toluene) or complex hydrocarbon is ingested or the material is contaminated by heavy metals, pesticides, or other toxins. Activated charcoal and cathartics are *not* indicated.

   d. Signs and symptoms of hydrocarbon ingestion include coughing, choking, hemoptysis, tachypnea, dyspnea, cyanosis, rales, rhonchi, and wheezes. Somnolence is the chief neurologic manifestation (probably related to hypoxia and acidosis). High fever is common and does not correlate with infection. Respiratory symptoms almost always begin within 6 hours of ingestion.

   e. All patients should be observed for at least 6 hours. A CXR is indicated only for those patients who are symptomatic; 90% of abnormal x-ray studies become abnormal within 4 hours. The x-ray study may show evidence of aspiration pneumonia, patchy densities, consolidation, hyperinflation, atelectasis, and pneumatoceles.

   f. All symptomatic patients should be admitted; there may be rapid deterioration over 24-48 hours.

   g. Treatment is supportive. Steroids are not effective, and prophylactic antibiotics are not indicated. Even in patients with fever and leukocytosis, bacterial pneumonia is unusual.

   h. The course usually lasts 3-8 days. There may be fever up to 8-10 days. The CXR may show pneumatoceles 2-3 weeks after ingestion.

3. Iron
   a. Toxicity: Ingested dose of elemental iron 20-60 mg/kg, mild symptoms; 60-100 mg/kg, moderate-to-severe; 100-180 mg/kg, life-threatening; >180 mg/kg, lethal
   b. A serum iron level obtained within 2-4 hours of ingestion is the best predictor of potential toxicity.
      1) >300 μg/dL: Intoxication likely
      2) 300-500 μg/dL: Mild toxicity
      3) 500-1000 μg/dL: Moderate-to-severe toxicity
      4) >1000 μg/dL: Life-threatening toxicity
   c. Diagnosis
If the clinical picture is consistent with iron poisoning, ingestion can be confirmed by the following:
      1) History: Always assume that the maximum number of tablets missing has been ingested. Most prenatal vitamins contain 60 mg of elemental iron per tablet.
      2) Obtain an abdominal x-ray examination for iron tablets and fragments.
      3) Combine 2 ml gastric fluid and 2 gtt 30% H_2O_2 with 0.5 ml of deferoxamine solution (500-mg ampule) in 4 ml distilled water. The color will vary from light orange to dark red with increasing amounts of iron.
      4) Give one IM dose of deferoxamine (Desferal) 50 mg/kg up to 1 g. Pink (vin rose) urine (compared with baseline urine) indicates that the serum iron level exceeds the TIBC and is high enough to produce toxicity.
   d. Clinical features
There are four phases with iron poisoning:
      1) 0.5-1 hour after ingestion: Hemorrhagic gastroenteritis (vomiting and bloody diarrhea), fever, metabolic acidosis, hyperglycemia, coagulation defects, shock, coma
NOTE: If signs and symptoms of toxicity do not appear within 4-6 hours, the process is unlikely to progress.
      2) 6-24 hours: Period of relative improvement (may be the calm before the storm!)
      3) 24-48 hours: Delayed profound shock, acidosis, pulmonary edema, hepatic failure, hypoglycemia, bleeding diathesis, renal shutdown, coma
      4) 1-2 months: Gastric scarring, pyloric obstruction, bowel stricture, cirrhosis
   e. Management

1) Perform gastric lavage with half-normal saline solution, 1% sodium bicarbonate, or deferoxamine (2 g) added to 1.5% bicarbonate solution; 100-150 ml of 1% sodium bicarbonate should be left in the stomach. Phosphate lavage, activated charcoal, and PO deferoxamine *are not indicated.* An abdominal x-ray study should be obtained after lavage to check for retained fragments and tablets in the stomach. If positive, a whole-bowel lavage should be considered.
2) Supportive care
   a) Correction of fluid and electrolyte abnormalities and acidosis
   b) Maintenance of intravascular volume: Blood, colloid, pressors
   c) Correction of clotting abnormalities
3) Support of ventilation
4) Follow CBC, LFTs, clotting studies, electrolytes, ABGs, renal function
5) Chelation therapy with IV or IM deferoxamine; indications include the following:
   a) Ingested dose of iron >25 mg/kg
   b) Clinical evidence of severe toxicity
   c) Serum iron exceeds TIBC (positive deferoxamine provocation test)
   d) Serum iron exceeds 300 µg/dL 2-4 hours after ingestion

NOTE: WBC >15,000 and blood glucose >150 mg/dL correlate with serum iron >300 µg/dL and suggest severe toxicity.

6) Chelation protocol (with deferoxamine)
   a) IM: 90 mg/kg/dose (up to 1 g) q8h up to a maximum of 6 g in 24 hours
   b) IV: 15 mg/kg/h by slow infusion in a solution of 100-200 ml D_5W (this is the preferred route if the patient is hypotensive). The dose may be repeated q6h depending on urine color and the patient's clinical status.
   c) Chelation therapy is continued until the vin rose color disappears from urine or the serum iron level is less than TIBC.
   d) Exchange transfusion or hemodialysis may be indicated if the serum iron level >1000 µg/dL or if the patient shows evidence of severe toxicity or renal shutdown.

4. Salicylate
   a. Clinical picture
      1) Nausea, vomiting, abdominal pain, fever, hyperpnea, tinnitus, coma, convulsions, hyperglycemia (early), hypoglycemia (late),

TABLE 12-2.
Estimation of Toxicity for Acetylsalicylic Acid

ASA dose ingested (mg/kg)	Expected toxicity
<150	None
150-300	Mild-to-moderate
300-500	Serious
>500	Potentially lethal

oliguria, bleeding diathesis. Severe poisoning is associated with seizures, coma, and respiratory and cardiovascular failure.

2) Respiratory alkalosis (early), metabolic acidosis (late)

3) May be confused with diabetic ketoacidosis, Reye's syndrome, encephalitis, and other ingestions

4) Positive ferric chloride test (burgundy color change after 5-10 gtt of 10% ferric chloride are added to urine that has been boiled for 1-2 minutes); positive phenistix test

b. Estimation of toxicity (Table 12-2)

1) In an acute ingestion the Done nomogram (Fig. 12-3), which is based on the serum salicylate level at least 6 hours after ingestion, gives a useful estimate of potential severity but is not as important as the patient's clinical status; it is not useful in chronic poisoning.

2) In an acute overdose, the peak serum level is as follows:

<35 mg/dL: No symptoms
35-70 mg/dL: Mild-to-moderate symptoms
70-100 mg/dL: Severe symptoms
>100 mg/dL: Potentially fatal

c. Management

1) Decontamination by emesis/lavage. Lavage can be effective as long as 4-6 hours after ingestion.

2) Administration of activated charcoal and cathartic. Multiple doses may enhance salicylate clearance, even beyond what is achieved by urinary alkalinization.

3) Hospitalization is indicated if the patient is symptomatic or if the peak serum level exceeds 50 mg/dL.

4) IV replacement of fluid/electrolyte deficits (aim for urine output of 3-6 ml/kg/h). Start with 10-15 ml/kg/h for the first 2 hours and then adjust.

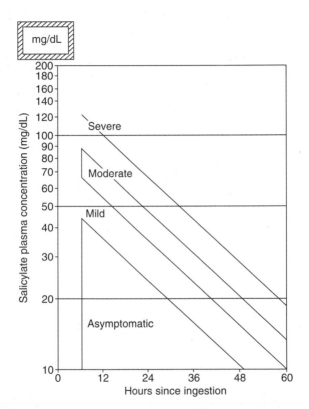

FIG 12-3. Nomogram relating serum salicylate concentration and expected severity of intoxication at varying intervals following ingestion of a single dose of salicylate. (From Done AK: *Pediatrics* 26:800, 1960.)

5) Alkalinize the urine; give sodium bicarbonate 1-2 mEq/kg as a loading dose followed by 1-2 mEq/kg q2-4h to maintain urine pH >8. Add 35-40 mEq/L of potassium to IV fluids. Follow urine pH and volume, plasma pH, serum glucose, LFTs, electrolytes, and PT.

NOTE: Monitor for hypocalcemia, which can occur with prolonged alkalosis secondary to diuresis.

6) Administer vitamin K if PT is prolonged.
7) Hemodialysis and hemoperfusion are rarely needed. Indications include chronic overdose, renal failure, unresponsive acidosis, intractable seizures, coma, and a serum salicylate level >100 mg/dL.

5. Theophylline
   a. Manifestations include agitation, tremors, obtundation, seizures, sinus tachycardia, nausea, arrhythmias, vomiting, hypokalemia, and hyperglycemia. The risk of life-threatening events increases with younger age.
   b. Difference in *acute* vs. *chronic* overdose: Patients with chronic intoxication are at a higher risk for seizures and arrhythmias at lower serum concentrations.
      1) In an *acute* overdose, serious toxicity is unlikely with a serum theophylline level <100 µg/ml.
      2) In a *chronic* overdose, serious toxicity can occur at levels <40 µg/ml.
   c. Treatment
      1) Vigorous GI decontamination by activated charcoal and cathartic
      2) Activated charcoal can bind the drug within the GI tract, prevent enterohepatic reabsorption, and increase drug clearance from within the vascular compartment.
      3) Charcoal can be given as multiple intermittent oral doses or as a continuous nasogastric infusion (0.5 g/kg/h) that is interrupted for one dose of cathartic and continued until the serum level is in the nontoxic range.
      4) Hemodialysis or hemoperfusion is indicated if the serum level is >80-100 µg/ml in acute overdose, >40 µg/ml in chronic intoxication, or if the patient fails to respond to supportive care.
      5) Seizures should be treated with IV diazepam or phenobarbital.
      6) Arrhythmias can be treated with lidocaine or propranolol.

6. Tricyclic antidepressants
   a. The manifestations of TCAs are those of autonomic dysfunction:

fever, dry mouth, tachycardia, flushing, dilated pupils, excitation along with confusion, arrhythmias, hallucinations, hypotension, ataxia, seizures, and coma. The triad of anticholinergic signs, acute alteration of mental status, and sinus tachycardia suggests tricyclic poisoning. Prolongation of the QRS complex (>100 msec) has been correlated with severe overdoses: >100 msec, seizures; >160 msec, ventricular arrhythmias. However, this finding excludes a substantial portion of patients with CNS toxicity and includes many patients who never develop serious problems.

b. Serum drug levels are not usually helpful in acute ingestions; treatment should be based on the clinical picture and QRS duration.

c. Avoid emesis and gastric lavage (risk of arrhythmia). Even if the patient is alert, *do not give syrup of ipecac.*

d. Administer activated charcoal and a cathartic; repeat q2-4h as indicated.

e. All symptomatic patients should be admitted to an intensive care unit for supportive management and cardiac monitoring.
   1) Support of BP and cardiac output
   2) IV diazepam, lorazepam (Ativan), or phenobarbital for seizures
   3) Correction of acidosis and electrolyte disturbances. Bicarbonate is probably the single most effective therapy for TCA overdose.
   4) Management of arrhythmias

f. Physostigmine is contraindicated, and dialysis usually is not indicated.

g. A depressed level of consciousness (Glasgow Coma Scale score <8) predicts serious complications of TCA overdose. Significant complications almost always occur within 3.5 hours of ingestion. Patients who remain awake after 6 hours of observation in the ED are at low risk for serious complications.

E. HOUSEHOLD PRODUCT INGESTION

Be suspicious of household product ingestion if any of the following are true:

1. 1-5–year-old with a previous history of ingestion
2. Nonfebrile illness; multisystem involvement without obvious explanation
3. Unusual odor, stains on clothing, burns around mouth or on oral mucosa, lip or tongue swelling, dysphagia, drooling
4. Unexplained hematemesis

NOTE: Caustics can cause severe burns to the esophagus or stomach in the absence of other symptoms.

F. MUNCHAUSEN SYNDROME BY PROXY (see p. 41)

1. Accidental ingestion *may not be* accidental. Some children may be abused by the administration of drugs. In many cases the abuse continues while the patient is in the hospital. The abuser is often pleasant, cooperative, and appreciative.
2. Be suspicious if any of the following are true:
   a. Child <1 or >5 years of age
   b. More than one ingestion episode
   c. Bizarre clinical manifestations. Such poisonings may have an insidious onset or an inexplicable presentation.
   d. Presence of risk factors for abuse

G. ANOREXIA NERVOSA

1. Adolescents with anorexia nervosa are at a particularly high risk for intentional self-poisoning, some as a result of purging attempts.
2. Common agents include psychotherapeutic drugs, cathartics, and analgesics; multiple toxins may be involved.
3. Management may be complicated by the following:
   a. Unreliable history and a delay in seeking medical attention
   b. Presence of underlying electrolyte disturbances
   c. Underlying GI abnormality (e.g., delayed gastric emptying)

BIBLIOGRAPHY

Anas N et al: Criteria for hospitalizing children who have ingested products containing hydrocarbons, *JAMA* 246:840, 1981.

Anderson AC: Iron poisoning in children, *Curr Opin Pediatr* 6:289, 1994.

Arena JM: Hydrocarbon poisoning: current management, *Pediatr Ann* 16:879, 1987.

Banner W Jr, Tong TG: Iron poisoning, *Pediatr Clin North Am* 33:393, 1986.

Boehnert MT, Lovejoy FH: Value of the QRS duration versus serum drug level in predicting seizures and ventricular arrhythmias after an acute overdose of tricyclic antidepressants, *N Engl J Med* 313:474, 1985.

Braden NJ et al: Tricyclic antidepressant overdose, *Pediatr Clin North Am* 33:287, 1986.

James LP et al: A comparison of cathartics in pediatric ingestions, *Pediatrics* 96:235, 1995.

Klein BL, Simon JE: Hydrocarbon poisoning, *Pediatr Clin North Am* 33:411, 1986.

Kornberg AE, Dolgin J: Pediatric ingestions: charcoal alone versus ipecac and charcoal, *Ann Emerg Med* 20:648, 1991.

Kulig K et al: Management of acutely poisoned patients without gastric emptying, *Ann Emerg Med* 14:562, 1985.

Meadow R: Munchausen by proxy, *Arch Dis Child* 57:92, 1982.

Nejman G et al: Gastric emptying in the poisoned patient, *Am J Emerg Med* 8:265, 1990.

Riggs BS et al: Current status of aspirin and acetaminophen intoxication, *Pediatr Ann* 16:886, 1987.

Rodgers GC, Jr, editor: *Handbook of common poisonings in children,* ed 3, Evanston, Ill, 1994, Committee on Accident and Poison Prevention, American Academy of Pediatrics.

Rodgers GC, Jr, Matyunas NJ: Gastrointestinal decontamination for acute poisoning, *Pediatr Clin North Am* 33:261, 1986.

Rumack BH: Acetaminophen overdose in children, *Pediatr Clin North Am* 33:691, 1986.

Shannon M, Lovejoy FH: Effect of acute versus chronic intoxication on clinical features of theophylline poisoning in children, *J Pediatr* 121:125, 1992.

Snodgrass WR: Salicylate toxicity, *Pediatr Clin North Am* 33:381, 1986.

Woolf AD: Poisoning in children and adolescents, *Pediatr Rev* 14:411, 1993.

Woolf AD, Gren JM: Acute poisonings among adolescents and young adults with anorexia nervosa, *Am J Dis Child* 144:785, 1990.

NEONATAL PROBLEMS *13*

A. BLOODY STOOLS

1. The differential diagnosis includes bacterial enterocolitis, Meckel's diverticulum, intussusception, GI duplication, Hirschsprung's disease, milk protein allergy, polyps, rectal injury (thermometer), and anal fissure (most common cause of bloody stool in a well-looking infant).
2. Evaluation
   a. Meticulous exam of the anal canal for fissures
   b. Stool exam for leukocytes (methylene blue), culture (enteric pathogens, *Campylobacter*), and *Clostridium difficile* toxin
   c. Meckel scan
   d. Radiographic studies
   e. Milk protein precipitins
   f. Endoscopy/biopsy
3. Treatment depends on the specific diagnosis. For anal fissures, give a stool softener such as malt soup extract 1-2 tsp tid, and clean the perianal area with water following bowel movements.

B. BREAST ENGORGEMENT

Breast engorgement secondary to the transfer of maternal hormones is physiologic in neonates. It is usually bilateral and may be associated with breast secretions. Peak enlargement (1-3 cm) may not be reached until 4-6 weeks and may persist for several months. No treatment is indicated.

C. BREAST INFECTION

1. Breast infection is most common during weeks 2 and 3 and presents as *unilateral* firm swelling with tenderness and warmth. Systemic manifestations, except for low-grade fever, are rare.
2. It may be helpful to aspirate material for Gram's stain and culture; infection usually results from *Staphylococcus aureus*.
3. Admit patient for IV antistaphylococcal therapy. Incision and drainage may be needed.

D. CEPHALHEMATOMA

1. Cephalhematoma is a traumatic subperiosteal hemorrhage that usually involves a parietal bone. Predisposing factors are large head size, prolonged labor, vacuum extraction, and forceps delivery (most important).
2. Firm swelling is fixed at suture lines without discoloration of overlying skin; it may not become apparent until hours to days after birth. An underlying linear skull fracture is present in 1%-5% of cases, but routine skull x-ray studies are not indicated (obtain only with CNS signs and symptoms).
3. Spontaneous resolution occurs over weeks; 1%-2% calcify. No treatment is required, but watch for jaundice and anemia (rare).

E. CLEFT PALATE

1. A cleft palate ranges from a frank defect in the hard and soft palate to an occult submucous cleft to a bifid uvula; associated defects are noted in approximately 15% of affected infants. It may be part of Pierre Robin malformation sequence (micrognathia, glossoptosis, U-shaped cleft of the soft palate, risk of obstructive apnea).
2. A neonate with a cleft palate is at high risk for problems with sucking, feeding, and weight gain.
   a. Breast-feeding, although not impossible, requires extraordinary effort on the part of the mother to express milk; a breast pump may be helpful.
   b. For bottle feeding, use a long, soft lamb's nipple, or enlarge the opening of a soft rubber nipple by cross-cutting with a surgical blade; each of these nipples empties by gravity.
   c. Refer immediately to a multidisciplinary craniofacial team for early treatment and counseling.

F. CONSTIPATION

1. Constipation is defined by stool consistency (hard and dry) and not frequency. The number of stools can be variable, ranging from 8-10/d to one q3-4d, even in nursing infants.
2. Causes of constipation include inadequate milk intake and switching from breast to bottle. Consider hypothyroidism, hypotonia, and Hirschsprung's disease. A rectal exam is indicated; look for anal fissures, a tight anal sphincter, and a lack of stool in the rectum (Hirschsprung's disease).

NOTE: Almost all cases of Hirschsprung's disease are symptomatic by 4 weeks of age.

3. If specific causes are ruled out, treat with 1-2 tsp malt soup extract tid, 4-6 oz of glucose water/d, or the occasional use of glycerine suppositories.

G. FRACTURED CLAVICLE
1. A fractured clavicle is present in 1.5%-3.0% of vaginal deliveries, with right > left (2:1). Predisposing factors are large size, shoulder dystocia, and traumatic delivery.
2. Findings include swelling/fullness over the fracture site, crepitus, decreased arm movement, and irritability during arm movement; however, 80% have no symptoms and only minimal physical findings. It is often diagnosed when callus is detected at 3-6 weeks of age. Radiography is not usually indicated.
3. No specific treatment is needed; if both ends of the bone are in the same room, good healing will occur. Advise parents to avoid tension on the affected arm.

H. HYPOSPADIAS
1. With hypospadias, the urethral meatus is on the ventral surface of the glans (87%), the penile shaft (10%) or, in severe cases, on the perineum (3%). It is often accompanied by ventral curvature of the penis (chordee) or a hooded prepuce.
2. Familial tendency; 7% of patients have a brother or father with hypospadias. Some cases may be related to maternal exposure to progestins at 8-14 weeks' gestation.
3. Examine carefully for other anomalies, especially genital (micropenis, cryptorchidism). Additional diagnostic studies are not indicated in infants who have mild hypospadias without other abnormalities. Patients with urinary tract symptoms, a family history of reflux, multiple anomalies, or ambiguous genitalia should have a complete evaluation for other GU abnormalities.
4. Management
   a. Circumcision withheld
   b. Surgical repair at 6-12 months, usually after a short course of testosterone

I. OMPHALITIS
1. During the first week, faint erythema of the rim of the umbilical stump is common and of no consequence.
2. Omphalitis is defined by the following:
   a. Foul-smelling discharge

b. Periumbilical erythema, induration, and tenderness to palpation
c. Purulent or serosanguineous drainage
3. Treatment
   a. With purulent discharge or periumbilical involvement, use oral or parenteral antibiotics on the basis of culture and sensitivity.
   b. In the absence of periumbilical spread, use a topical antibiotic containing neomycin, polymyxin, and bacitracin.

NOTE: With serous umbilical secretion, need to rule out a vitelline duct or urachal remnant.

NOTE: A wet malodorous stump with minimal inflammation can be seen with group A β-hemolytic streptococcus infection.

J. PYLORIC STENOSIS
1. Pyloric stenosis usually appears at 3-6 weeks of age but has been observed from birth to 4 months of age; it is more common in first-born males.
2. Signs and symptoms include persistent and progressive vomiting (usually projectile, occasionally bloody, *never* bilious), failure to thrive, palpation of a tumor ("olive") in the epigastrium just to the right of midline, visible peristaltic waves, and metabolic alkalosis.
3. Diagnosis is based on clinical findings, which can be confirmed by ultrasound. An upper GI study is usually unnecessary.
4. Treatment consists of hydration, correction of metabolic alkalosis, and pyloromyotomy.

K. RASHES
1. Acropustulosis: Recurrent crops of pruritic vesiculopustules on the hands and feet, which last 7-10 days and recur every few weeks to months over the first 2-3 years. Gram's stain reveals numerous PMNs and occasional eosinophils. The etiology is unknown, and there is no specific therapy. Antihistamines and short courses of moderate- or high-potency topical steroids to the palms and soles may provide temporary relief.
2. Bullous disease: Several varieties of epidermolysis bullosa have their onset in the neonatal period, with bullae involving the skin and mucous membranes. Bullae often occur at sites of trauma. Any bullous lesions (blistering) in the neonatal period require immediate dermatologic consultation.
3. Café-au-lait spots: Discrete tan macules that appear at birth or during childhood in 10%-20% of normal individuals; may involve any site on the skin surface. In the neonatal period, the presence of six or more

lesions larger than 0.5 cm, especially when associated with axillary freckling, is highly suggestive of classic NF. In children with NF, café-au-lait spots may increase in size and number during first few years of life. Café-au-lait spots are also seen in McCune-Albright syndrome, epidermal nevus syndrome, Bloom syndrome, ataxia-telangiectasia, and Russell-Silver syndrome.

4. Erythema toxicum: Evanescent papules, vesicles, and pustules on an erythematous base occur on the face, forehead, chest, trunk, and extremities (*not* the palms and soles) of a high percentage of full-term neonates. They usually appear between 24 and 72 hours but may be seen at birth. A Wright's or Giemsa stain of contents reveals sheets of eosinophils. Peripheral eosinophilia is seen in 7%-15% of cases. The condition resolves over 3-5 days without therapy.

5. Miliaria (prickly heat): Pruritic, erythematous 1-2–mm papulovesicular lesions with predilection for the face and clothed areas of the body. A Gram's stain of the contents is negative. This condition may occur during the first few weeks of life. Treatment consists of less heat, less clothing, and cool soaks.

6. Neonatal lupus syndrome: Lesions consist of an erythematous, oval (discoid), slightly atrophic plaque with scaling. The condition may appear from birth up to 12 weeks. It is primarily localized to the head (periorbital areas) and neck but may spread. It may be associated with anemia, leukopenia, and thrombocytopenia; 15% have congenital A-V block. Serum is positive for antibodies to Ro antigen. Most cases are transient, with resolution of skin lesions by 6 months, but some may progress to subacute or acute SLE.

7. Pustular melanosis: Appears at or shortly after birth as brownish 3-4–mm vesicles and pustules on the neck, face, palms, and soles. Within a few days the pustules shed, leaving pigmented macules with scaling. Wright's stain reveals PMNs. Lesions tend to recur in crops but gradually resolve by 3-4 months without scarring. It is seen mainly in darker-pigmented infants. The etiology is unknown, and there is no treatment.

8. Pustulosis (neonatal impetigo)
   a. Pustulosis involves small vesicles to larger bullae that rupture easily and leave a red, moist, denuded base that crusts over. It occurs in periumbilical and diaper areas, appears at 7-10 days of age, and usually results from *Staphylococcus aureus*.
   b. Obtain a Gram's stain and culture of fluid; start an oral antistaphylococcal agent (cephalexin). Lesions usually clear in 5-7

days. Most patients can be treated at home. It is rarely associated with systemic manifestations.

NOTE: It is important to report all cases of pustulosis to the nursery of origin; the condition may be a harbinger of a staphylococcus outbreak in the nursery.

L. STRIDOR

1. Stridor is a harsh sound produced by turbulent airflow through a partial obstruction. It is a description, not a disease entity, and it may be inspiratory, biphasic, or expiratory. Differential diagnosis includes the following:
   a. Laryngomalacia, tracheomalacia
   b. Subglottic stenosis
   c. Vascular ring
   d. Laryngeal ring, laryngeal cleft
   e. Subglottic hemangioma
   f. Vocal cord paralysis (unilateral or bilateral)
   g. GER with aspiration

NOTE: Laryngomalacia and vocal cord paralysis are the most common causes of stridor in the neonate.

2. Evaluation
   a. History: Onset and duration, aggravating and alleviating factors, quality of cry, hoarseness, cough, color change, relation to feeding and position (Table 13-1)
   b. Examination: Facial and chest configuration, retractions, nasal flaring, cyanosis. Define the portion of the respiratory cycle affected by the stridor.
      1) Inspiratory: Above glottis (i.e., supraglottic larynx, pharynx, or nose)

TABLE 13-1.
Symptoms Associated with Site of Airway Obstruction*

Site of obstruction	Inspiratory stridor	Expiratory stridor	Feeding problems	Abnormal cry
Nose	++		++	+
Oropharynx	++		++	+
Supraglottic	++		++	++
Glottis/subglottic	++	++		++
Trachea		++		

*+, Mild; ++, moderate-to-severe.

2) Biphasic: Glottic or subglottic lesion

3) Expiratory: Intrathoracic tracheobronchial tree

Auscultate for the location of loudest stridor and abnormal or asymmetric breath sounds. Examine for neck masses, tongue abnormalities, and cutaneous hemangiomas.

   c. Diagnostic studies (Table 13-2)
3. Treatment
   a. If there is stridor with airway compromise, the first step is establishment of a stable airway with endotracheal intubation. A tracheostomy may be needed.
   b. Subsequent treatment is guided by the specific cause.

M. THRUSH
1. Oral candidiasis, which has peak incidence during the second week of life
2. Cheesy white plaques on an erythematous base over gingiva, tongue, palate, and buccal mucosa that cannot be removed easily
3. Often associated with candidal diaper rash
4. Treatment: Nystatin suspension 100,000-200,000 U PO qid × 7-10 days

NOTE: In a breast-fed infant, it may help to have the mother apply nystatin (Mycostatin) cream to the areola/nipple area. If thrush is

TABLE 13-2.
Diagnostic Tests for Infants with Stridor*

	Neck/ airway x-ray films	Airway fluoro- scopy	Barium esopha- gram	Fiberoptic laryngo- scopy	Operative laryngo- scopy, broncho- scopy
Laryngomalacia	–	–	–	++	++
Tracheomalacia	–	+	–	–	++
Subglottic stenosis	+	+	–	–	++
Vascular ring	–	+	+	–	++
Laryngeal web	–	–	–	++	++
Laryngeal cleft	–	–	+	+	++
Vocal cord paralysis	–	–	–	++	++
Subglottic hemangioma	+	+	–	–	++

*–, Usually not diagnostic; +, often suggests diagnosis; ++, diagnostic procedure of choice.

recurrent or refractory to treatment, consider a work-up for endocrinopathy or immunodeficiency (?AIDS).

N. TORTICOLLIS

1. When a head tilt is recognized in the early neonatal period, the usual cause is congenital muscular torticollis. It occurs in 0.4% of live births and affects male infants more than female infants. It may be noted at birth and is almost always obvious by 2-4 weeks of age.
2. Clinically, the head is tilted toward the involved side, and the face is turned toward the opposite side. A firm, nontender, discrete fusiform mass ("tumor") that is 1-3 cm in diameter may be palpable in the body of the sternomastoid. It may increase in size gradually over the first month but then regresses; by 4-6 months it is usually no longer palpable.
3. The cause is unknown; it may be secondary to an intrauterine positional deformity or an intrauterine or perinatal compartment syndrome.
4. The differential diagnosis includes congenital anomalies of the cervical vertebrae, vertebral dislocation, cystic hygroma, and a branchial cleft cyst.
5. Treatment consists of passive stretching exercises and positioning. Surgery (open bipolar tenotomy) is indicated if torticollis persists beyond 1 year of age or if there is residual craniofacial deformity or a 30% loss of range of motion.

NOTE: Associated musculoskeletal disorders such as talipes equinovarus, metatarsus adductus, and hip dysplasia occur in up to 20% of cases.

O. UMBILICAL GRANULOMA

1. The umbilical cord usually separates by 8-10 days (2-3 days later if cesarean section) and heals within 3-5 days. Delayed separation and/or mild infection may result in a moist granulating area at the base of the cord with slight mucoid discharge. Treat with alcohol swabs several times a day.
2. Occasionally there may be a persistence of reddish-pink, soft, granular, meaty tissue (granuloma) protruding from the base of the umbilicus. Treatment consists of a single application of silver nitrate cautery; be careful to swab only over the area of granuloma.
3. If there is persistent drainage of fluid or (?) stool from the umbilicus, consider a patent omphalomesenteric duct or urachus.

NOTE: A marked delay in cord separation may be a clue to granulocyte dysfunction.

P. UMBILICAL HERNIA
1. An umbilical hernia is a central fascial defect resulting from incomplete closure of the umbilical ring; it may be pinpoint to >5 cm. It is easily reduced. Incarceration is possible but rare. It is common in black infants and premature infants and is also associated with hypotonia (e.g., Down syndrome, hypothyroidism).
2. Most close spontaneously by 2-3 years of age. Surgery is not indicated unless they are >5 cm or are still large past 5 years of age. Pressure or adhesive dressings with coins and metallic or plastic objects are popular but useless (may lead to contact dermatitis).

NOTE: Surgical repair probably is needed if there is progressive enlargement of the skin over the umbilicus until a downward-pointing proboscis is formed.

Q. VAGINAL DISCHARGE/BLEEDING
1. During the first week of life, a thick, milky-white vaginal discharge and vaginal bleeding (a result of estrogen withdrawal) are common; only reassurance is indicated.
2. Older infants may develop labial adhesions secondary to mild irritation (see p. 162).

R. VOMITING
1. Vomiting involves forceful expulsion of the GI contents as compared with regurgitation, which is more passive and effortless; 80% of all infants under 3 months of age regurgitate feedings at least once a day. Persistent regurgitation without other signs or symptoms usually represents uncomplicated GER.
2. Etiology
   a. Nonbilious vomiting
      1) Overfeeding
      2) Milk/formula protein sensitivity
      3) Infection (sepsis, urinary tract infection, meningitis)
      4) Necrotizing enterocolitis
      5) Pyloric stenosis
      6) Electrolyte/metabolic abnormalities
      7) Hirschsprung's disease
      8) Lactobezoars
   b. Bilious vomiting: Congenital anomalies (malrotation, atresia,

stenosis, webs, annular pancreas, persistent omphalomesenteric duct)
3. Management
   a. Review of feeding history; examination for signs of infection; serum electrolytes
   b. Plain abdominal x-ray examination with upright and cross-table lateral
   c. Upper GI series to R/O obstructive anomalies
   d. Abdominal ultrasound to R/O pyloric stenosis
   e. Passage of gastric tube if obstruction is suspected
   f. Prompt surgical consultation if there is bilious vomiting or hematemesis

BIBLIOGRAPHY

Davids JR et al: Congenital muscular torticollis: sequela of intrauterine or perinatal compartment syndrome, *J Pediatr Orthop* 13:141, 1993.

Fanaroff A, Martin RJ: *Neonatal-perinatal medicine,* St Louis, 1992, Mosby.

Findlay RF, Odom RB: Infantile acropustulosis, *Am J Dis Child* 137:455, 1983.

Holinger LD: Etiology of stridor in the neonate, infant, and child, *Ann Otol Rhinol Laryngol* 89:397, 1980.

Joseph PR, Rosenfeld W: Clavicular fractures in neonates, *Am J Dis Child* 144:165, 1990.

Tunkel DE, Zalzal GH: Stridor in infants and children: ambulatory evaluation and operative diagnosis, *Clin Pediatr* 31:48, 1992.

Watson R: Neonatal lupus syndrome, *Pediatr Ann* 15:605, 1986.

Yasunaga S, Rivera R: Cephalhematoma in the newborn, *Clin Pediatr* 13:256, 1974.

Yip WC et al: Sonographic diagnosis of infantile hypertrophic pyloric stenosis: critical appraisal of reliability and diagnostic criteria, *J Clin Ultrasound* 13:329, 1985.

NEUROLOGY

14

A. ALTERED MENTAL STATUS

1. Altered mental status includes any change in sensorium or behavior; it is manifest in extreme cases by stupor/coma and hyperirritability and in milder cases by confusion, sleepiness, aggressive behavior, and decreased school or social performance.

2. Important historical information includes the following:
   a. A complete description of the altered sensorium (e.g., acute vs. gradual onset, duration, waxing and waning vs. steady progression)
   b. Previous mental status
   c. Possible precipitating events, trauma, psychologic stressors, medication, or illicit drug use
   d. Signs of illness, especially fever, headaches, visual disturbances
   e. Chronic medical condition or preexisting neurologic problem
   f. History of depression or a change in school or social performance

3. The PE must be thorough. Special emphasis should be placed on the neurologic exam, fundoscopic assessment, nuchal rigidity, and skin findings (e.g., herpetic lesions, bruises). Note any odor on the breath that might suggest an ingestion or a metabolic disturbance, such as diabetic ketoacidosis.

4. Causes of altered mental status
   a. CNS infection (meningitis, encephalitis)
   b. CNS mass (usually a gradual onset of symptoms)
   c. CNS hemorrhage (may be acute or gradual and may be preceded by headache) or infarct
   d. CNS trauma
   e. Medication/drug overdose
   f. Alcohol and illicit drug use, including secondhand exposure to "crack" cocaine
   g. Hypertensive encephalopathy
   h. Hypoglycemia
   i. Diabetic ketoacidosis
   j. Reye's syndrome

   k. Depression

   l. Ictal/post-ictal states

5. Laboratory tests are dictated by the history, PE, and type of mental status change.

   a. For the comatose, stuporous, and hyperirritable patient, CBC, electrolytes, glucose, ammonia, BUN, LFTs, and a toxicology screen should be obtained.

   b. If vital signs are stable and there are no localizing neurologic signs or evidence of increased ICP, an LP should be considered (CSF sent for glucose, protein, Gram's stain, cell count, culture/ELISA). Consider obtaining an opening pressure.

   c. A CT scan should precede the LP in a patient who is unstable or has localized neurologic signs.

6. Treatment is directed toward the underlying cause of the altered mental status.

B. HEADACHE

1. Headache is a common presenting complaint, especially in the older pediatric age group and in febrile children.

2. Important historical information includes the following:

   a. Location, day(s) and time(s) of occurrence, frequency, duration, precipitating factors, ameliorating factors, and associated symptoms (e.g., fever, neck pain, scotoma, photophobia, nausea, vomiting). Is the headache acute or chronic, progressive or nonprogressive? (See Fig. 14-1.)

   b. Does the patient have a chronic medical condition or take medications on a long-term basis?

   c. Is there a family history of headaches? If so, who has them and what are they like?

   d. Does the patient have a history of head trauma, seizures, cranial surgery, allergies, decreased vision or hearing, pain on chewing? Has the headache ever awakened him or her from sleep?

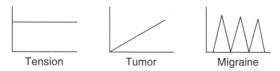

     Tension   Tumor   Migraine

FIG 14-1. Pain course over time.

e. Is the patient stressed? Have there been changes in his or her personality, school performance, or growth?

3. The PE should be complete. Place emphasis on the skull, eyes, ears, teeth, temporomandibular joints, sinuses, and neurologic exam. Look for areas of tenderness, asymmetry, and bruits.

4. No single laboratory test is mandatory for the patient with a headache. Laboratory tests and radiographic studies are dictated by the results of the history and PE. A CT scan or MRI is not indicated unless abnormal neurologic findings are present.

5. Frontal headaches may result from viral illnesses (especially when accompanied by fever), sinus infection, sinus edema (resulting from exposure to allergens or noxious environmental stimuli such as smoke), stress, or fatigue.

   a. The presence of pain on palpation over the sinuses and a purulent nasal discharge suggests sinusitis; an x-ray examination confirms the diagnosis.

   b. The presence of suborbital edema/cyanosis, edematous bluish nasal turbinates, and watery ocular/nasal discharge suggests allergic disease.

6. Facial pain may result from dental disease, middle ear disease, temporomandibular joint dysfunction, or maxillary sinusitis.

7. Pain in the temples or neck pain (tightness) may result from stress (especially if the pain occurs during stressful situations) or depression.

8. Frontal or occipital headaches may be associated with intracranial disease (bleeding, tumor, abscess, pseudotumor cerebri), especially if the pain occurs with arising in the morning, is relieved by vomiting, and is accompanied by visual field or acuity changes or alterations in mental status, mood, motor function, or sensation.

9. Generalized (or poorly localized) headaches may result from fatigue, stress, migraines, medications such as sympathomimetics, illicit drugs such as amphetamines, encephalitis (often associated with sensorium changes), meningitis (usually associated with positive Kernig's and Brudzinski's signs), severe anemia, hypertension, hyperventilation, hypoglycemia, hypoxia, hypercapnia, carbon monoxide poisoning, and trauma.

10. A severe headache may herald a subarachnoid bleed, especially if the patient is confused or unconscious.

11. Migraine headaches are "classically" paroxysmal, either bilateral or unilateral, and are preceded by an aura or accompanied by nausea and vomiting. However, not all patients have this classic presentation.

Younger children may have abdominal pain and vomiting. A family history of migraine is helpful.

12. Treatment of uncomplicated headaches includes analgesics and rest.
    a. Headaches resulting from bacterial processes respond to antibiotic therapy of the underlying disease.
    b. Headaches resulting from allergen exposure respond to the elimination of the offending agent. Antihistamines may be useful if other histamine-mediated symptoms are present.
    c. Headaches resulting from stress or depression respond to the elucidation and resolution of the psychic conflict. Biofeedback techniques may be useful.
    d. Headaches resulting from intracranial mass lesions or bleeding are usually treated surgically.
    e. Once a migraine headache has been firmly established, it cannot be resolved easily; ice packs, remaining in a dark and quiet place, or biofeedback may be useful. If vomiting is a problem, promethazine (Phenergan) or prochlorperazine (Compazine) may be helpful. Propranolol 1-2 mg/kg/d up to 4 mg/kg/d for children ≥12 years of age can prevent episodes or abort a headache if taken early in its course. Propranolol should be avoided in those with asthma, diabetes mellitus, and heart disease. Another useful drug in adolescents is amitriptyline; it is most useful in those with migraines, muscle contraction headaches, and headaches associated with depression. For adolescents, the starting dose is 25 mg hs.

    Dihydroergotamine mesylate (DHE 45), a serotonin antagonist, may be useful for symptomatic and abortive treatment of severe or intractable migraines in adolescents. The serotonin receptor agonist sumatriptan succinate (Imitrex) is useful for adult migraine and cluster headaches, but its safety and efficacy in young children are unknown. Other helpful modalities for all ages include regular sleep and meal schedules, elimination of any foods that seem to be associated with headaches, biofeedback, and counseling.

C. HEAD TRAUMA

1. Evaluation: The main objective is to sort out patients who have treatable complications (e.g., intracranial bleeding, depressed fractures) from those who do not; doing so can be difficult.
    a. The history should include a detailed description of the type of trauma (e.g., fall, blow), loss of consciousness and duration, amnesia (especially retrograde), lethargy, vomiting, seizures,

vision difficulties, and a history of other medical problems (especially a shunt). Many patients have a period of sleepiness, headaches, and vomiting a few times without sequelae. Consider the possibility of child abuse.

b. The PE should be complete and include vital signs (increased ICP causes ↓ HR, ↑ BP, irregular respirations); look for direct signs of trauma (e.g., soft-tissue swelling, hematoma, skull depression, lacerations). Give particular attention to the following:

1) Fundus: Retinal hemorrhage; papilledema (usually a *late* sign of ↑ ICP). Do not use mydriatics to dilate pupils.
2) Tympanic membrane: Blood behind eardrum, CSF discharge
3) Ecchymosis behind ear (Battle's sign), or orbital (raccoon sign)
4) Nose: CSF rhinorrhea
5) Neck exam: Make sure cervical spine is not injured. If in doubt, stabilize head with sandbags and obtain cervical spine x-ray studies.
6) Skin: Check for signs of abuse.
7) Neurologic exam: Emphasize level of consciousness (probably the most important observation) and general mental state; serial observations are mandatory.
   a) Eyes: Unequal pupils signify compression of the third nerve by a herniating temporal lobe.
   b) Diplopia: Sixth nerve (to lateral rectus) is particularly vulnerable to ↑ ICP.
   c) Motor: Use of arms and legs normal? Ataxic gait?
   d) Reflexes: Symmetric? Toes turn down?

c. X-ray studies

1) Skull x-ray studies are expensive, overused, and of limited usefulness. In general, fractures are poor predictors of intracranial injury.
   a) Patient treatment is rarely affected by skull x-ray examination findings.
   b) Although skull x-ray studies may be indicated in the following clinical circumstances, a CT scan is preferable: age <1 year, unconsciousness >5-10 minutes, gunshot wound or skull penetration, V-P shunt in place, palpable scalp depression, CSF discharge from ear or nose, blood in middle ear, Battle's sign, raccoon eyes, lethargy, coma, stupor, or focal neurologic signs. Most patients with minor head trauma need *no* imaging studies.

2) Cervical spine stabilization and an x-ray study are indicated if the head injury is severe, such as in an automobile accident. Cervical abrasions and upper spine tenderness suggest a neck injury.

d. A CT scan is indicated if intracranial bleeding is suspected (e.g., patient with persistent or progressing neurologic signs). In infants and toddlers, a subdural hemorrhage indicates abuse, whereas an epidural hemorrhage makes a diagnosis of abuse less likely.

e. An MRI is superior to a CT scan for visualizing diffuse axonal (shear) injury and subarachnoid hemorrhage. It is also useful for detecting traumatic hematomas of varying duration, brain ischemia, or edema.

f. An EEG is not indicated in the initial evaluation or in uncomplicated cases.

2. Management

a. The patient may be sent home when the level of consciousness and neurologic function are back to normal.

b. If the exam and level of consciousness are normal, give the parent instructions for home care. The level of alertness should be evaluated every few hours for the first 24 hours. The parent should also look for evidence of blood or clear fluid from the nose or ear; an inability to use limbs properly; difficulty speaking, hearing, or seeing; seizures; repeated vomiting; or behavior changes. The parent should note any fever, headaches, or change in mental status or behavior during the next 2 weeks, and the child should return if such problems develop.

c. The patient is usually hospitalized if any of the following are true:

1) Any sign of deterioration

2) Clear-cut neurologic signs

3) Prolonged loss of consciousness

4) The level of function does not return promptly to normal (sometimes the patient may be sent home if parents are reliable, overall exam results are reassuring, and neurology consult agrees)

5) Fracture across area of middle meningeal artery or a depressed skull fracture

d. Seizure in the first 24 hours after the injury is not an automatic admission, nor is a skull fracture.

e. If there are any questions, get a neurology consult.

f. Give parents written instructions for follow-up at home, including the information in Point b).

D. ACUTE INCREASED INTRACRANIAL PRESSURE: EMER- GENCY DEPARTMENT MANAGEMENT

1. Signs and symptoms include headache, nausea, vomiting, spectrum of altered mental status, and papilledema.
   a. Note vital signs and any change suggestive of ↑ ICP (↓ HR, slow respirations, ↑ BP with widening pulse pressure).
   b. The patient with severe ↑ ICP may be delirious and thrashing about or may be completely obtunded.
2. Causes include trauma, infection, metabolic (Reye's syndrome), tumor, hypoxic/ischemic damage, and shunt malfunction.
3. Priorities are to establish and maintain appropriate ventilation and perfusion and to decrease ICP.
   a. Elevation of head-of-bed to 30 degrees, midline positioning of head, and maintenance of normal body temperature should be accomplished.
   b. Provide controlled intubation and hyperventilation. Hyperventila- tion is the most rapid means to decrease ICP. If the patient is obtunded, intubation should neither be difficult nor require premedication (e.g., muscle relaxants). If the patient is thrashing about, diazepam (Valium) 0.1-0.2 mg/kg by IV push or lidocaine 1.5 mg/kg IV should be adequate to allow intubation; neither drug increases ICP.

NOTE: Do not use pancuronium (Pavulon) because doing so prevents assessment of neurologic status during the first critical hours. Succinyl- choline may lead to fatal hyperkalemia. Diazepam (Valium) is a safe "relaxant" to use in the ED until the patient can be transferred to an intensive care unit.

   c. Hypertonic agent: Mannitol 0.5-1.0 g/kg IV over 10-20 minutes helps decrease cerebral edema and thereby decreases ICP; it is useful in initial emergency management.
      or
   d. Diuretic: Furosemide 1-2 mg/kg/dose IV (max 6 mg/kg) q6-12h has both a diuretic and independent effect on decreasing ICP (probably by decreasing CSF production).

E. CENTRAL NERVOUS SYSTEM INFECTIONS

1. CNS infections include bacterial meningitis, aseptic meningitis, encephalitis, and brain abscesses.
   a. Patients with these processes may have nuchal rigidity, headache, behavior changes, seizures, sensorium changes, focal neurologic signs, or fever.

    b. Depending on the etiologic agent, other signs may be present (e.g., rash, vomiting, diarrhea, pneumonia).

2. Important information includes a history of immune compromise, antibiotic use, immunizations, travel, animal/insect exposure, and the duration and character of any of the signs listed under Point 1. With a confused or comatose patient, drug ingestion must also be considered.

3. A complete PE is mandatory, with special emphasis on the neck (nuchal rigidity), skull (trauma, tenderness, split sutures), skin (rash, especially petechiae/purpura), and the neurologic exam (e.g., focal findings, sensorium, orientation, cranial nerves). Check for lymphadenopathy (generalized or local). Optimally, the fundi should be visualized (to R/O papilledema) before an LP is performed.

4. Laboratory tests are usually crucial.

    a. Spinal fluid is examined for cell count, protein, glucose (compare with a simultaneous serum glucose), and organisms (Gram's stain).

    b. CIE and latex particle agglutination tests of CSF, blood, and urine may help to rapidly diagnose *Haemophilus influenzae, Streptococcus pneumoniae, Neisseria meningitidis,* and group B streptococcus infections.

    c. Blood and urine cultures should be obtained.

    d. Serum electrolytes, BUN, creatinine, and a CBC with differential and smear may be helpful.

    e. If an ingestion is suspected, a toxicology screen is indicated.

    f. LP is contraindicated if there are focal findings (e.g., if a brain abscess is suspected) because herniation is possible. Instead, an emergent CT scan is indicated.

5. Causes

    a. Bacterial meningitis: *H. influenzae, S. pneumoniae, N. meningitidis,* group B streptococcus, *Listeria* organisms, *Staphylococcus aureus, Pseudomonas* organisms. The latter four occur in neonates.

    b. Aseptic meningitis, most commonly enterovirus

    c. Encephalitis: S/P measles, varicella, mumps, influenza, Epstein-Barr infection, herpes

    d. Abscesses: *S. aureus,* group A streptococcus, *H. influenzae,* anaerobes, gram-negative enteric bacteria, fungi

6. Treatment

    a. Bacterial meningitis: Cefotaxime 200 mg/kg/d ÷ q6h or ceftriaxone 100 mg/kg/d ÷ q12-24h. If *S. pneumoniae* or *N. meningitidis* is the etiologic organism, penicillin G 300,000 U/kg/d ÷ q4h is used (for multiply resistant pneumococci, use vancomycin 60 mg/kg/d ÷ q6h).

Follow vital signs and neurologic status carefully; fluid restrict (NPO × 24 hours, then oral and IV total fluids at 60%-75% maintenance) to prevent SIADH. Follow head circumference; may need CT scan to R/O subdural fluid accumulation if focal neurologic signs, focal seizures, or increasing head circumference occur.

For seizures: Phenobarbital (loading dosage 15-20 mg/kg no faster than 30 mg/min; maintenance dosage 3-5 mg/kg/d ÷ q12h) or phenytoin (Dilantin) (loading dosage 15-20 mg/kg in normal saline no faster than 50 mg/min; maintenance dosage 5-10 mg/kg/d ÷ qd or q12h). See Section G regarding status epilepticus.

b. Aseptic meningitis: If CSF cell count is confusing or contaminated with blood, may need to give cefotaxime 200 mg/kg/d ÷ q6h or ceftriaxone 100 mg/kg/d ÷ q12h for 3 days pending negative cultures. Fluid restrict to avoid SIADH, administer IV fluids and analgesics/antipyretics, and incline head-of-bed 30 degrees. For herpes encephalitis, give acyclovir/vidarabine; give phenobarbital/phenytoin (Dilantin) for seizures.

c. Brain abscess: Surgery or aspiration via burr holes; fluid restriction; ceftazidime 50 mg/kg q8h or ceftriaxone 50 mg/kg q12h and nafcillin or oxacillin 200 mg/kg/d ÷ q4-6h (or vancomycin 10 mg/kg q6h for methicillin-resistant *S. aureus*); dexamethasone 10-12 mg loading dose followed by 0.1-0.2 mg/kg/dose IV q4h. If ICP is severely elevated, incline head-of-bed to 30 degrees. Provide mannitol 0.5-1.0 g/kg/dose over 20 minutes, intubation, paralysis, hyperventilation to keep Pco_2 23-25 mm Hg, ICP monitoring, pentobarbital coma 10-15 mg/kg IV over 1-2 hours followed by 1-3 mg/kg/h to maintain a blood level of 30-40 μg/dL. Provide phenobarbital 15-20 mg/kg loading dose followed by 3-5 mg/kg/d or phenytoin (Dilantin) 15-20 mg/kg loading dose followed by 5-10 mg/kg/d to control seizures.

d. Bacterial meningitis (*H. influenzae* and pneumococcal): dexamethasone 0.6 mg/kg/d ÷ qid × 4 days

F. RETT SYNDROME

1. Characterized by the following:
   a. Female gender
   b. Normal prenatal/perinatal period and normal development in the first 6-18 months of life

    c. Normal head circumference at birth with deceleration of head growth between 6 months and 4 years of age

    d. Early behavioral, social, and psychomotor regression with evolving communication dysfunction and dementia

    e. Loss of purposeful hand skills between 1 and 4 years of age

    f. Hand wringing/clapping/washing stereotypies between 1 and 4 years of age

    g. Gait apraxia and truncal apraxia/ataxia between 1 and 4 years of age

2. Four stages of Rett syndrome

    a. Stage 1: Onset of slowing of development, some hypotonia

    b. Stage 2: Obvious loss of acquired skills, onset of hand stereotypies, loss of contact with environment and autistic affect, evolving dementia, loss of speech and purposeful hand use, screaming episodes, sleep disturbances

    c. Stage 3: Seizures, disappearance of autistic affect, prominent hand stereotypies and jerky apraxic movements, disappearance of screaming episodes, improvement of sleep, onset of apnea spells, loss of gross motor skills, hypertonia

    d. Stage 4: Spasticity; muscle wasting; immobility; cool, mottled extremities; cachexia; constipation; profound mental retardation

3. Incidence is 0.4-1.0 per 10,000 girls.

4. Etiology is unknown, but a genetic cause seems likely.

5. Various CNS biochemical abnormalities have been noted; EEG is abnormal.

6. Life span per se is not shortened.

7. Referral to a pediatric neurologist is in order.

G. SEIZURES, FEBRILE SEIZURES, AND STATUS EPILEPTICUS

1. Seizures are a common problem in children; approximately 3.5% of children have at least one seizure by 15 years of age. Most have a single seizure or recurrent seizures over a limited time. Only a small percentage (1%) have epilepsy.

2. Causes of seizures

    a. Neonatal: Hypoxic-ischemic insult, CNS bleed, infection, CNS malformation, metabolic derangement

    b. Infants >28 days: Infection, dehydration, fever (>6 months of age), inborn errors of metabolism, electrolyte imbalance, birth injury, CNS trauma, malformations

    c. Children: Head trauma; noncompliance with, change of, or

inadequate dose of anticonvulsant medication; intercurrent infection in a known seizure patient; toxin ingestion (do not forget lead); tumor; fever (up to 6 years of age)

3. Initial evaluation of nonfebrile seizure

   a. Assess whether a real seizure occurred (choking spell or breath-holding spell?). Is the child ictal or post-ictal? Any seizure activity (lateralization, eye deviation, focal vs. generalized)?

   b. Prior seizures? Medications? Fever? Other signs of illness? Aura? Circumstances preceding the seizure? Precipitating event? History of drug abuse or ingestion? Trauma (remember occult trauma such as abuse)? Presence of preexisting neurologic disease?

   c. Vital signs

   d. Exam (quick and pertinent): Assess neurologic (pupils, response, signs and symptoms of ↑ ICP, fontanelle), cardiovascular (BP, perfusion), respiratory (cyanosis, irregular breathing, ineffective ventilation). Note breath odor, rash, signs of trauma, liver size, signs of infection (sepsis, meningitis). *Keep reassessing*—status may change quickly!

   e. Initial laboratory evaluation
      1) Dextrostix or Chemstrip
      2) Electrolytes, Ca, glucose, BUN, CBC, anticonvulsant levels (if applicable)
      3) Toxicology screen on blood and urine (+ vomitus, if indicated)
      4) Sepsis work-up, including LP, may be indicated
      5) Consider need for LFTs, Mg, Pb, NH_4^+
      6) CNS imaging (CT scan or MRI) may be indicated

   f. Treatment
      1) After a complete assessment, decide if the patient needs an antiepileptic drug and, if so, the drug most appropriate for the seizure type. These decisions are best made in conjunction with a pediatric neurologist.
      2) When initiating therapy, perform the following procedures:
         a) Start with a single drug and begin with the lowest dose needed to achieve a therapeutic serum level. Increase the dose as needed to achieve a clinical response.
         b) Switch to a second drug if the first is not effective.
         c) If monotherapy fails, add a second drug.
      3) It is important to monitor serum drug levels and evaluate for drug toxicities.
      4) Most children with recurrent seizures remain on an anticonvulsant medication for at least a 2-year seizure-free period.

4. Febrile seizures
   a. Two to five percent of all children will develop a febrile seizure. Although most are simple seizures, a minority are complex.
   b. Onset: Most seizures occur between 6 weeks and 6 years of age, with a peak between 1 and 3 years. There is a 50% recurrence rate if onset is before 1 year of age.
   c. Duration: 50% <5 minutes, 75% <20 minutes, 2%-3% >30 minutes
   d. Type: Typically generalized tonic-clonic, but 15% are focal. Usually only one seizure occurs during any febrile illness.
   e. Most occur with a temperature >39° C and at the onset of fever. A seizure that occurs after a fever has been present for >24 hours is more likely to be associated with a significant infection.
   f. Evaluation
      1) LP is indicated if any of the following are true:
         a) Any suspicion of meningitis
         b) Abnormal postseizure neurologic exam
         c) History of illness for several days before seizure
         d) Slow recovery from febrile seizure
      2) CBC, electrolytes, glucose, Ca, Mg, CNS imaging, and EEG are not indicated with simple febrile seizures.
   g. Treatment
      1) Give lorazepam for acute control of status epilepticus (dosages are given later in this section).
      2) Reduce fever with tepid water sponging and rectal acetaminophen.
   h. Consider long-term prophylaxis with phenobarbital or valproic acid *only* if the patient has multiple risk factors as follows:
      1) Prior history of abnormal neurologic or neurodevelopmental exam
      2) Family history of nonfebrile seizures
      3) Seizure duration >15 minutes
      4) Seizure with focal component or associated with transient or persistent neurologic abnormalities
      5) More than one seizure during the same illness within a 24-hour period

NOTE: There is no evidence that prophylaxis reduces the risk of subsequent nonfebrile seizures and no evidence that recurrent febrile seizures, even when complex, increase a child's risk for epilepsy or neurodevelopmental problems.

5. Status epilepticus
   a. Status epilepticus describes seizure activity that lasts ≥ 30 minutes or in which there is incomplete recovery between recurrent seizures.
   b. Immediate management includes the following:
      1) Maintain airway and maximize ventilation (oral airway or intubation); provide oxygen as indicated.
      2) Suction secretions and insert NG tube to prevent aspiration.
      3) Establish IV access.
      4) If febrile, provide tepid sponging and rectal acetaminophen.
      5) Check Dextrostix; if hypoglycemia is present, give IV bolus of $D_{25}W$ 3-4 ml/kg followed by continuous glucose infusion of D_5, 0.25 normal saline or D_{10}, 0.25 normal saline.
      6) IV anticonvulsant therapy
         a) Lorazepam 0.05-0.1 mg/kg (max 5 mg). One dose usually stops status in 2-3 minutes. The half-life is 10-12 hours. Lorazepam may be less likely than diazepam to cause respiratory depression and hypotension, but both can occur, especially if the patient has been taking a barbiturate.
         b) Diazepam 0.05-0.3 mg/kg (max 5 mg in infants and 10 mg in older children) at a rate of 1 mg/min by IV push; may repeat in 15 minutes. The rectal route can be used if IV access is a problem.
            (1) Advantage: Rapidly effective
            (2) Disadvantage: Respiratory and cardiovascular depression, especially if the patient has been taking a barbiturate. In addition, the drug is quickly redistributed throughout the body, and seizures may recur as redistribution occurs.
            (3) After initial therapy with lorazepam or diazepam, the patient needs to be placed on a long-acting anticonvulsant such as phenytoin or phenobarbital.
   c. Phenytoin 15-20 mg/kg (max 1 g) is administered slowly in normal saline at 1-3 mg/kg/min (not to exceed 50 mg/min).
      1) Advantage: Phenytoin does not alter mental status (useful in patients with head trauma) and has a longer half-life than benzodiazepines.
      2) Disadvantage: Seizures do not respond as quickly as with benzodiazepines; when given parenterally, need to monitor ECG for arrhythmia.

d. Phenobarbital 15-20 mg/kg (max 300 mg) is administered by IV no faster than 30 mg/min. If seizures continue, may give second dose of 10 mg/kg after 20 minutes. The disadvantage is slow onset of action compared with benzodiazepines (takes up to 15 minutes to cross blood-brain barrier).

H. SHUNT MALFUNCTION

1. Anything that goes wrong with a patient with a shunted hydrocephalus results from a shunt problem until proven otherwise. Shunt obstruction and shunt infection (usually a result of *S. aureus* or *Staphylococcus epidermidis*) are common.
2. Signs and symptoms of acute obstruction include headache, irritability, lethargy, vomiting, acute strabismus, eye movement dysfunction, bulging fontanelle, and behavior change. If present, evaluate as an emergency.
3. Shunt infection may or may not be accompanied by fever. Most shunt infections occur within 2 months of initial shunt placement.
4. Do not waste time pumping the device; doing so may result in misleading information. Perform a general/neurologic evaluation and call a neurosurgeon for probable tap of pump device. Imaging studies may or may not have diagnostic value depending on the study selected, the age of the child, and the acuity of the obstruction.

I. SYNCOPE

1. Syncope is the sudden, transient loss of consciousness (seconds to a minute or more) as a result of cerebral hypoperfusion or anoxia.
2. Important historical information includes the following:
   a. A complete description of the episode and antecedent events or patient's feelings (e.g., palpitations, dizziness, nausea, lightheadedness)
   b. A history of similar events and their precipitating factors
   c. Presence of aura or ictal stereotypic movements during the episode (R/O seizure)
   d. Cardiac symptoms (exertional dyspnea, palpitations)
   e. History of cardiac, endocrine, CNS, pulmonary disease
   f. Chronic medication use
   g. Family history of syncopal episodes
3. The PE is usually normal. It should be complete with special emphasis on cardiac (murmurs, arrhythmias, tachyarrhythmias) and neurologic assessment, especially the patient's mental state and recollection of the event.

4. Causes of syncope
   a. Vasovagal: Preceded by light-headedness, dizziness, diaphoresis, and pallor. This type of syncope may be preceded by physical discomfort, emotionally charged situations, or fright (e.g., seeing blood).
   b. Hysteria: The clue is that the patient is seemingly unconcerned about the event.
   c. Hyperventilation: Prolonged deep breathing intentionally or unintentionally during stress may lower Pco_2 enough to cause syncope. Other symptoms include chest tightness, weakness, and light-headedness.
   d. Breath-holding: Usually precipitated by injury or anger. There may be cyanosis following crying or there may be pallor and collapse without antecedent crying.
   e. Cardiac lesions: Aortic stenosis, pulmonic stenosis, truncus arteriosus, transposition of the great vessels, tetralogy of Fallot, pulmonary hypertension, carotid sinus syncope
   f. Cardiac arrhythmias: Paroxysmal atrial tachycardia, atrioventricular block, paroxysmal ventricular fibrillation, long QT syndrome (episodes precipitated by physical or mental exertion), mitral valve prolapse (chest pain may also be present)
   g. Postural hypotension
   h. Prolonged coughing
   i. Micturition
   j. Severe anemia
   k. Antihypertensives/antihistamines
   l. Hypoglycemia
   m. Cerebellar or brainstem tumor
5. History and PE guide the choice of laboratory tests.
   a. Most individuals with a simple faint require no laboratory evaluation, except perhaps a Dextrostix.
   b. An ECG is in order if there is a history of recurrent faints or "seizures" or if there are cardiac symptoms. Holter monitoring may also be helpful.
   c. The patient's BP should be measured in the supine, sitting, and standing positions.
6. For most patients with syncope, treatment is usually reassurance.
   a. Patients with hyperventilation should be taught to breathe into a paper bag (to increase Pco_2) during episodes.
   b. Patients with transient hypoglycemia should be encouraged to not skip meals.

c. Patients with chronic or recurrent hypoglycemia are managed as described in Hypoglycemia (p. 82).

d. Individuals with postural hypotension should be instructed to go slowly from a supine to a standing position.

e. Correction of anemia, discontinuation of offending medications, and therapy for tumors should aid patients with these causes.

f. Individuals with cardiac processes should be managed together with a cardiologist, especially if there are episodes of syncope during exercise.

J. TICS AND TOURETTE'S SYNDROME

1. A tic is a sudden, involuntary, repetitive, rapid, random, nonrhythmic, purposeless, and highly stereotypic movement. The stereotypic nature differentiates it from chorea, myoclonus, athetosis, dystonia, and hemiballism. Other than the tics, affected children generally have a normal exam.

2. The etiology of tics is not well understood.
   a. Dopamine may play a role because drugs that increase dopamine metabolites suppress tics, whereas drugs that decrease dopamine levels worsen symptoms.
   b. Psychologic factors play some role because tics tend to increase when a child is stressed and tend to be precipitated by traumatic events.

3. Tics may be transient (duration of weeks) or chronic (duration >12 months).

4. Average age of onset is 7 years, and there is a male predominance.

5. Tics may occur singly or in groups. A child with a simple tic disorder has only one type of tic at any one time, but this tic may be replaced serially by other tics.

6. Tics typically wax and wane in severity. There is usually an ability to voluntarily suppress tics for minutes to hours, and they disappear during sleep.

7. Types of tics include the following:
   a. Motor: Commonly involve the head, face, and neck (eye blinking, eye rolling, mouth twitching, head bobbing, facial grimacing, shoulder shrugging). Individuals may also display hopping, jumping, skipping, squatting, twisting, compulsive touching, and ritualistic acts.
   b. Vocal: Coughing, sniffing, throat clearing, high-pitched cries, screams, barking, hiccuping, belching, echolalia, palilalia (repeating one's own words), coprolalia (involuntary utterance of obscenities), and animal sounds

    c. Complex: Multiple motor and vocal tics simultaneously; usually begins with a single tic

8. Tourette's syndrome represents a subset of tic disorders that usually has its onset between 2 and 15 years of age (mean age 7 years). The incidence is 5 per 1000, with a 3:1 male predominance.

    a. Historically, the child has multiple motor tics and multiple vocal tics that have waxed and waned for >1 year.

    b. The tics wax and wane over weeks; the child can suppress them temporarily, but the syndrome itself lasts for years or even a lifetime.

    c. Familial clustering of affected individuals is common. A genetic etiology is likely (perhaps an autosomal dominant with variable expression).

    d. Some investigators believe the syndrome may be precipitated or exacerbated by the use of methylphenidate (Ritalin) and other stimulants used for attentional problems commonly associated with Tourette's syndrome.

9. No laboratory abnormalities have been detected in patients with tics or Tourette's syndrome. The PE is normal except for the tics.

10. Treatment

    a. Simple tics: Because of the side effects of the medications used to control tics, transient tics that are not socially objectionable should be permitted to spontaneously abate. Counseling of the patient and parent is necessary, but psychotherapy and medication are unnecessary and do not hasten resolution.

    b. Complex tic disorder and Tourette's syndrome

        1) Management in consultation with a pediatric neurologist is essential.

        2) No drug is curative or alters the long-term prognosis. Medication only suppresses symptoms so that a child is better able to function.

        3) For chronic tics and Tourette's syndrome, haloperidol (starting with 0.25-0.5 mg hs, with 0.5 mg incremental increases q4-5d until the desired effect is achieved) has been used with success. The usual dosage requirement is 2.0-2.5 mg/d. Side effects include lethargy, dysphoria, depression, and diminution of cognitive functioning. Extrapyramidal side effects (dystonia, tardive dyskinesia) have also been reported.

        4) Pimozide (starting with 1 mg hs, with 1 mg increases q5-7d until relief of tic or side effects). The usual dosage requirement is 5-6 mg/d. Do not exceed 10 mg/d in children and 20 mg/d in adolescents and adults. Side effects include lengthening of

the QT interval, sedation, impaired motivation, dysphoria, phobia, weight gain, ocular changes, dry mouth, gynecomastia or lactation, akathisia, and decreased libido. However, these effects occur less commonly than with haloperidol.

5) Clonidine has been statistically less efficacious than haloperidol and pimozide in reducing tics but has fewer side effects and improves other symptoms such as hyperactivity. The starting dosage is 0.05 mg/d, with increases of 0.05 mg q2wk. The usual daily dose is 0.125-0.3 mg. Sedation and orthostatic hypotension are the most common side effects.

c. Counseling (psychotherapy) of the patient and parent is necessary. Educational and social counseling is also important.

BIBLIOGRAPHY

Headache

Elser J: Easing the pain of childhood headaches, *Contemp Pediatr* 8:108, 1991.

Olness K, MacDonald J: Recurrent headaches in children: diagnosis and treatment, *Pediatr Rev* 8:307, 1987.

Prensky A: Differentiating and treating pediatric headaches, *Contemp Pediatr* 1:12, 1984.

Rothner AD: A practical approach to headaches in adolescents, *Pediatr Ann* 20:200, 1991.

Singer H, Rowe S: Chronic recurrent headaches in children, *Pediatr Ann* 21:369, 1992.

Head trauma

Duhaime AC et al: Head injury in very young children, *Pediatrics* 90:179, 1992.

Goldstein B, Powers K: Head trauma in children, *Pediatr Rev* 15:213, 1994.

Hennes H et al: Clinical predictors of severe head trauma in children, *Am J Dis Child* 142:1045, 1988.

Kaufman B, Dacey R: Acute care management of closed head injury in childhood, *Pediatr Ann* 23:18, 1994.

Masters S et al: Skull x-ray examination after head trauma, *N Engl J Med* 316:84, 1987.

Rivara F: Epidemiology and prevention of pediatric brain injury, *Pediatr Ann* 23:12, 1994.

Rivara F et al: Poor prediction of positive computed tomographic scans by clinical criteria in symptomatic pediatric head trauma, *Pediatrics* 80:579, 1987.

Steinbok P et al: Management of simple depressed skull fractures in children, *J Neurosurg* 66:506, 1987.

Tecklenburg F, Wright M: Minor head trauma in the pediatric patient, *Pediatr Emerg Care* 7:40, 1991.

Increased intracranial pressure

Bergman I: Increased intracranial pressure, *Pediatr Rev* 15:241, 1994.

Central nervous system infections

Burg F, Ingelfinger J, Wald E, editors: *Gellis and Kagan's current pediatric therapy,* ed 14, Philadelphia, 1993, WB Saunders.

Committee on Infectious Disease: Dexamethasone therapy for bacterial meningitis in infants and children, *Pediatrics* 86:130, 1990.

Kennedy W et al: The role of corticosteroid therapy in children with pneumococcal meningitis, *Am J Dis Child* 145:1374, 1991.

Kornberg A et al: Should corticosteroids be used in the treatment of bacterial meningitis? *Pediatr Emerg Care* 7:234, 1991.

Lebel M et al: Dexamethasone therapy for bacterial meningitis, *N Engl J Med* 319:963, 1989.

McCracken G: Current management of bacterial meningitis in infants and children, *Pediatr Infect Dis J* 11:169, 1992.

McCracken G et al: Consensus report: antimicrobial therapy for bacterial meningitis in infants and children, *Pediatr Infect Dis J* 6:501, 1986.

Rautonen J et al: Prognostic factors in childhood acute encephalitis, *Pediatr Infect Dis J* 10:441, 1991.

Saez-Llorens X et al: Brain abscess in infants and children, *Pediatr Infect Dis J* 8:449, 1989.

Wildin S, Chonmaitree T: The importance of the virology laboratory in the diagnosis and management of viral meningitis, *Am J Dis Child* 141:454, 1987.

Rett syndrome

Kozinetz C et al: Epidemiology of Rett syndrome, *Pediatrics* 91:445, 1993.

Moeschler J et al: Rett syndrome: natural history and management, *Pediatrics* 82:1, 1988.

Seizures, febrile seizures, and status epilepticus

Burg F, Ingelfinger J, Wald E, editors: *Gellis and Kagan's current pediatric therapy,* ed 15, Philadelphia, 1996, WB Saunders.

Camfield C, Camfield P: Febrile seizures: an Rx for parent fears and anxieties, *Contemp Pediatr* 10:26, 1993.

Consensus Development Panel: Febrile seizures: long-term management of children with fever-associated seizures, *Pediatr Rev* 2:209, 1987.

Farwell J: Febrile seizures, *Pediatr Ann* 20:25, 1991.

Freeman J: What have we learned from febrile seizures? *Pediatr Ann* 21:355, 1992.

Freeman J, Vining P: Decision making and the child with febrile seizures, *Pediatr Rev* 13:298, 1992.

Freeman J, Vining P: Decision making and the child with afebrile seizures, *Pediatr Rev* 13:305, 1992.

Mikati M: The newer antiepileptic drugs: carbamazepine and valproic acid, *Pediatr Ann* 20:34, 1991.

Papazian O: Common epileptic syndromes in children, *Pediatr Ann* 20:15, 1991.

Selbst S: Office management of status epilepticus, *Pediatr Emerg Care* 7:106, 1991.

Shinnar S, Ballaban-Gil K: An approach to the child with the first unprovoked seizure, *Pediatr Ann* 20:29, 1991.

Shunt malfunction

Key C et al: Cerebrospinal fluid shunt complications: an emergency medicine perspective, *Pediatr Emerg Care* 11:265, 1995.

Meirovitch J et al: Cerebrospinal fluid shunt infections in children, *Pediatr Infect Dis J* 6:921, 1987.

Piatt J: Physical examination of patients with cerebrospinal fluid shunts: is there useful information in pumping the shunt? *Pediatrics* 89:470, 1992.

Syncope

Hardy C: Syncope and chest pain: to worry or not? *Contemp Pediatr* 11:19, 1994.

Pratt J, Fleisher G: Syncope in children and adolescents, *Pediatr Emerg Care* 5:80, 1989.

Ruckman R: Cardiac causes of syncope, *Pediatr Rev* 9:101, 1987.

Tics and Tourette's syndrome

Barabas G: Tourette's syndrome: an overview, *Pediatr Ann* 17:391, 1988.

Erenberg G: Pharmacologic therapy of tics in childhood, *Pediatr Ann* 17:395, 1988.

Frantz D: Tremor in childhood, *Pediatr Ann* 22:60, 1993.

Golden G: Movement disorders: sorting the benign from the serious, *Contemp Pediatr* 4:77, 1987.

Golden G: Tic disorders in childhood, *Pediatr Rev* 8:229, 1987.

Ostfeld B: Psychological interventions in Tourette syndrome, *Pediatr Ann* 17:417, 1988.

Pranzatelli M: Miscellaneous movement disorders in childhood, *Pediatr Ann* 22:65, 1993.

Roddy S: Bad habit, simple tic, or Tourette syndrome, *Contemp Pediatr* 6:22, 1989.

Shapiro A, Shapiro E, Fulop G: Pimozide treatment of tic and Tourette disorders, *Pediatrics* 79:1032, 1987.

Shelov S: Tourette syndrome: abstract, *Pediatr Rev* 13:37, 1992.

Singer H: Tic disorders, *Pediatr Ann* 22:22, 1993.

OPHTHALMOLOGY   *15*

A. CONJUNCTIVITIS (PINK EYE)

1. Evaluation: Conjunctivitis must be differentiated from a more serious ocular inflammation (e.g., keratitis, iritis).
   a. Conjunctivitis: Diffuse redness of conjunctiva (more prominent on palpebral surface); associated with watery or purulent discharge; usually no photophobia; minimal pain; near-normal vision; normal pupillary and red reflexes. Causes are bacterial, viral, allergic, or chemical.
   b. Keratitis: Acute inflammation of the cornea associated with extreme pain, tearing, and photophobia. Causes are bacteria, viruses, fungi, and ultraviolet light (e.g., sun, sunlamps).

   NOTE: Do not miss corneal ulcers or lacerations; a clue might be an irregular corneal light reflex. Corneal injury may precede keratitis. The patient may have combined keratoconjunctivitis.

   c. Iritis: Red eye with tearing, circumlimbal injection (not seen in conjunctivitis), photophobia, pain, and little or no discharge. The pupil may be smaller and ± irregular; red reflex may be lost. Vision is often blurred. Refer to ophthalmologist if iritis or keratitis is suspected.

2. Diagnosis and therapy
   a. Neonatal
      1) Chemical
         a) Secondary to silver nitrate drops or antibiotic ointment
         b) Begins during the first 24-48 hours and clears in the next 24-48 hours; no treatment needed
      2) Bacterial
         a) There are a wide variety of gram-positive and gram-negative organisms, but by far the most serious is *Neisseria gonorrhoeae.*
         b) Gonococcal conjunctivitis presents as bilateral purulent eye drainage 2-6 days after birth. It is especially likely in settings of inadequate prenatal care and maternal substance abuse.
         c) Diagnosis is confirmed by Gram's stain and culture.

d) Treatment options
   (1) IM or IV ceftriaxone 25-50 mg/kg/d as a single dose × 7 days. Use cautiously in infants at risk for hyperbilirubinemia.
   (2) IM or IV cefotaxime 100 mg/kg/d in two divided doses × 7 days
   (3) IV penicillin G 100,000 U/kg/d in two divided doses × 7 days
   (4) Buffered saline eye flushes
   (5) Mother and sexual partner(s) should be referred for evaluation and treatment.
3) *Chlamydia trachomatis* (inclusion blennorrhea)
   a) Most common identifiable cause of neonatal conjunctivitis; incubation period 5-14 days
   b) Presents as mild hyperemia with scant discharge to severe hyperemia, copious purulent discharge, pseudomembrane formation, and chemosis
   c) Diagnosis
      (1) Giemsa stain of conjunctival scrapings showing basophilic cytoplasmic inclusions
      (2) Direct fluorescent antibody test (e.g., MicroTrak)
      (3) DNA probes
      (4) Enzyme immunoassay
      (5) Culture
   d) Treatment
      (1) PO erythromycin estolate or ethylsuccinate 50 mg/kg/d in four divided doses × 14 days
      (2) No need for topical therapy
      (3) Treatment should be offered to mother and sexual partner(s), even if they are asymptomatic.
4) Viral: Isolated HSV infection is rare in neonates. It usually occurs in association with infection at other sites.
b. Older infants and children
   1) Bacterial
      a) Presents as unilateral or bilateral purulent exudate and crusting of lashes. It is often associated with otitis media in infants and toddlers.
      b) The most common pathogens are nontypable *Haemophilus influenzae*, *Streptococcus pneumoniae*, and *Staphylococcus epidermidis*. *Staphylococcus aureus* is probably not a common pathogen except after trauma or surgery.

c) Diagnosis is based on the clinical presentation. Gram's stain is helpful, but cultures are not routinely indicated.
d) Treatment
    (1) Topical polymyxin-bacitracin ointment, 10% sodium sulfacetamide drops, gentamicin drops, polymyxin B–trimethoprim drops
    (2) Although bacterial conjunctivitis is self-limited, topical therapy is associated with faster symptom resolution and bacterial eradication.

NOTE: The use of an oral antibiotic such as amoxicillin may prevent the subsequent development of otitis media in young children who have only conjunctivitis.

2) Viral
    a) Often bilateral with watery discharge, ± photophobia. It may be associated with preauricular adenopathy and pharyngitis.
    b) Most cases result from adenovirus.
    c) Treatment is not usually indicated, but it is often difficult to differentiate a viral from a bacterial etiology; if in doubt, a short course of topical antibiotic is the best course of action.

NOTE: Epidemic keratoconjunctivitis (adenovirus type 8 and others) is extremely contagious. To minimize spread, thorough hand-washing and contact precautions are imperative for family members, as well as day care, school, and medical personnel.

    d) Primary HSV infection may involve the eyelid, conjunctiva, and cornea.
        (1) HSV infection usually presents as unilateral follicular conjunctivitis with preauricular adenopathy, photophobia, tearing, and blurred vision; there may be satellite vesicular lesions. Recurrent HSV infection usually presents as dendritic keratitis.
        (2) Diagnosis is by Tzanck smear and culture.
        (3) Treatment (in conjunction with ophthalmologist)
            (a) Trifluorothymidine 1% solution (Viroptic) applied q2h while awake × 10-15 days
            (b) Vidarabine (Vira-A) or idoxuridine 0.5% ointment for lid involvement

NOTE: Topical steroids are contraindicated for conjunctivitis if there is any possibility of HSV infection.

3) Allergic
    a) Bilateral conjunctivitis with itching, redness, periorbital

edema, tearing, ± photophobia. There is usually a seasonal pattern with other atopic manifestations; there may be a secondary bacterial infection.

  b) Treatment
    (1) Decongestants: Naphazoline (Vascocon-A, Naphcon-A, or Albalon-A drops)
    (2) Ketorolac (Acular), levocabastine (Livostin), lodoxamide 1% (Alomide)
    (3) Systemic antihistamine
    (4) Attempt to identify and eliminate the allergen (a topical antibiotic may be the culprit).

NOTE: Vernal conjunctivitis is a severe form of allergic conjunctivitis, which produces giant papillae of the conjunctivae and may be associated with photophobia and keratitis. The mast-cell stabilizers lodoxamide (Alomide) 1% ophthalmic solution (1-2 gtt qid) or cromolyn 4% provide effective prophylaxis.

  4) Chronic conjunctivitis (>2 weeks)
    a) In young infants, the usual cause is nasolacrimal duct obstruction or chlamydia infection.
    b) In older children, consider allergy, blepharitis, *Chlamydia* organisms (sexually active teenagers), chemical irritants (chlorine, mascara, antibiotic eyedrops), retained foreign body, contact lens cleansing and wetting solution, and Parinaud's oculoglandular syndrome.
    c) Corneal problems, uveitis, and glaucoma may produce a red eye and be confused with conjunctivitis.
  5) Refer a patient with conjunctivitis to an ophthalmologist when any of the following are present:
    a) History of ocular injury or recent eye surgery
    b) Loss of visual acuity or significant pain
    c) Use of contact lenses
    d) Vesicles or ulceration
    e) Chronic or recurrent episodes

B. ORBITAL CELLULITIS

1. Orbital cellulitis is an infection of the orbital contents posterior to the orbital septum. It usually (90%) represents contiguous infection from the adjacent sinus, especially the ethmoid sinus.
2. Etiology: *S. aureus,* group A streptococcus, *S. pneumoniae, H. influenzae* type B
3. Onset is often insidious and is characterized by lid edema, chemosis, proptosis, pain on eye movement, decreased ocular mobility, and

decreased visual acuity. Marked proptosis, globe displacement, and impaired vision indicate abscess formation.

4. Treatment
   a. Admit patient for IV antibiotic therapy directed at the pathogens listed previously, including resistant *S. pneumoniae.*
   b. Obtain ophthalmology consult, blood culture, culture of any aspirated material (from abscess or sinus), and a CT scan of the orbit and sinuses.
   c. Surgical drainage of the sinus or orbital abscess may be necessary.

C. PERIORBITAL CELLULITIS (PRESEPTAL CELLULITIS)

1. Periorbital cellulitis is an acute onset of unilateral eyelid edema, erythema, a well-demarcated purplish hue *(H. influenzae),* tenderness of the overlying skin, and fever. The eye itself is usually normal. Differential diagnosis includes insect bite and chemosis secondary to severe conjunctivitis.
2. It may result from hematogenous spread (*H. influenzae* type B, *S. pneumoniae*) or local trauma *(S. aureus).*
3. Blood culture and CIE of tears and urine may help identify the organism; obtain a CT scan of the sinuses if no source is evident.
4. Treatment
   a. Treatment usually requires IV antibiotic therapy.
   b. Oral antibiotics may be adequate in mild cases.

NOTE: There is a 1%-2% incidence of bacterial meningitis in children who have orbital and periorbital cellulitis. An LP is indicated if there are signs and symptoms of meningeal irritation.

D. STYE (HORDEOLUM)

A stye is an infection (usually *S. aureus*) of one of the sebaceous glands along the lid margin. It causes a small, red, tender swelling that often suppurates and drains spontaneously.

1. Treatment consists of applying warm moist compresses × 15 minutes qid and continuing until several days after clinical resolution.
2. A local ophthalmic ointment (bacitracin, erythromycin) may be helpful.
3. Systemic antibiotics and incision and drainage are rarely indicated.

E. CHALAZION

A chalazion is a sterile granulomatous inflammation of a meibomian gland (one of numerous sebaceous glands in the eyelid tarsus). It results in a slow-growing, firm, nodular swelling that most often points on the conjunctival aspect of the lid and usually causes little discomfort.

1. If the chalazion becomes secondarily infected (inflamed and tender), apply warm, moist compresses × 15 minutes qid; continue until 1 week after clinical resolution.
2. If a chalazion persists for many months, it can be injected with a steroid (triamcinolone) or incised with evacuation of its contents by an ophthalmologist.

F. CHEMICAL BURNS

Burns from strong acids and (especially) strong alkalis can be devastating.

1. Profuse irrigation of the eye with tap water should be instituted as soon as possible. If a family member calls with such an injury, instruct that person to irrigate the eye immediately at home (being careful to retract both lids) and then bring the patient to the ED.
2. In the ED, apply 1-2 gtt of a topical anesthetic, proparacaine HCl 0.5% (Ophthetic), to the eye to facilitate irrigation with an elevated bottle of normal saline and an IV tubing set. This procedure is a convenient way to provide a controlled and copious flow of irrigation fluid. Swab the upper and lower fornices to remove foreign material. Litmus paper touched to the conjunctival surface should register in the neutral range when irrigation is satisfactory.
3. Refer to an ophthalmologist for assessment of the extent of injury.

G. CORNEAL ABRASIONS AND FOREIGN BODIES

Corneal abrasions and foreign bodies are usually unilateral. Perform a fluorescein stain. Otherwise, refer to an ophthalmologist.

1. If the abrasion is large or over the central cornea, refer to an ophthalmologist.
2. A simple abrasion with no suspicion of a retained foreign body is treated with a single application of erythromycin or bacitracin ointment and a tight eye patch × 24-48 hours.
3. Foreign bodies require prompt removal by an ophthalmologist, usually followed by a local antibiotic and patching.

H. BLUNT OCULAR TRAUMA (BLACK EYE OR SHINER)

With blunt ocular trauma, a complete eye and retinal exam is indicated, including an eye movement test to detect injury to the inferior rectus muscle. Look for a blow-out fracture of the orbital floor, retinal detachment, hyphema, a dislocated lens, and traumatic iritis. Refer to an ophthalmologist if there is any suspicion of these complications, and always if vision is reduced.

I. PENETRATING OCULAR TRAUMA

A perforation site can usually be seen with the naked eye. Another sign is distortion of the pupil. Apply a metal shield over the eye, and do *not* put pressure on the eye. Refer to an ophthalmologist.

NOTE: Do not forget to measure visual acuity during the initial evaluation of a patient with ocular trauma. Use the Snellen chart, Allen picture cards, or the "E" game. For children under 2 years of age, observe the ability to reach for a small object using only the damaged eye.

J. DACRYOSTENOSIS

Dacryostenosis results from congenital nasolacrimal duct obstruction and is characterized by excessive tearing in the involved eye and crusting of the lids on awakening. There may also be mild conjunctival injection and a purulent discharge. Symptoms usually begin in the first few days to weeks of life, and 90% of cases remit during the first 8-12 months.

1. Treatment involves massaging the lacrimal sac bid and applying sulfacetamide 10% drops, polymyxin B–trimethoprim drops, or erythromycin ointment if purulent drainage is present.
2. Probing of the nasolacrimal duct is indicated if the obstruction persists >8-12 months.

K. DACRYOCYSTITIS

Dacryocystitis represents delayed canalization of the nasolacrimal duct with superimposed infection characterized by swelling, tenderness, and erythema below the medial canthus.

1. Treat with IV or PO antibiotics effective against *S. aureus, H. influenzae,* and *S. pneumoniae.*
2. Warm compresses may speed resolution.
3. Once inflammation has diminished, lacrimal drainage system probing may be performed.

L. BLEPHARITIS

Blepharitis represents an inflammatory condition of the eyelid margin.

1. Blepharitis presents as erythema of the lid with flaking scales along the lid margin, inspissated plugs of fibrinous exudate encircling the eyelashes, and breakage and possible loss of eyelashes; it may lead to chalazion formation.
2. It is usually associated with seborrhea. Other causes include HSV infection and lice infestation. There may be secondary bacterial infection *(S. aureus, S. epidermidis).*
3. Treatment

a. Lid hygiene, debridement with diluted (1:1) tearless baby shampoo, topical antibiotic
b. For severe pruritus, a short-term course of topical steroid (dexamethasone phosphate 0.05%) may be helpful.

BIBLIOGRAPHY

Baker JD: Treatment of congenital nasolacrimal system obstruction, *J Pediatr Ophthalmol Strabismus* 22:34, 1985.

Bodor FF et al: Bacterial etiology of conjunctivitis: otitis media syndrome, *Pediatrics* 76:26, 1985.

El-Mansoury J et al: Results of late probing for congenital nasolacrimal duct obstruction, *Ophthalmology* 93:1052, 1986.

Friedlander MH et al: Diagnosis of allergic conjunctivitis, *Arch Ophthalmol* 102:1198, 1984.

Gigliotti F: Acute conjunctivitis, *Pediatr Rev* 16:203, 1995.

Gigliotti F et al: Efficacy of topical antibiotic therapy in acute conjunctivitis in children, *J Pediatr* 104:623, 1984.

Hammerschlag MR: Neonatal conjunctivitis, *Pediatr Ann* 22:346, 1993.

Hammerschlag MR et al: Enzyme immunoassay for diagnosis of neonatal chlamydia conjunctivitis, *J Pediatr* 1076:741, 1985.

Knox DL: Uveitis, *Pediatr Clin North Am* 34:1467, 1987.

Lavrich JB, Nelson LB: Disorders of the lacrimal system apparatus, *Pediatr Clin North Am* 40:767, 1993.

Lohr JA: Treatment of conjunctivitis in infants and children, *Pediatr Ann* 22:359, 1993.

MacEwen CJ, Yang JD: Epiphora in the first year of life, *Eye* 5:596, 1991.

Newell FW: *Ophthalmology: principles and concepts,* ed 5, St Louis, 1982, Mosby.

Ogawa GSH, Gonnering RS: Congenital nasolacrimal duct obstruction, *J Pediatr* 119:12, 1991.

Persaud D, Moss WT, Munoz JL: Serious eye infections in children, *Pediatr Ann* 22:379, 1993.

Rettig PJ: Chlamydial infections in pediatrics: diagnostic and therapeutic considerations, *Pediatr Infect Dis J* 5:158, 1986.

Robb RM: Probing and irrigation for congenital nasolacrimal duct obstruction, *Arch Ophthalmol* 104:378, 1986.

Sandstron KI et al: Microbial causes of neonatal conjunctivitis, *J Pediatr* 105:706, 1984.

ORTHOPEDICS

16

Paul D. Sponseller

A. BOWLEGS (GENU VARUM)

1. Infants are physiologically bowlegged because of their intrauterine position; however, this physiologic state corrects itself by 18-24 months of age. The child's knee then develops decided valgus before assuming the mild valgus of adulthood (Fig. 16-1). The degree of bowleggedness is appreciated on examination by bringing the medial malleoli together and measuring the distance between the knees. Parents of children with *physiologic* bowing are often reassured if shown the graph in Fig. 16-1.

2. If correction has not begun by 24 months of age or if the degree of bowing is >20 degrees, x-ray studies of the lower limbs to rule out Blount disease or rickets (see Points 3 and 4) should be obtained. Physiologic bowing generally corrects by 2-3 years of age. Some orthopedists recommend the use of splints, braces, or shoe bars.

3. Blount disease (tibia vara) is the defective formation of the medial corner of the proximal tibial epiphysis, perhaps as a result of epiphyseal overload caused by early or excessive weight-bearing in a child with severe physiologic bowing. There are two variants, infantile and adolescent.

   a. The infantile variant occurs between 1 and 4 years of age.

      1) Initially, infants with Blount disease are indistinguishable from infants with physiologic bowing.

      2) However, after 2-3 years of age, the x-ray studies of children with Blount disease demonstrate angulation beneath the medial proximal epiphysis (Fig. 16-2), metaphyseal irregularities, proximal tibial breaking, and proximal epiphyseal wedging.

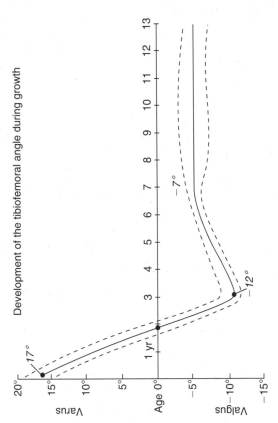

Development of the tibiofemoral angle during growth

FIG 16-1. "Bowed legs" and "knock knees." Note broad variation with age. Varus corrects to neutral at approximately 20 months of age and changes to valgus by 3 years of age, with slight valgus persisting to adulthood.

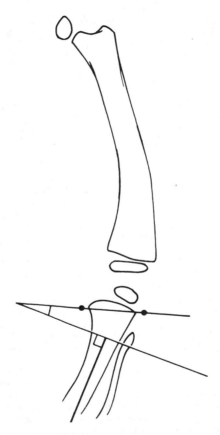

FIG 16-2. In early Blount disease, the metaphyseal-diaphyseal angle is >11 degrees.

3) Bracing with a valgus-producing brace may be effective if the condition is detected between 18 and 24 months of age.

4) Surgery is usually indicated after 3-4 years of age.

b. The adolescent variant develops in obese children (>8 years of age) or in adolescents whose legs have been in slight varus; it is much less common and milder (<20-degree bowing) than the infantile variant. Previous epiphyseal injury may be present. Spontaneous regression may occur; however, progressive cases require surgery.

4. Rickets represents deficient mineralization of the growing skeleton. The most common cause worldwide is deficient dietary vitamin D. The most common cause in the United States is familial hypophosphatemia.

B. DEVELOPMENTAL DYSPLASIA OF THE HIP

1. With DDH, the hip is dislocated as the femoral head is displaced from the shallow acetabulum. Two common factors in its causation are ligamentous laxity and intrauterine breech position. The male-to-female ratio is 1:4-6. Genetic predisposition seems likely.

2. Infants with DDH usually (but not universally) have the following:

   a. A positive Barlow's sign (hip is dislocatable by flexion, adduction, and axial pressure) (Fig. 16-3) and a positive Ortolani's sign (as the flexed hip is slowly abducted, the femoral head shifts into the acetabulum, producing a "soft clunk") (Fig. 16-4). These maneuvers should be performed on one hip at a time.

   b. After age 3-6 months when muscle contractures develop, the Barlow and Ortolani tests become negative. Thigh-fold asymmetry, leg-length discrepancy (which is best observed when the infant is in the supine position and the hips and knees are flexed to 90 degrees), and limitation of hip abduction on the affected side are then seen (Fig. 16-5).

3. Older children with untreated DDH have a characteristic gait. Because the abductor muscles on the affected side are shortened and weakened, the opposite side of the pelvis drops during the stance phase on the affected side (Trendelenburg gait). Children with bilateral DDH have wide-set hips, a double Trendelenburg (waddling) gait, and exaggerated lumbar lordosis.

4. X-ray studies during the neonatal period are not necessarily diagnostic but become so as the infant ages. Ultrasound of the hips, performed by an experienced pediatric sonographer, may be diagnostic.

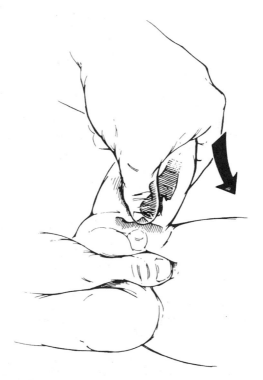

FIG 16-3. Barlow's test. Flexion-adduction and axial pressure elicit laxity or a "clunk" in an abnormal hip in a child up to 3-5 months of age.

5. Successful treatment of DDH in the neonatal period is most reliably achieved by the use of a Pavlik harness; this device holds the hip in reduction (hyperflexion [90-100 degrees] with no more than 60 degrees of abduction), allows the infant to be diapered and cleaned, and permits some movement by the infant.

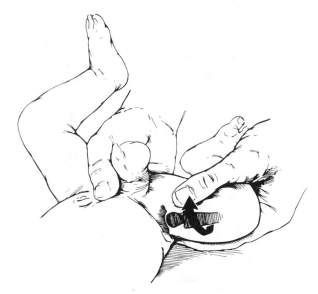

FIG 16-4. Ortolani's test involves reduction of the dislocated hip by abduction in the flexed position. Examine only one hip at a time. This test is useful in children up to 3-5 months of age.

    a. Extremes of flexion and abduction must be avoided because such extremes are associated with avascular necrosis and severe hip deformity.

    b. Infants 6-18 months of age at diagnosis usually require traction, reduction under arthrographic control, and subsequent casting. Open surgery may be needed if closed reduction is not possible. Avascular necrosis may still occur.

    c. Children 18-48 months of age at diagnosis require surgery (muscle release, open reduction, and pelvic or femoral osteotomy) to obtain a stable hip. Avascular necrosis is a more common complication.

    d. Children older than 48 months of age at diagnosis require more extensive surgical intervention. The risks and benefits of surgery with potential complications must be carefully discussed.

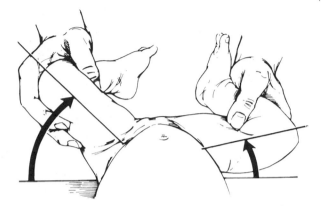

FIG 16-5. In the older child with fixed dysplasia and in whom Barlow's and Ortolani's signs cannot be elicited, the main signs are limited abduction and apparent shortening.

C. IN-TOEING (FEMORAL ANTEVERSION AND INTERNAL TIBIAL TORSION)

1. In evaluating the child who is in-toeing, the following three common conditions should be considered: metatarsus adductus (see Section H), which is usually seen before 1½ years of age; internal tibial torsion, 1½-4 years of age; and femoral anteversion, 3-8 years of age. These conditions can be sorted by a systematic exam (Fig. 16-6). The angle of the foot in walking should be noted. The child should be placed in the prone position, and the thigh-foot angle, shape of the foot, and hip rotation should be checked.
2. Tibial torsion measures 0-20 degrees at birth; with growth, derotation occurs until the adult configuration of 0-40 degrees (average 20 degrees) of *external* tibial torsion is reached.
   a. The angle is measured as follows: The knee is flexed to 90 degrees. The medial and lateral malleoli are palpated; in a neonate, the malleoli may be parallel or the medial malleolus may lie posterior to the lateral malleolus; in the adult, the medial malleolus is anterior to the lateral one.
   b. The angle may also be measured (with the child in the prone

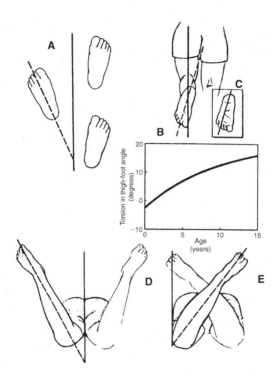

FIG 16-6. Steps in assessing rotational abnormality. **A,** Angle of the foot during walking should be observed. **B,** Thigh-foot angle reflects tibial torsion and becomes more external with age. **C,** Bleck's line indicates the degree of forefoot adduction. Heel bisector should normally fall between the second and third toe. Here it falls lateral, indicating metatarsus adductus. Hip rotation occurs if internal rotation (**D**) is significantly greater than that of external rotation (**E**). Anteversion or capsular tightness contributes to in-toeing.

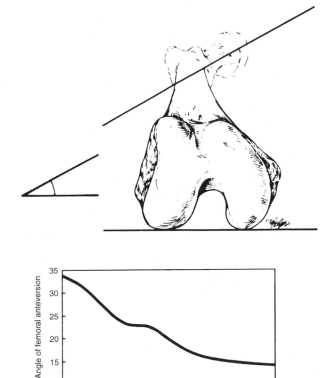

FIG 16-7. Definition of anteversion and its normal variation.

position and the knee flexed) by estimating the angle between the foot axis and the long axis of the thigh (see Fig. 16-6).
3. Growth alone corrects the vast majority (99%) of cases of tibial torsion by 3-4 years of age.

a. Night splints (Denis Browne splints) currently are believed to be of no real benefit.
b. Shoe modifications are of no value.
c. Rarely (1 per 1000 cases) is surgery needed.
4. Excessive femoral anteversion occurs when the femoral neck is rotated forward or anteriorly more than usual from the femoral shaft (Fig. 16-7). When the child stands, the leg rotates internally to accommodate the femoral head into the acetabulum. The underlying cause of excessive femoral anteversion is unknown. The child with femoral anteversion may have internal rotation of the leg, flexible flat feet, genu recurvatum, and increased lumbar lordosis. On examination with the child in the prone position, internal rotation markedly exceeds external rotation (up to 90 degrees vs. 30 degrees); normally, external exceeds internal rotation.
5. Treatment consists of reassurance. By 8 years of age, 99% of all children with this condition experience resolution. Even if it persists, anteversion generally results in no functional hindrance.
a. Surgery is necessary for the 1% of children with severe deformity (internal hip rotation ≥80 degrees, external rotation ≤15 degrees, severe gait deformity, and absence of compensatory external tibial torsion).
b. Braces and cables have no influence on femoral anteversion.

D. JOINT PAIN AND JOINT SWELLING
1. Arthritis vs. arthralgia
   a. Arthritis: Swelling of a joint or limitation of motion accompanied by heat, pain, and tenderness
   b. Arthralgia: Subjective complaint of joint pain or tenderness without swelling or limitation of motion
   c. Joint swelling can occur secondary to the following:
      1) Periarticular soft-tissue swelling (angioneurotic edema, tenosynovitis)
      2) Thickened synovium (JRA, hemophilia)
      3) Joint effusion (septic arthritis, Lyme disease, acute rheumatic fever, transient synovitis, JRA, trauma)
      4) Bony enlargement (traumatic arthritis)
2. General: Joint complaints are common in children. In most cases the problem is transient and is the result of trauma or strenuous activity. The patient needs to be evaluated for evidence of tendonitis, myositis, myalgia, and muscular or ligamentous strain. Pain and loss of motion can result from changes at musculoskeletal sites

other than joints. Bone, muscle, nerve, and referred pain can be confused with arthritis.

3. Evaluation

a. History: Which joints are involved? Characteristics (large joints, small joints; monarticular, polyarticular, symmetric, migratory, duration)? Systemic manifestations (fever, rash, weight loss, stool abnormalities)? Response to antiinflammatory drugs? Family history? Recent trauma, new activities, immunizations, exposure to infections (e.g., hepatitis, rubella, gonorrhea, mononucleosis)?

b. PE should be complete but should focus on bone, joint, muscle, and nerve status. Useful findings include rash (JRA, HSP, serum sickness, gonococcal infection, Lyme disease, Kawasaki disease, inflammatory conditions), hepatosplenomegaly, lymphadenopathy, eye changes on slit-lamp exam, and a positive joint exam. Look for evidence of hypermobility.

c. Laboratory studies: These studies should be based on the findings of the history and PE.

1) CBC: Leukocytosis favors an infectious or inflammatory cause.

2) ESR and CRP elevations favor an infectious or inflammatory cause. A highly elevated ESR is *not* usually seen in traumatic, mechanical orthopedic problems.

3) ANA and rheumatoid factor are helpful if positive but are not very sensitive tests.

4) Synovial fluid exam and culture; blood, throat, and stool cultures; monospot test; and antibody titers (EBV, parvovirus, *Borrelia* organisms) are helpful in selected patients with suspected infection. In patients with acute monarticular arthritis, an elevated ESR or CRP, temperature >38.5°C, and leukocytosis are independent predictors for the diagnosis of septic arthritis. In a patient whose symptoms exceed 2 weeks, a low CRP, absence of fever, and elevated IgG are independent predictors for the diagnosis of JRA.

5) Perform bone marrow aspiration in patients with suspected malignancy.

6) U/A: HSP

d. Imaging

1) An x-ray examination is indicated in patients with suspected orthopedic problems (e.g., trauma, Legg-Calvé-Perthes disease, slipped capital femoral epiphysis), osteoid osteoma, and malignancy.

2) Radionuclide joint and bone scans may be useful (e.g., malignancy, diskitis, osteoid osteoma, toddler's fracture, Legg-Calvé-Perthes disease). Bone scintigraphy is useful with occult bone and periosteal injuries (child abuse, sports injuries) and *may* differentiate among septic arthritis, cellulitis, and osteomyelitis.

3) Ultrasound of the hip is useful for joint effusion (transient synovitis) and thickened synovium.

4) CT scan may localize a foreign body in a patient with monarticular arthritis.

e. Arthroscopy: Useful for evaluating traumatic or mechanical joint problems

4. Differential diagnosis

a. Trauma and orthopedic conditions

1) Child abuse

2) Femoral neck anteversion

3) Legg-Calvé-Perthes disease

4) Osgood-Schlatter disease

5) Osteochondritis dissecans

6) Osteoid osteoma

7) Slipped capital femoral epiphysis

8) Sports injuries

9) Subluxation or chondromalacia of patella (patella-femoral pain syndrome)

b. Inflammatory conditions

1) Acute rheumatic fever

2) Allergic reactions, serum sickness

3) Connective tissue disorders (e.g., SLE)

4) Inflammatory bowel disease

5) JRA

6) Psoriatic arthritis

7) Vasculitis: HSP, Kawasaki disease, periarteritis

c. Infections and postinfections

1) Antecedent enterobacterial infections (*Salmonella, Shigella,* and *Yersinia* organisms)

2) Gonococcal infections

3) Lyme disease

4) *Mycoplasma* organisms

5) Osteomyelitis

6) Periarticular cellulitis

7) Septic arthritis

8) Viral infections (hepatitis, mononucleosis, parvovirus, rubella)
d. Miscellaneous
   1) Foreign body synovitis, arthritis
   2) Hypermobility syndromes
   3) Inflammatory bowel disease
   4) Malignancy
   5) Neuropathic arthropathy
   6) Psychogenic conditions
   7) Sickle-cell disease
   8) Transient synovitis of the hip
e. Diagnostic tips
   1) Fever and ESR are the most useful screening parameters. An elevation of either suggests an inflammatory or infectious origin.
   2) A normal ESR and the absence of fever are strongly *against* an inflammatory or infectious cause but may be seen in pauciarticular JRA.
   3) In monarticular disease, a positive joint exam in association with fever or an elevated ESR suggests septic arthritis or osteomyelitis.
   4) A positive joint exam *not* associated with fever or an elevated ESR suggests an orthopedic problem but may also occur with JRA, SLE, and psoriatic arthritis.
   5) A rash is predictive of inflammatory disorders.
5. Specific disorders
   a. Gonococcal arthritis: There are two forms; GU infection is usually asymptomatic with both.
      1) Multiple large (knees, wrists, and ankles) and small joints are involved, often in association with fever, chills, and skin lesions. The blood culture may be positive.
      2) Monarticular arthritis with minimal systemic signs and symptoms: Blood culture is negative, but organisms may be recovered from a joint effusion and from skin lesions. It may present as repeated episodes of tenosynovitis coincident with menses.
   b. Hypermobility syndrome: May occur with a number of syndromes or as a distinct clinical entity. Along with evidence of hypermobility, the patient usually has recurrent episodes of self-limited arthralgias involving multiple joints. Episodes may last for several days to several weeks.
   c. JRA: After excluding other possibilities, consider JRA in patients

with arthritis that lasts more than 6 weeks. JRA may present in one of three forms as follows:

1) Systemic: Multiple joints and prominent constitutional symptoms (rash, spiking fevers); 10%-15% of patients

2) Polyarticular: >4 joints; often symmetric and often involves the hands; minor systemic manifestations; 15% of patients

3) Pauciarticular: ≤4 joints; systemic involvement rare; young girls (<4 years of age) with pauciarticular disease and + ANA are at high risk for uveitis; 70% of patients

4) Conditions often confused with JRA include soft-tissue pain resulting from myalgia, malignancy, hypermobility syndromes, infectious arthritis, "growing pains," and psychogenic pain. Misdiagnosis is especially common in patients with monarticular disease. ANA and rheumatoid factor screens are helpful if positive but are not very sensitive.

NOTE: The diagnosis of JRA should be considered in children with chronic joint swelling, even in the absence of pain; 25% of children with pauciarticular JRA report no pain.

    d. Lyme disease

1) Lyme disease is a tickborne, immune-mediated, inflammatory response to the deer tick–borne spirochete, *Borrelia burgdorferi*. It is reported in most states, but distinct foci are in the Northeast, upper Midwest, and coastal California and Oregon. The onset of illness is generally from May to November, with the peak in June to July.

2) Typically, clinical features occur in 3 stages, but there is considerable overlap, and features of late Lyme disease may develop without any history of early disease. Only one third of patients remember a previous tick bite.

    a) Stage 1 (early localized infection): Occurs 2-30 days after the bite. Erythema migrans appears at the site of the bite; it starts as an erythematous papule or macule that develops into an expanding (at least 5 cm) erythematous annular lesion with central clearing. It is most common on the lower extremities but may occur on the face and axillae. It is often accompanied by fever and mild constitutional symptoms. Some children with Lyme disease have a history of an antecedent flulike illness *without* erythema migrans.

    b) Stage 2 (early disseminated infection): Occurs 1-4 months after the bite; multiple erythema migrans–like cutaneous lesions; asymmetric oligoarthritis; neurologic involvement (cranial nerve palsies, aseptic meningitis, encephalitis); cardiac involvement (myocarditis, A-V block)

   c) Stage 3 (late persistent infection): Occurs weeks to 2 years after the bite; arthritis, encephalopathy, and neuropathy occur. Arthritis often starts abruptly with swelling, pain, redness, and ± effusion of large joints, especially the knee; however, small joints of the hands and feet may be involved. The swelling is often out of proportion to the degree of pain. Attacks may last from days to months, with frequent recurrences during the first year after onset. Arthritis may be accompanied by fatigue, but fever and other systemic symptoms are unusual; 10% of patients develop chronic arthritis.

3) Diagnosis

   a) Most clinical manifestations of Lyme disease are nonspecific and may be present in a variety of other diseases. The condition is overdiagnosed, mostly as a result of the misuse and misinterpretation of serologic tests.

   b) The diagnosis should be based on a careful clinical and epidemiologic evaluation. Serologic testing should be performed *only* when the clinical evaluation suggests the diagnosis. Serologic test results should never be the sole criteria for the diagnosis of Lyme disease. In endemic areas there may be a high incidence of seropositive results among individuals who have never had clinically apparent disease.

   c) Confirmation of the diagnosis is based on the demonstration of *Borrelia* antibodies by ELISA. Specific IgM antibodies appear 3-4 weeks after infection begins, peak after 6-8 weeks, and decline. Specific IgG antibodies appear 6-8 weeks after the onset of infection, peak after 4-6 months, and may remain elevated indefinitely.

NOTE: Early treatment may blunt the antibody response. Once the IgG antibody has developed, antimicrobial treatment may result in a decline in titer, but the antibody is usually detectable for several years.

   d) Serologic testing performed in reference laboratories (CDC, State Health Department) is reliable. Commercially available serologic testing kits have poor sensitivity and specificity (high percentage of false-positive results because of cross-reacting antibodies) and are not reliable.

   e) Immunoblotting (Western blot) is a useful way to validate positive or equivocal ELISA results.

       f) Serologic testing is not indicated for patients with definite erythema migrans. The patient should be treated for Lyme disease irrespective of the serologic test results.

       g) In patients with early disseminated disease and possible CNS involvement, an LP should be performed and the CSF should be tested for *Borrelia* antibodies.

       h) Serologic confirmation should be obtained for patients with suspected late persistent infection. A negative result makes the diagnosis unlikely; a positive result does not definitively establish Lyme disease as the cause of the illness but merely establishes that the patient was at some time infected with *B. burgdorferi*.

4) Treatment

    a) Early localized infection, mild carditis or arthritis, isolated Bell's palsy

       (1) <9 years of age: Penicillin V potassium or amoxicillin, 1-2 g/d or 25-50 mg/kg/d in divided doses

       (2) >9 years of age: Doxycycline 100 mg bid, tetracycline 250 mg qid, or amoxicillin 500 mg tid

       (3) The duration of treatment is 10-30 days depending on manifestations and the clinical response.

       (4) Although it may be less effective, erythromycin 30 mg/kg/d ÷ qid is an acceptable alternative for patients who are allergic to penicillin.

    b) Severe carditis or persistent arthritis

       (1) Penicillin G 300,000 U/kg/d (max 20 million U) IV × 14-30 days
         or

       (2) Ceftriaxone 75-100 mg/kg/d (max 2 g) IV × 14-30 days

    c) Neurologic involvement: Ceftriaxone 75-100 mg/kg/d (max 2 g) IV × 14-30 days

    d) Relapses can occur and require retreatment with the same or other antibiotics.

NOTE: In Lyme-endemic areas, patients who have fever and fatigue within a month after a deer-tick bite should be considered for empiric antimicrobial treatment.

5) Prognosis

    a) Among untreated patients, 80% develop arthritis or neurologic or cardiac complications.

    b) Most treated children are disease-free after a year of follow-up, irrespective of the stage of infection at the time of treatment. However, such patients may have subsequent episodes of erythema migrans.

6) Prevention

a) In endemic areas, wear clothing with long sleeves and long pants. Inspect children and pets daily for ticks.

b) Remove ticks by grasping with a fine tweezer close to the skin and pulling gently after a tick bite.

c) Antibiotic prophylaxis is not indicated.

e. Malignancies: The patient may have localized or diffuse bone pain or "arthritis" as an early sign of unrecognized malignancy (leukemia, neuroblastoma). There may be true arthritis secondary to bony, capsular, or periosteal lesions. In acute leukemia, pain tends to involve few joints, is evanescent, and is often out of proportion to the findings of the exam. Night pain, pain without stiffness, nonarticular bone pain, and a refusal to walk should always raise suspicion of leukemia. X-ray studies, radionuclide scans, and bone marrow aspirates are eventually diagnostic but may not become positive for many months.

f. Mechanical problems: Complaints are often chronic, and the diagnosis is suggested by the history. In the absence of fever and an elevated ESR, a positive joint exam suggests an orthopedic disorder. An x-ray examination and MRI may be helpful.

g. Parvovirus-associated arthritis: In children, infection with human parvovirus B19 may be associated with arthritis.

1) Patients have fever, anorexia, malaise, fatigue, pauciarticular or polyarticular arthritis/arthralgia; large joints (especially knee) >small joints. One third of the patients have a rash.

2) The diagnosis is suggested by the elevation of IgM anti–human parvovirus B19 antibody titer. ESR is usually normal; RA factor is not present. Imaging studies may show joint effusion or synovial thickening.

3) The duration of joint symptoms is generally brief; most resolve within 4 months. However, some children may develop chronic arthritis and fulfill the criteria for JRA.

h. Septic arthritis

1) For a patient with acute monarticular arthritis, an elevated ESR or CRP, a temperature >38.5° C, and leukocytosis are highly suggestive of septic arthritis. Cultures of blood and joint fluid are mandatory.

2) The hip, knee, and ankle are the most commonly affected joints.

3) Beyond 2 years of age, septic arthritis is usually associated

with trauma or skin infection *(Staphylococcus aureus)*; under 2 years of age, it is usually associated with URI symptoms (*S. aureus, Streptococcus pneumoniae, Haemophilus influenzae* type B). The introduction of HIB vaccine should reduce the frequency of infection caused by *Haemophilus* organisms.

4) Bone scintigraphy can occasionally be useful in differentiating septic arthritis from osteomyelitis and periarticular cellulitis.

E. KNOCK KNEES (GENU VALGUM)

1. Most children are slightly knock-kneed at 3-5 years of age; excessive knock knee may develop in late childhood or adolescence. With genu valgum, the medial malleoli cannot touch when the knees are touching. The child may walk and run awkwardly but does not experience pain.
2. Genu valgum may be any of the following:
   a. Apparent: Fat thighs, hypotonia, lax joints
   b. Pathologic: Paralytic disorders, JRA, rickets, trauma, bone infections
   c. Physiologic (idiopathic): Accounts for the vast majority of cases
3. The diagnosis of idiopathic genu valgum should be made by an x-ray examination of the child's legs while he or she is standing (feet straight ahead). This examination excludes some of the pathologic causes of the disorder.
4. Idiopathic genu valgum resolves spontaneously with growth. Fewer than 1% of children who are affected develop degenerative arthritis of the knee. Surgery may be needed in severe cases (i.e., >8 cm between medial malleoli) but is rare.

F. LEGG-CALVÉ-PERTHES DISEASE

1. Legg-Calvé-Perthes disease is avascular necrosis of the femoral head.
   a. The male-to-female ratio is 6:1.
   b. The etiology is unknown.
   c. Affected children are slightly shorter than their peers and have delayed maturation.
   d. Routine childhood trauma may bring an asymptomatic child to attention.
2. The disease lasts 1-3 years in most children. There are five stages, which are listed as follows:
   a. Prenecrosis, in which there is vascular compromise
   b. Necrosis (3-6 months), in which the affected section of bone dies with microfracture formation

    c. Revascularization (6-12 months), in which the dead bone is resorbed and replaced with cartilage

    d. Reossification (18-36 months), in which the deformed femoral head reossifies

    e. Remodeling, in which there is some improvement of the joint

3. The affected child has a limp, ± intermittent pain in the hip or thigh, and decreased hip motion (especially rotation and abduction).

4. The radiographic picture varies by the stage of the disease. There may be a widened joint space (growth failure), a lucent crescent under the femoral head margin, distortion of the femoral neck and head (shortened neck, flattened head), or loss of density in the metaphysis. A bone scan may quantify the amount of avascularity.

5. Treatment consists of restoring range of motion and maintaining the softened portion of the femur within the acetabular mold; doing so may require bed rest and is often combined with Buck's traction if the range of motion is limited. If there is minimal involvement of the femoral head (<50%) or if the child is under 6 years of age, observation alone is appropriate; check for maintenance of range of motion. If there is >50% involvement or if the child is older, an abduction brace or surgery may be used to set the femoral head within the acetabulum.

G. LIMP

1. A limp can be painless or painful.

    a. The causes of *painless* limp include an alteration in muscle tone, strength, or joint function. Specifically, these alterations include the following:

        1) Neurologic problems: Flaccid paralysis, spasticity, ataxia, spinal diseases such as masses or herniated disks

        2) Muscle disease: Muscular dystrophy, arthrogryposis

        3) Joint disorders: Contractures, hyperextensible joints, developmental dysplasia of the hip

        4) Bone disorders: Knock knees, leg-length discrepancies, Blount disease, tibial torsion, slipped capital femoral epiphysis, coxa vara, epiphyseal dysplasias, spondylolisthesis

        5) Hysteria or mimicry

        6) Generally, painless limps are insidious in onset. The child is not acutely ill. The cause is usually apparent from the PE, which must include a careful neurologic assessment to rule out intraspinal disorders.

    b. Causes of *painful* limp include the following:

        1) Trauma: Local, especially foot lesions or foreign bodies,

ligamentous strains and sprains, tendonitis, tendon tears, muscle bruises, fractures, injections, or patellar subluxation in adolescent girls

2) Infections: Septic joint, osteomyelitis, pyomyositis, intervertebral disk inflammation or infection, epidural abscess

3) Intraabdominal processes: Appendicitis, retroperitoneal mass, ileal adenitis

4) Inflammatory disorders: Toxic synovitis, rheumatic fever, JRA, SLE, other collagen-vascular disorders

5) Aseptic necrosis, osteochondritis, other orthopedic conditions: Legg-Calvé-Perthes disease, Osgood-Schlatter disease, chondromalacia patellae, osteochondritis dissecans, SCFE

6) Neoplasms: Leukemia, malignant and benign bone tumors

7) Hematologic disorders: Hemophilia with hemarthrosis, sickle-cell disease (hand-foot-and-mouth syndrome), phlebitis, scurvy

8) Miscellaneous: HSP, serum sickness, inflammatory bowel diseases

2. The painful limp may have an acute or gradual onset; the child may be febrile (infectious processes) or afebrile. Depending on the cause, the child may have GI symptoms or dermatologic findings.

a. The history should address all of these issues, with particular emphasis on the onset, progression, duration, aggravating factors, and measures to relieve the pain.

b. Other symptoms of illness should be elicited; ask about chronic conditions, medication use, previous orthopedic injury, or surgery.

c. Do not forget child abuse.

3. The PE should be complete.

a. The affected limb's appearance, joints, symmetry with mate, and range of motion (active and passive) should be assessed.

b. The limbs should be systematically palpated for tenderness because a minor buckle fracture may be subtle. The most commonly involved areas are the distal tibia and calcaneus. Palpation is also a good way to localize a possible osteomyelitis.

c. The skin and other joints should be carefully examined.

d. A meticulous abdominal and rectal exam must be performed to rule out an abdominal process.

4. Laboratory tests are dictated by the history and physical findings.

a. An x-ray examination of the entire limb may be useful to identify and localize the problem.

b. If the child appears ill, a CBC with differential, ESR, and blood culture are in order.

c. A suspicious joint needs to be tapped. If abuse is suspected, a radiographic trauma series may be in order.

5. Treatment of the limp is directed at the underlying disorders, most of which have been discussed elsewhere in this chapter.

H. METATARSUS ADDUCTUS

1. In metatarsus adductus, the bones of the forefoot are deviated medially on the bones of the midfoot at the tarsometatarsal joint; it is most prominent at the first joint. The sole of the foot is laterally convex and medially concave; the fifth metatarsal may be subject to excessive weight-bearing forces. When the child stands, the hindfoot may be in a valgus position. Metatarsus adductus may be supple or fixed. Genetic and intrauterine forces may play roles in its occurrence.

2. Supple metatarsus adductus implies that the deviation is easily correctable with passive manipulation of the foot.
   a. Children with this variant usually require either no treatment or simple stretching exercises.
   b. At diaper changes, the parent holds the heel in one hand and with the other hand gently exerts laterally directed pressure against the first metatarsal.
   c. Straight-last or outflare shoes worn day and night may also be beneficial.

3. Rigid metatarsus adductus in children often does not correct spontaneously; passive correction is impossible. This condition requires a serial cast or brace correction; if begun in the first through sixth month of life, correction usually occurs in 1-2 months. Serial casting may be effective up to 1-2 years of age but is ineffective after 2 years. After the deformity has been corrected by casts, holding casts, or straight-last or outflare shoes are used until there is no chance of recurrence. Symptomatic children older than 2 years of age usually require surgery to correct their defects.

I. OSGOOD-SCHLATTER DISEASE

1. Osgood-Schlatter disease consists of a painful enlargement of the tibial tuberosity as a result of a vigorous quadriceps pull in a growing child. The inflammation at the patellar tendon insertion accounts for the symptom of pain below the kneecap, especially after physical activity or kneeling. The examiner can elicit this pain by pressing on the tibial tuberosity at the patellar tendon insertion. An x-ray examination is unnecessary if the presentation is classic. The x-ray

examination shows soft-tissue swelling and an irregular, prominent tubercle; ossicles may be present in the tendon.
2. The disease is self-limited; symptoms cease when the proximal tibial epiphysis closes (14-16 years of age).
   a. Mild cases can be managed by rest, quadriceps and hamstring stretching, restriction of activity, antiinflammatories, and ice packs. After the pain subsides, activity can be resumed gradually.
   b. Crutches, knee immobilization, or casting may be necessary in more severe cases.

J. OSTEOMYELITIS

1. Acute osteomyelitis occurs either through hematogenous spread, from direct inoculation of bacteria as a result of trauma, or via spread from a contiguous nidus of infection. Chronic osteomyelitis is a result of inadequately treated acute osteomyelitis.
2. If the spread is by bloodstream, the initial occult bacteremia occurred days to weeks before the onset of symptoms. There may be a history of trauma to the affected limb. Penetrating trauma can introduce bacteria from skin, clothing, shoes, or the instrument of trauma.
3. The femoral and tibial metaphyses are the most commonly involved bones, but any bone can be affected. Children younger than 2 years of age are more likely than older children to have a bone infection spread into the contiguous joint space.
4. *S. aureus* is the most common bacterial pathogen, followed by gram-negative rods, group A streptococcus, and *H. influenzae*. *Pseudomonas aeruginosa* is an important cause of osteomyelitis of the foot, especially if a puncture wound occurred through a sneaker. *Salmonella* organisms are an important cause of osteomyelitis in patients with hemoglobinopathies.
5. Important historical information includes the nature of the bone/limb symptoms and the history of trauma, fever, or constitutional symptoms. Does the child limp or refuse to bear weight altogether (if the leg is involved)? Does the child refuse to use the limb (leg or arm)? What type of trauma occurred and when? Has the child been irritable? Does the child have a hemoglobinopathy?
6. The PE should be complete, but particular attention should be given to the affected limb. Is it swollen, bruised, red, hot, tender? Will the child actively use the extremity? Will he or she allow the examiner to passively move it? Is the child febrile?
7. Laboratory tests to assist in the diagnosis include a CBC with differential (WBC ↑ with shift to the left), ESR (usually ↑), and blood

culture. Aspiration of material from the involved bone can provide a definitive diagnosis of the offending organism.

8. Radiographic studies of the affected bone may demonstrate only soft-tissue findings within 3-4 days of symptom(s) onset. These findings include swelling, edema, and alterations in fat lines and planes between muscles.

9. After 7-10 days of symptoms, the x-ray study shows periosteal elevation, lytic lesions, and sclerosis.

10. A technetium 99m bone scan may show increased uptake at the involved site as early as 1-2 days into the illness. However, the incidence of false-negative findings is high (25%), and increased uptake is also seen in trauma, cellulitis, neoplasms, and septic arthritis.

11. Differential diagnosis
    a. Cellulitis
    b. Septic joint
    c. Soft-tissue injury secondary to trauma
    d. Fracture
    e. Tumor

12. Treatment
    a. Oxacillin 150 mg/kg/d IV ÷ q6h *or* (if penicillin allergy) cefazolin 50-100 mg/kg/d ÷ q8h *or* (if penicillin and cephalosporin allergy) clindamycin 10-40 mg/kg/d ÷ q8h. Remember, however, that there is cross-sensitivity to the cephalosporins among *some* individuals with "cillin" allergies (penicillin skin testing can be helpful). IV therapy is given for 3-7 days until clinical improvement is noted. After that, the patient's drug regimen can be changed to oral therapy: dicloxacillin 25-50 mg/kg/d ÷ q6h *or* cephalexin 100 mg/kg/d ÷ q6h *or* clindamycin 10-40 mg/kg/d ÷ q8h.
    b. *Pseudomonas* organisms should be covered if the suspected infection is in the sole of the foot, especially if the patient had been wearing rubber-soled shoes at the time of the injury; treat with IV ticarcillin 200-300 mg/kg/d ÷ q4-6h and gentamicin 5-7.5 mg/kg/d ÷ q8h.
    c. In a neonate or a patient with a hemoglobinopathy, *Salmonella* organisms may be the cause; treat with IV ampicillin 200 mg/kg/d ÷ q4h *and* gentamicin 7.5 mg/kg/d ÷ q8h. In neonates, nafcillin and cefotaxime can be used; in patients with sickle-cell disease, cefotaxime or ceftriaxone can be used.
    d. Surgical drainage may also be needed.
    e. Before oral therapy is considered, patients with *S. aureus*

osteomyelitis usually are treated with IV antibiotics until ↓ temperature, ↓ ESR, and ↓ local inflammation (usually 5-7 days).

  f. If the patient does not respond to IV staphylococcus coverage, consider other organisms and change therapy accordingly.

  g. After the patient has shown a good response to IV antibiotics, oral antibiotics can be substituted: dicloxacillin 25-50 mg/kg/d ÷ q6h, cephalexin 100 mg/kg/d ÷ q6h, or clindamycin 10-40 mg/kg/d q6h. Total treatment (IV and PO) lasts *at least* 3 weeks and perhaps as long as 6 weeks. Good compliance must be ensured.

  h. During treatment, serum bactericidal or antibiotic levels are monitored. A bactericidal titer of 1:8 or a β-lactam concentration of >20 μg/ml is desirable. Titers and levels are measured 45-60 minutes after a dose of (oral) suspension and 1.5-2 hours after ingestion of a capsule or tablet.

  i. Involve an orthopedist early. The patient may also require physical therapy.

K. SCOLIOSIS

1. Scoliosis is a lateral curvature of the spine. Most cases are idiopathic, but there are also congenital and neuromuscular causes.
   a. Girls are more commonly affected than boys.
   b. The usual onset is after 9-10 years of age for girls and after 11-12 years of age for boys.
2. Screening for scoliosis should begin at 6-7 years of age (Fig. 16-8).
   a. Look at the standing child from behind for asymmetry of the arm/trunk angles, shoulder lines, and flank creases.
   b. Place your hands on the iliac crests to detect differences in leg lengths.
   c. Have the child bend at the waist as he or she extends the arms in front with the palms together (a diving position). As the child bends to touch the toes, observe the horizontal plane of each set of ribs to determine on which side an elevation occurs.
NOTE: The elevation is on the convex side of the curve, and the depression is on the concave side.
   d. Observe the patient from the side during the bending test to determine if there is kyphosis (an abnormal angling of the spine rather than a rounded contour).
3. Worsening of scoliotic curves is associated with the following:
   a. Younger age (<12 years) at diagnosis, especially if the curve is severe
   b. Location of the curve, with thoracic and thoracolumbar curves the most likely to progress

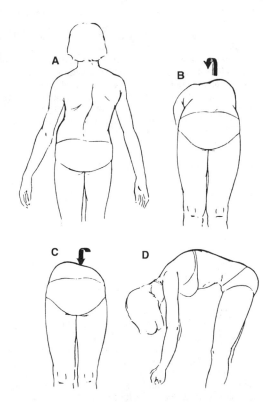

FIG 16-8. Screening for spinal deformities. **A,** Scoliosis may be demonstrated by subtle or striking elevation of one shoulder, a trunk shift, and waistline asymmetry. **B,** Forward bending with the hands clasped and the knees straight may reveal a thoracic prominence on the convex side, even if the standing exam appears normal. **C,** Further forward bending shows any lumbar curve (usually opposite of the thoracic curve). **D,** Always look from the side to see a focal kyphosis.

    c. Severity of the curve, with those ≥30-40 degrees the most likely
      to progress
    d. Skeletal immaturity, as measured by the ossification of the iliac
      apophysis
    e. Gender, with small curves in boys much less likely to progress
4. Refer the child for an x-ray examination or an orthopedic consult if
    the angle of trunk rotation (i.e., the angle between the horizontal plane
    and a plane across the posterior trunk at the point(s) of *maximum*
    deformity) is >6 degrees or if the vertebral angulation (Cobb
    measurement) is >20-25 degrees. If a smaller curve is present, the
    child should still be followed up with bend tests or x-ray
    examinations until growth ceases.

L. SLIPPED CAPITAL FEMORAL EPIPHYSIS
1. SCFE is an abrupt or gradual displacement of the proximal femoral
    epiphysis on the femoral neck.
    a. The male-to-female ratio is 2-3:1, and it most commonly occurs
      during preadolescence or adolescence.
    b. The cause is unknown, but the following factors have been
      implicated: obesity, growth spurts, hormonal factors, an intrinsi-
      cally defective growth plate, genetic predisposition, and trauma.
2. The child may have an acutely painful limp and pain in the groin,
    thigh, or knee. Hip motion is painful and limited (especially
    abduction and internal rotation). Flexing the involved hip causes
    external rotation. Alternatively, the child may have a gradual onset of
    intermittent pain and limping.
3. The x-ray examination of SCFE may show a widened growth plate
    of the proximal femur on the affected side.
    a. In true cases, the x-ray study demonstrates the altered position of
      the femoral head on the neck.
    b. Medial and posterior displacement of the femoral head with
      apparent loss of height can be seen, especially by drawing a line
      along the lateral aspect of the femoral neck.
    c. Because many slips are posterior, a cross-table lateral x-ray
      examination is mandatory.
4. Treatment of SCFE is directed toward preventing further slippage,
    avascular necrosis, premature degenerative arthritis, and further gait
    deterioration.
    a. The patient with suspected SCFE should be forbidden to walk.
    b. Urgent fixation of the slip may be achieved through screw insertion
      or an open bone graft.

M. SUBLUXED RADIAL HEAD

1. With a subluxed radial head, the radial head temporarily loses contact with the capitellum, and the annular ligament surrounding the radial neck becomes partially interposed between joint surfaces (Fig. 16-9).
    a. This series of events occurs when a young child's forearm or wrist is jerked with longitudinal and pronational forces.

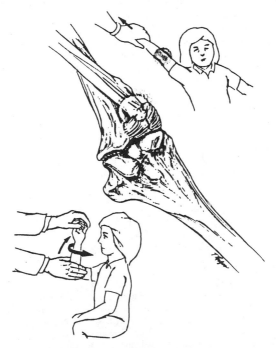

FIG 16-9. A "pulled" or "nursemaid's" elbow is a partial tear of the annular ligament of the radial head; it can be reduced by flexion and supination.

b. The child holds his or her arm in extension and actively resists attempts to flex it.

c. X-ray studies are normal.

2. Treatment consists of hypersupination of the forearm with the elbow held in flexion; once the child's ligament is released, he or she begins to use the arm again. Some orthopedists recommend a posterior splint for 10 days to allow healing of the ligament, especially if the subluxation is recurrent. Parents and siblings should be educated about the mechanism of injury and discouraged from jerking the arm.

N. TORTICOLLIS

1. Torticollis (wryneck, tilted neck) may be congenital (vertebral anomalies, tumors, intrauterine malposition, birth trauma) or acquired (vertebral column or spinal cord tumors, inflammatory disorders such as cervical adenitis or intervertebral diskitis, or trauma such as cervical subluxation or neck muscle strain). The most common cause is neck muscle strain acquired during play, participation in sports, or an awkward sleeping position.

2. In a child with torticollis, the head is tilted toward the affected side. The sternocleidomastoid muscle is shortened as a result of muscle spasm.

3. Because torticollis may be secondary to subluxation or dislocation of the facets of the atlantoaxial joint, anteroposterior, lateral, and open-mouth odontoid x-ray studies should be obtained if suspicion is high.

4. Treatment of torticollis resulting from neck strain consists of warm soaks, analgesics, mild antiinflammatory agents, and a soft cervical collar. Treatment of torticollis resulting from atlantoaxial subluxation consists of rest and cervical traction; a soft collar may provide relief after reduction. Surgery is rarely necessary.

O. TRANSIENT SYNOVITIS

1. Toxic or transient synovitis is an acute inflammation of the hip in a child 2-12 years of age. Boys are more commonly affected than girls. The cause is unknown, but the episode may follow a URI or trauma.

2. The child with transient synovitis may have a limp; groin, hip, thigh, and knee pain are also reported. The limp is characterized by a shortened stance on the affected side, with guarding or spasm of the muscles around the hip joint. Severely affected children may refuse to walk. All symptoms are of an acute onset. On examination, the

child has limited active and passive range of motion at the hip as a result of muscle guarding.

3. Laboratory tests are indicated if the child is febrile or if there is suspicion that he or she has a septic joint. In toxic synovitis, the CBC with differential and ESR are normal or only mildly elevated; although the soft-tissue planes around the hip may be distorted, the hip x-ray examination is normal. Ultrasound may show a small amount of joint effusion. Aspiration of the joint under fluoroscopy should be performed if a septic hip cannot be ruled out by examination and CBC/ESR. With toxic synovitis, the joint fluid is sterile as opposed to the fluid from a septic joint, which has WBCs and may have organisms on Gram's stain.

4. Hospitalization may be necessary if the child has a high fever or severe symptoms.
   a. If the child is not hospitalized, serial examinations of the hip should be performed every day or every few days because synovitis may herald osteomyelitis, neoplasm, Legg-Calvé-Perthes disease, or SCFE.
   b. Toxic synovitis usually resolves in 3-5 days; prolonged symptoms should prompt reconsideration of the diagnosis.
   c. Treatment consists of rest, analgesics, and restricted activity; severely affected patients may benefit from light traction.

BIBLIOGRAPHY

General

Staheli LT: *Fundamentals of pediatric orthopedics,* New York, 1996, Raven Press.

Bowlegs

Renshaw T: *Pediatric orthopedics,* Philadelphia, 1986, WB Saunders.
Scoles P: *Pediatric orthopedics in clinical practice,* ed 2, Chicago, 1988, Mosby.

Developmental dysplasia of the hip

Aronsson D et al: Developmental dysplasia of the leg, *Pediatrics* 94:201, 1994.
MacEwen G, Millet C: Congenital dislocation of the hip, *Pediatr Rev* 11:249, 1990.

Mosca V: Pitfalls in diagnosis: the hip, *Pediatr Ann* 18:12, 1989.

Renshaw T: *Pediatric orthopedics,* Philadelphia, 1986, WB Saunders.

Rosendahl D et al: Ultrasound screening for developmental dysplasia of the hip in the neonate, *Pediatrics* 94:47, 1994.

Scoles P: *Pediatric orthopedics in clinical practice,* ed 2, Chicago, 1988, Mosby.

Staheli L: Management of congenital hip dysplasia, *Pediatr Ann* 18:24, 1989.

In-toeing

Craig C, Goldberg M: Foot and leg problems, *Pediatr Rev* 14:395, 1993.

Renshaw T: *Pediatric orthopedics,* Philadelphia, 1986, WB Saunders.

Rosman M: When parents ask about in-toeing, *Contemp Pediatr* 4:116, 1987.

Scoles P: *Pediatric orthopedics in clinical practice,* ed 2, Chicago, 1988, Mosby.

Joint pain and joint swelling

American Academy of Pediatrics: Treatment of Lyme borreliosis, *Pediatrics* 88:176, 1991.

Baltimore R, Shapiro E: Lyme disease, *Pediatr Rev* 15:167, 1994.

Barton LL, Dunkle LM, Habib FH: Septic arthritis in childhood: a 13-year review, *Am J Dis Child* 141:898, 1987.

Biro F, Gewanter HL, Baum J: The hypermobility syndrome, *Pediatrics* 72:701, 1983.

Brewer EJ, Jr: Pitfalls in the diagnosis of juvenile rheumatoid arthritis, *Pediatr Clin North Am* 33:1015, 1986.

Feder HM, Jr et al: Early Lyme disease: a flu-like illness without erythema migrans, *Pediatrics* 91:456, 1993.

Gerber MA, Shapiro ED: Diagnosis of Lyme disease in children, *J Pediatr* 121:157, 1992.

Kummano I et al: Clinical signs and laboratory tests in the differential diagnosis of arthritis in children, *Am J Dis Child* 141:34, 1987.

Nocton JJ et al: Human parvovirus B19–associated arthritis in children, *J Pediatr* 122:186, 1993.

Ostrov BE: Differentiation of systemic juvenile rheumatoid arthritis from acute leukemia near the onset of disease, *J Pediatr* 122:595, 1993.

Prose NS, Abson KG, Berg D: Lyme disease in children: diagnosis, treatment and prevention, *Semin Dermatol* 11:31, 1992.

Rose CD et al: The overdiagnosis of Lyme disease in children residing in an endemic area, *Clin Pediatr* 33:663, 1994.

Salazar JC et al: Long-term outcome of Lyme disease in children given early treatment, *J Pediatr* 122:591, 1993.

Schaller JG: Arthritis as a presenting manifestation of malignancy in children, *J Pediatr* 81:793, 1972.

Schaller JG: Arthritis in children, *Pediatr Clin North Am* 33:1565, 1986.

Sherry DD et al: Painless juvenile rheumatoid arthritis, *J Pediatr* 116:921, 1990.

Welkon CJ et al: Pyogenic arthritis in infants and children, *Pediatr Infect Dis J* 5:669, 1986.

Knock knees

Renshaw T: *Pediatric orthopedics,* Philadelphia, 1986, WB Saunders.

Scoles P: *Pediatric orthopedics in clinical practice,* ed 2, Chicago, 1988, Mosby.

Legg-Calvé-Perthes disease

Bunnell W: Legg-Calvé-Perthes disease, *Pediatr Rev* 7:299, 1986.

Renshaw T: *Pediatric orthopedics,* Philadelphia, 1986, WB Saunders.

Scoles P: *Pediatric orthopedics in clinical practice,* ed 2, Chicago, 1988, Mosby.

Thompson G et al: Legg-Calvé-Perthes disease, *Ciba Clin Symp* 38(1):1-25, 1986.

Limp

MacEwen G, Dehne R: The limping child, *Pediatr Rev* 12:268, 1991.

Renshaw T: The child who has a limp, *Pediatr Rev* 16:458, 1995.

Sherry D: Limb pain in childhood, *Pediatr Rev* 12:39, 1990.

Singer J: The cause of gait disturbance in 425 pediatric patients, *Pediatr Emerg Care* 1:7, 1985.

Tunnessen W: *Signs and symptoms in pediatrics,* Philadelphia, 1983, JB Lippincott.

Metatarsus adductus

Craig C, Goldberg M: Foot and leg problems, *Pediatr Rev* 14:395, 1993.

Renshaw T: *Pediatric orthopedics,* Philadelphia, 1986, WB Saunders.

Rosman M: When parents ask about in-toeing, *Contemp Pediatr* 4:116, 1987.

Scoles P: *Pediatric orthopedics in clinical practice,* ed 2, Chicago, 1988, Mosby.

Osgood-Schlatter disease

Scoles P: *Pediatric orthopedics in clinical practice,* ed 2, Chicago, 1988, Mosby.

Osteomyelitis

Barkin R, editor: *Emergency pediatrics,* ed 3, St Louis, 1990, Mosby.

Gold R: Diagnosis of osteomyelitis, *Pediatr Rev* 12:292, 1991.

Krugman S et al: *Infectious diseases of children,* ed 9, St Louis, 1992, Mosby.

Scoliosis

Berweick D: Scoliosis screening, *Pediatr Rev* 5:238, 1984.

Keim H, Hensinger R: Spinal deformities, *Ciba Clin Symp,* vol 41(4):1-32, 1989.

Marsh J: Screening for scoliosis, *Pediatr Rev* 14:297, 1993.

McLain R, Karol L: Conservative treatment of the scoliotic and kyphotic patient, *Arch Pediatr Adolesc Med* 148:646, 1994.

Renshaw T: *Pediatric orthopedics,* Philadelphia, 1986, WB Saunders.

Scoles P: *Pediatric orthopedics in clinical practice,* ed 2, Chicago, 1988, Mosby.

Slipped capital femoral epiphysis

Ledwith C, Fleisher G: Slipped capital femoral epiphysis without hip pain leads to missed diagnosis, *Pediatrics* 89:660, 1992.

Renshaw T: *Pediatric orthopedics,* Philadelphia, 1986, WB Saunders.

Scoles P: *Pediatric orthopedics in clinical practice,* ed 2, Chicago, 1988, Mosby.

Subluxed radial head

Nichols H: Nursemaid's elbow: reducing it to simple terms, *Contemp Pediatr* 5:50, 1988.

Quan L, Marcuse E: The epidemiology and treatment of radial head subluxation, *Am J Dis Child* 139:1194, 1985.

Renshaw T: *Pediatric orthopedics,* Philadelphia, 1986, WB Saunders.

Torticollis

Caputo A et al: The sit-up test: an alternative clinical test for evaluating pediatric torticollis, *Pediatrics* 90:612, 1992.

Renshaw T: *Pediatric orthopedics,* Philadelphia, 1986, WB Saunders.

Scoles P: *Pediatric orthopedics in clinical practice,* ed 2, Chicago, 1988, Mosby.

Transient synovitis

Haueisen D et al: The characterization of "transient synovitis of the hip" in children, *J Pediatr Orthop* 6:11, 1986.

Renshaw T: *Pediatric orthopedics,* Philadelphia, 1986, WB Saunders.

Scoles P: *Pediatric orthopedics in clinical practice,* ed 2, Chicago, 1988, Mosby.

OTOLARYNGOLOGY 17

A. ALLERGIC RHINITIS
Allergic rhinitis is the most common cause of chronic nasal congestion in children.
1. Cause
   a. In young children, causes are usually perennial: dust mite, molds, and animal dander.
   b. In older children (>4 years of age), causes are often seasonal: tree/grass pollens in the spring, ragweed in the fall. Environmental history is crucial; *play detective!*
   c. A family history of atopy often exists.
   d. Symptoms often are aggravated by smoking, pollutants, and temperature and humidity changes.
2. Signs and symptoms
   a. Sneezing, nasal congestion and pruritus, clear watery discharge, conjunctival erythema, nasal speech, mouth breathing, snoring, malaise
   b. "Allergic salute," "allergic shiners"
   c. PE shows pale, bluish, boggy nasal mucosa and enlarged turbinates. With perennial symptoms, otitis, epistaxis, circles under the eyes, and follicular hypertrophy of the pharynx may be seen.
3. Differential diagnosis
   a. Foreign body: Unilateral purulent discharge with odor
   b. Anatomic: Septal deviation
   c. Chronic infection: Sinusitis, adenoiditis (purulent nasal discharge, low-grade fever, malaise, anorexia)
   d. Chronic use of topical agents (rhinitis medicamentosa)
   e. Vasomotor (nonallergic, noninfectious): Thin discharge, unimpressive, no history of allergy, negative skin tests; may be eosinophilic or noneosinophilic
   f. Nasal polyposis: R/O cystic fibrosis
4. Diagnostic aids
   a. A Hansel stain of nasal secretions is *very helpful.*
      1) Blow nose into plastic or wax paper wrap.

2) Spread secretions on a glass slide and dry overnight.
3) Stain for 30 seconds with Hansel stain.
4) Add distilled water for 30 seconds.
5) Wash with water.
6) Decolorize with methanol or 95% ethyl alcohol.
7) Dry and examine under oil.

>10% eosinophils suggests allergy; sheets of PMNs and bacteria suggest bacterial infection.

b. Skin tests or RAST for patients not responding to usual treatment
c. Sinus x-ray studies or CT scan to rule out sinusitis

5. Treatment
   a. Avoid suspected allergens (especially control animal dander and household dust mites).
   b. Antihistamines: Start dosage low and increase to tolerance or effect; terfenadine (Seldane) and astemizole (Hismanal) are associated with less drowsiness.
   c. Oral decongestants
      1) Pseudoephedrine
      2) Phenylpropanolamine
   d. Topical intranasal agents
      1) Adrenergics (phenylephrine) for short-term use
      2) Cromolyn sodium 4% spray for prophylaxis only
      3) Steroids (beclomethasone, flunisolide, and others): Very useful; not well absorbed from the mucosa; may be irritating
   e. Immunotherapy for treatment failures, especially when clinical history and skin tests concur; best for seasonal, pollen-related allergy

B. EPISTAXIS

Peak age 4-10 years; boys > girls; usually from anterior portion of nasal septum

1. Cause
   a. Young children: Trauma, inflammation
   b. Older children: Dryness, crusting, "picking"

NOTE: In teenage girls, epistaxis may be associated with menses; in teenage boys, it may be associated with angiofibroma.

   c. Blood dyscrasia or clotting abnormalities are rare but need to be considered with chronic or recurrent episodes.

2. Diagnosis
   a. Careful exam to identify bleeding point
   b. CBC, clotting studies with recurrent episodes

3. Management
   a. Compression of anterior nasal septum ≈10 minutes with gauze soaked with 1:1000 epinephrine may be helpful.
   b. With persistent bleeding, use silver nitrate cautery and/or packing (Gelfoam, petrolatum gauze).
   c. Consult an ENT specialist if the bleeding is profuse or if the site is not located.
   d. In cases caused by dryness, crusting, or "picking," humidification, local petrolatum, and well-trimmed fingernails can be helpful.

C. FOREIGN BODIES
1. Ear
   a. Foreign bodies in the ear can be almost anything; at Johns Hopkins Hospital, roaches, paper toy parts, earring parts, hair beads, and erasers occur in that order of frequency.
   b. Presentation: Pain, decreased hearing, discharge, "digging at ear"
   c. Management: 90% of objects can be removed in the office or ED with simple equipment. Parents should be cautioned against trying to remove objects at home. Cooperation is essential. Sedation and a topical anesthetic (2% lidocaine spray) may be helpful.
      1) If the object does not completely occlude the ear canal, use an ear loop, curette (friable objects), or forceps.
      2) Two choices for insects
         a) Fill ear canal with mineral oil.
         b) Irrigate the ear canal with 2% lidocaine, which usually causes the insect to flee but may be associated with vertigo.
   d. Consult an ENT specialist if the canal is swollen, if there is significant bleeding, or if the FB cannot be *easily* removed.

NOTE: A new hazard is the alkaline button battery, which can produce rapid tissue destruction on contact with moist tissue and can lead to perforation of the TM, destruction of ossicles, and ulceration of local tissues. Button batteries should be removed by an ENT specialist with the patient under sedation or general anesthesia.

2. Nose
   a. Cause: Hair beads, toy parts, paper, food, crayons, erasers
   b. Presentation: Pain, foul odor, discharge, bleeding. It can sometimes present as *generalized* body odor. Unilateral purulent or malodorous nasal discharge is *always* suggestive of an FB.
   c. Management: Most nasal FBs can be handled in the office or ED with simple equipment. Parents should be cautioned against trying to remove objects at home. Cooperation, a topical anesthetic (2%

lidocaine), and vasoconstriction are helpful. It is important not to push objects into the nasopharynx, where they can be aspirated by a struggling child.

1) Most objects can be removed with a small hook, loop, forceps, or nasal suction.

2) A cooperative child can be asked to apply positive pressure through his or her nose.

3) An unesthetic but effective technique involves occluding the nonobstructed nostril with digital pressure and blowing into the patient's mouth with a tight seal. This technique should be reserved for relatives and close friends.

4) Button batteries can rapidly cause tissue damage and need to be removed quickly!

3. Upper airway

  a. Laryngotracheal

    1) Presentation: Dyspnea, cough, stridor, and wheezing. A choking episode is observed in 90% of cases. It is commonly confused with croup. FB should always be considered in the differential diagnosis of croup, especially in the absence of URI symptoms.

    2) Diagnosis: Lateral neck and high KV x-ray studies of the airway may be helpful. The CXR is usually normal. If suspicious of an FB in the upper airway, refer to an ENT specialist for endoscopy.

    3) Management: Remove the FB via a rigid endoscope.

  b. Cricopharyngeal

    1) Presentation: Dysphagia, excessive salivation, pain in throat, FB sensation, tenderness on palpation over trachea

NOTE: There may be no clinical findings in many cases of cricopharyngeal FBs.

    2) Diagnosis: An intraoral exam, laryngoscopy, and high KV x-ray study of the airway may be helpful; a normal x-ray study is not helpful.

    3) Management: Remove the FB via a rigid endoscope.

4. Esophagus

  a. Causes: Mostly coins (especially pennies), followed by safety pins and straight pins; in 5% of cases there may be multiple FBs.

  b. Presentation: Symptoms include pain, FB sensation, coughing, choking, vomiting, dysphagia, and drooling.

  c. Diagnosis: Metallic FBs are easily diagnosed by AP and lateral x-ray examinations of the neck and chest. Hand-held metal detectors are also highly accurate and in experienced hands can be used as an alternative to x-ray studies.

d. Evaluation: Although somewhat controversial, all patients who come to the ED with a history of coin ingestion should be screened by an x-ray examination or a metal detector.

e. Management

1) Immediate removal is indicated if the child is symptomatic, if the coin is in the upper third of the esophagus, or if there is a history of esophageal disease or surgery.

2) Asymptomatic patients with a coin in the distal esophagus should be observed and given nothing by mouth. The coin should be removed if a repeat x-ray examination shows that it has not passed.

3) Methods of removal include rigid endoscopy with forceps extraction or flexible endoscopy with forceps extraction. The choice of technique depends on the location of the coin, duration of impaction, associated symptoms, and expertise of available personnel.

a) Use rigid endoscopy if there is a history of prolonged impaction, impaction of a sharp or irregular object, respiratory compromise, or a history of esophageal disease or surgery.

b) Use flexible endoscopy for recently impacted coins.

NOTE: A Foley catheter can be used for recently impacted coins in the proximal esophagus, and a dilating Bougie can be used for those in the distal esophagus. However, the use of these techniques is still highly controversial.

4) Once a coin enters the stomach, it is almost always passed spontaneously (average 5 days). Surgery is indicated only if there is a history of previous GI surgery (e.g., pyloric stenosis) or if the patient becomes symptomatic (e.g., severe pain, vomiting).

5) Button batteries

a) Button batteries (most often from hearing aids, toys, watches) can cause tissue injury secondary to liquefaction necrosis (alkali leakage) or electrochemical burns, especially if lodged in the esophagus. There is a risk of mercury absorption from fragmented mercuric oxide cells.

b) Prompt radiographic evaluation is indicated to determine the location of all ingested button batteries.

c) Esophageal batteries should be removed immediately via an endoscope and under direct observation. The Foley catheter technique is contraindicated because of the risk of perforation.

d) Large batteries (>15 mm) in the stomach can be observed safely for up to 48 hours; if not passed, endoscopic removal is indicated.

e) Asymptomatic patients with small battery (<15 mm) ingestion do not require a follow-up x-ray examination once the battery is past the esophagus.

f) Once beyond the pylorus, button batteries are usually passed without incident; passage can be confirmed by stool inspection. Surgery is indicated only if the patient develops signs of perforation or obstruction.

g) Ipecac is contraindicated for button batteries in the stomach. The efficacy of antacids and H_2 blockers is unproven. Blood mercury levels are indicated only if it is observed that the mercuric oxide cell has split in the GI tract.

D. HOARSENESS

1. Acute: Sudden voice change that lasts only a few days
   a. Etiology: Acute inflammation of vocal cords secondary to viral URI or vocal abuse such as screaming, shouting, or singing
   b. Treatment: Humidification, gargles, hot/cold liquids

2. Chronic: Voice change that lasts several weeks
   a. Causes: Vocal abuse or misuse, "screamer's nodes" (nodules on vocal cords), tumors (rare) such as laryngeal papillomas, psychogenic condition, trauma (postintubation), allergic laryngitis, gastroesophageal reflux, hypothyroidism
   b. Treatment: Symptomatic, voice therapy. Endoscopic removal of nodules is rarely indicated. Referral to an ENT specialist and laryngoscopy are indicated if hoarseness persists beyond a few weeks, is recurrent, or is accompanied by stridor or increased respiratory effort. Depending on airway findings, a plain x-ray examination, CT scan, or MRI evaluation of the airway and surrounding structures may be helpful.

E. OTITIS

1. Acute otitis media
   a. Symptoms: Ear pain, pulling at ear. There may be nonspecific findings of ± fever, irritability, poor feeding, vomiting, and diarrhea. AOM is usually associated with URI. During the first year of life, ≈50% of the episodes of AOM may be clinically asymptomatic.

b. Signs: The hallmark is tympanic immobility on pneumatic otoscopy.
   1) Erythema of TM: May be an early sign (crying alone may cause mild injection of TM)
   2) Absent or distorted landmarks: Thickened, inflamed TM, often bulging
   3) Asymmetry of appearance of TMs
   4) Otorrhea
c. Cause
   1) <3 months of age: Consider the usual pathogens *(Streptococcus pneumoniae, Haemophilus influenzae, Moraxella catarrhalis)* plus gram-negative organisms, *Staphylococcus aureus,* and *Chlamydia trachomatis* (in infants with otitis and afebrile pneumonia).
   2) >3 months of age: 30%-45% *S. pneumoniae,* 20% nontypable *H. influenzae,* 20% *M. catarrhalis.* The remainder results from a variety of bacteria, including group A streptococcus, viruses, and (?)mycoplasma; 15%-30% of *H. influenzae* strains and 90%-100% of *M. catarrhalis* strains isolated from middle ear fluid are β-lactamase producers. An increasing percentage of *S. pneumoniae* isolates are now penicillin and multidrug resistant. Young age, day care, hospitalization, and prior antibiotic exposure are risk factors for colonization and infection with resistant strains.
   3) *H. influenzae* is the usual pathogen in the "otitis-conjunctivitis syndrome."
   4) Bullous myringitis: Bullae on TM, often hemorrhagic and painful. Causes include bacterial, viral, and (uncommonly) mycoplasma. Treat as acute bacterial otitis media.
   5) Viral agents have been identified in approximately 40% of cases of AOM.
d. Laboratory studies
   1) With acute otorrhea, the drainage culture usually identifies the middle ear bacterial pathogen; however, the culture may also grow canal flora.
   2) NP culture *does not* predict middle ear bacteriology.
   3) TC is indicated in a child with accompanying exudative pharyngitis.
   4) Tympanocentesis to obtain middle ear fluid for Gram's stain and C&S is indicated for neonates, patients with severe otalgia and

toxicity, those with a failure to respond to appropriate antimicrobial therapy, those with suppurative complications, and those with immunodeficiency.

e. Treatment

1) Neonates: Consider a full sepsis work-up and admission because of the risk of sepsis and meningitis. Broad-spectrum IV antibiotic coverage with ampicillin + gentamicin, or ampicillin + cefotaxime is indicated. Preferably, tympanocentesis for C&S should be performed before initiating therapy.

2) >3 months of age (several approaches to therapy): Although many cases of AOM resolve spontaneously, a clear-cut advantage for antimicrobial therapy has been demonstrated. The choice of antibiotic should be individualized on the basis of the patient's age, recent history of otitis, drug treatment history, associated illness, and community bacterial susceptibility patterns.

a) For most patients, amoxicillin 40 mg/kg/d ÷ tid × 10 days remains the first-line drug for the initial treatment of AOM.

b) If there is no response within 48-72 hours, switch to a drug effective against β-lactamase producers: amoxicillin + clavulanate potassium (Augmentin) 40 mg/kg/d ÷ tid × 10 days; cefixime (Suprax) 8 mg/kg/d in 1-2 divided doses × 10 days; erythromycin ethylsuccinate + sulfisoxazole (Pediazole) 50 mg/kg/d erythromycin ÷ qid × 10 days; cefuroxime axetil (Ceftin) 125 mg bid (<2 years of age) or 250 mg bid (>2 years of age); TMP/SMZ (Bactrim, Septra) 8 mg/kg/d TMP, 40 mg/kg/d SMZ ÷ bid × 10 days.

NOTE: In some situations (older child, mild episode, relatively otitis-free past history, prompt symptomatic improvement), a shorter (i.e., 5-7–day) course of antimicrobial therapy may be adequate.

3) Do not use erythromycin, first-generation cephalosporins, sulfonamides, or penicillin; these drugs are not effective against *H. influenzae.*

4) Avoid TMP/SMZ in patients with associated exudative pharyngitis because group A streptococcus will not be adequately covered.

5) In infants with otitis and afebrile pneumonia, consider erythromycin and sulfisoxazole (Pediazole) to cover *C. trachomatis.*

6) In children with otitis and purulent conjunctivitis, consider a β-lactamase–resistant antibiotic to cover β-lactamase–producing *H. influenzae.*

     7) Antihistamines/decongestants: No evidence of efficacy

     8) Analgesics/antipyretics: Use prn for fever, pain. Auralgan otic drops (antipyrine, benzocaine, glycerin) may be effective as a local anesthetic for the ear canal or TM. Do not use if the TM has perforated or if there is discharge in the canal.

     9) A topical antibiotic suspension is not indicated for AOM with perforation and drainage.

   f. Follow-up: A recheck is indicated in the following situations:

     1) Lack of clinical response

     2) History of otitis media with effusion

     3) History of recurrent otitis media

     4) Children <3 years of age

2. Recurrent acute otitis media

   a. Recurrent AOM is defined as three episodes of AOM within 6 months or four episodes within 1 year; it often results from different pathogens.

   b. Evaluate for the underlying problem (e.g., allergy, immune defect, chronic sinusitis, adenoidal hypertrophy, anatomic defect in upper airway). Passive smoke exposure, day-care attendance, and bedtime bottle propping may be predisposing factors.

   c. Management: Antimicrobial prophylaxis with amoxicillin (20 mg/kg hs) or sulfisoxazole (50-75 mg/kg hs) × 6 months or through the winter-spring season. Continuous prophylaxis is probably more effective than intermittent prophylaxis; if this technique fails, referral to an ENT specialist is indicated for probable tympanostomy tube placement. Adenoidectomy may be indicated for patients with adenoidal obstruction, for those who fail after the use of tympanostomy tubes, and for patients >4 years of age with middle ear effusion.

   d. Children >2 years of age who continue to have recurrent episodes of AOM may benefit from the pneumococcal vaccine.

3. Otitis media with effusion: Also referred to as serous otitis, secretory otitis, "glue ear," nonsuppurative otitis media, or mucoid otitis media. It is defined as fluid in the middle ear *without* signs or symptoms of ear infection.

   a. Following treatment of AOM, middle ear effusion is present in 70% of patients at the 2-week follow-up, in 40% at 1 month, in 20% at 2 months, and in 10% after 3 months; it may also be picked up as an incidental finding in an asymptomatic patient. In approximately 50% of cases, pathogenic bacteria are recovered from middle ear fluid.

NOTE: Pneumatic otoscopy should always be used when evaluating the middle ear. Tympanometry can be used for confirmation.

  b. Predisposing factors: Mechanical obstruction (adenoidal hypertrophy, cleft palate), allergy, ciliary dyskinesia, barotrauma (diving, flying), passive smoke exposure, attendance at day care

  c. Symptoms: Decreased hearing, ear fullness, ear popping. Fever and ear pain are usually absent.

  d. Signs: Opaque, gray, thickened TM with decreased mobility; may be bulging (early) or retracted (late); ± air bubbles or air-fluid level behind TM; abnormal tympanogram; conductive hearing deficit

  e. Course: Most cases resolve spontaneously over several weeks to months but may be associated with a significant conductive hearing loss. Every child who has had fluid in both middle ears for a total of 3 months should undergo a hearing evaluation.

  f. Treatment

   1) Antibiotics: For patients with OME, a course of antibiotic with an agent effective against β-lactamase producers is indicated in the following circumstances:

    a) Unfavorable past history of otitis media

    b) Associated chronic URI (>2 weeks) that is not improving

    c) Tube placement being considered because of chronic OME (>3 months)

   2) Antihistamines, decongestants: No evidence of efficacy

   3) Steroids: The use of oral steroids is controversial. There are conflicting data on efficacy. Steroids may be indicated in selected patients before surgical approaches.

   4) Myringotomy and tympanostomy tube placement: Somewhat controversial but probably indicated if effusion persists >4-6 months in spite of medical therapy and if significant hearing loss (>20 dB in the better-hearing ear) is present. Myringotomy alone *is not* helpful. The main indication for tubes is to improve hearing and prevent a delay in auditory and language skills.

NOTE: Tympanostomy tubes are not benign. Complications include persistent otorrhea, tympanosclerosis, atrophy, residual perforation of TM, and cholesteatoma.

   5) Adenoidectomy: This approach is controversial but may be indicated in a patient who fails tympanostomy tube placement, a patient with evidence of obstructing adenoidal hypertrophy, or a child >4 years of age who has persistent OME.

NOTE: Adenoidectomy is contraindicated in patients with a cleft palate.

4. Chronic otitis media

  a. Chronic otitis media presents as intermittent/chronic foul-smelling otorrhea, hearing loss, or an abnormal otoscopic exam (granulation tissue, cholesteatoma) in patients with a history of recurrent AOM. This condition requires ENT consultation.

NOTE: Consider the possibility of ciliary dyskinesia in patients with recurrent/chronic draining otitis and evidence of lung infection. Only 50% of cases have situs inversus.

  b. Fluid aspirated through the perforated membrane may be helpful and should be sent for Gram's, potassium hydroxide, and acid-fast stains, as well as bacterial, fungal, and mycobacterial cultures. *Pseudomonas* and *S. aureus* are common pathogens.

  c. Treatment: A topical ophthalmic or otic suspension containing neomycin or polymyxins may be helpful, but parenteral antibiotics may be needed on the basis of C&S results. Definitive therapy involves surgical debridement of the middle ear space.

5. Otitis externa

  a. Otitis externa involves inflammation of the skin lining the auditory canal and is often secondary to trauma (e.g., from cotton swabs, bobby pins) or infection. It is also known as "swimmer's ear."

  b. Symptoms: Pain on pulling the pinna or tragus, itching, discharge

  c. Signs: Edematous, erythematous auditory canal with discharge

  d. Treatment

    1) Steroid-antibiotic drops (Cortisporin) 2-4 gtt in affected ear qid × 5-7 days. Use Cortisporin suspension, not solution, if PE tubes are in place. Cortisporin solution causes pain on contact with the middle ear. A cotton swab can be moistened with Cortisporin and inserted in the auditory canal q4h.

    2) Avoid swimming until the problem resolves.

F. PHARYNGITIS (including tonsillitis and tonsillopharyngitis)

1. Clinical features

  a. Signs and symptoms: Abrupt onset of fever, sore throat, malaise, headache, abdominal pain, and sandpapery rash (scarlet fever). Pharynx is at least erythematous, ± tonsillar hypertrophy, ± exudate, ± ulcerations, ± membranous covering, ± palatal petechiae, anterior cervical adenitis. Antibody rise against group A β-hemolytic streptococcus correlates best with enlarged, tender anterior cervical nodes.

b. Pharyngitis usually occurs in the winter-spring months.

c. The peak age is 5-15 years.

2. Etiology

a. Bacterial

1) Group A β-hemolytic streptococcus: The clinical picture is not reliable to diagnose "strep throat." Patients with strep throat may have fever (often very high), sore throat, headache, abdominal pain, and vomiting. The pharynx may appear erythematous or exudative; palatal petechiae and tender anterior cervical lymph nodes may be present. Diagnosis of strep throat is based on a positive culture or direct antigen screen and evidence of pharyngitis.

2) Other bacteria: GC (high index of suspicion, positive clinical history and PE); diphtheria (membranous pharyngitis, myocarditis), check immunization history.

b. Viral

1) Coxsackievirus (herpangina): Usually seen in summer and autumn; ulcers on soft palate, tonsils, pharynx. Also check soles and palms for vesicular lesions (hand-foot-and-mouth syndrome).

2) Epstein-Barr virus (infectious mononucleosis): May be associated with exudative or membranous pharyngitis, generalized lymphadenopathy, hepatosplenomegaly, rash, malaise, tender posterior cervical nodes, edema of the eyelids, or a nasal "twang" to voice

3) Adenovirus: Most common cause of nonstreptococcal pharyngitis; may be associated with abdominal pain, diarrhea, otitis media, rash (duration <3 days)

4) Herpes simplex virus: Both types I and II may produce pharyngitis ± tonsillar exudate. Ulcerations may appear 1-2 days after onset. The probable cause is herpes if signs of glossitis or gingivostomatitis are present.

5) Other viruses: Enterocytopathogenic human orphan, parainfluenza, influenza, RSV

NOTE: The presence of rhinorrhea, cough, hoarseness, and diarrhea favors a viral etiology.

c. Other organisms such as *Mycoplasma, Chlamydia*

3. Laboratory evaluation

a. A TC is the mainstay of diagnosis.

1) A single TC is 90%-97% sensitive. The swab should make

contact with both tonsillar regions and with the posterior pharyngeal wall.

2) Inoculate the swab on a 5% sheep-blood agar plate; it is helpful to place 0.04 unit bacitracin disk on the plate (95% of GABHS demonstrate a large zone of inhibition around the disk).

3) Anaerobic incubation may slightly increase the yield of GABHS, but its routine use is not justified or necessary.

NOTE: ≈15%-18% of children with infectious mononucleosis also have group A β-hemolytic streptococcus on TC.

b. A direct antigen screen (enzyme immunoassay) may be helpful. The test is very specific (few false-positive results), but false-negative results may be seen in up to 10%-40% of streptococcal infections. The usual strategy is to treat if the antigen screen is positive; perform a TC if the screen is negative. Optical immuno-assay screening tests may be more sensitive but need further evaluation.

c. CBC + differential + smear (lymphocytosis with atypical lymphs may be seen in ≈80% of patients with infectious mononucleosis). Platelets are decreased with some viral syndromes. Consider infectious mononucleosis when the TC is negative and severe pharyngitis persists. Perform a heterophile monospot test (may be negative before 5 years of age or during the first weeks of illness) or a specific serologic test for EBV antibodies.

4. Treatment

a. Antibiotics

1) Penicillin remains the drug of choice; a penicillin-resistant strain of GABHS has never been identified.

2) Treatment of GABHS pharyngitis decreases the risk of rheumatic fever but does not prevent poststreptococcal glomerulonephritis. Antibiotics shorten the duration and severity of symptoms if given early in the course. Although data are conflicting, immediate initiation of antibiotic therapy does not appear to increase the relapse or recurrence rate.

a) To ensure compliance: IM penicillin G benzathine as Bicillin C-R 900/300. It contains 900,000 U penicillin G benzathine and 300,000 U penicillin G procaine in a single-dose 2-ml injection.

b) For patients who will be compliant: PO penicillin V potassium × 10 days; 250 mg bid (<12 years of age) or 500 mg bid (>12 years of age). No benefit is shown for a tid or qid schedule (decreases compliance). A full 10-day course is mandatory.

c) For patients allergic to penicillin: Erythromycin ethylsuccinate 40 mg/kg/d ÷ qid × 10 days, or azithromycin 500 mg on day 1 followed by 250 mg on days 2-5. Tetracyclines and sulfonamides (including TMP/SMZ) are ineffective against GABHS infection.

NOTE: GABHS resistance to erythromycin is common in some countries (Japan, Finland) but is rare (<4%) in the United States.

d) If the patient has classic streptococcal symptoms, begin treatment while the TC is pending. If the patient is not highly symptomatic, it is best to withhold treatment until TC results are available (unless the patient is unlikely to return for follow-up).

e) The child may return to day care or school 24 hours after beginning the antibiotic.

b. Symptomatic treatment
1) Analgesics/antipyretics (ibuprofen more effective than acetaminophen)
2) Throat lozenges, throat spray

c. Posttreatment clinical and/or bacteriologic failures in 10%-20% of all cases
1) Failures may result from the presence of β-lactamase–producing organisms in the oropharynx, lack of compliance, or a GABHS carrier state (most common explanation). Some posttreatment failures may actually represent reinfection with the same or different serotypes.
2) The most difficult dilemma for the clinician is to determine whether a patient is having repeated episodes of acute GABHS pharyngitis or is a streptococcus carrier experiencing repeated episodes of viral illness. The streptococcus carrier state is likely if any of the following are true:
a) Clinical findings and season (summer) suggest a viral etiology
b) Lack of immediate clinical response to antibiotic therapy
c) Presence of GABHS between episodes
d) No serologic response to GABHS extracellular antigens
e) Same serotype for all isolates

NOTE: It is best to avoid culturing patients whose clinical findings suggest a viral etiology and who are likely to be streptococcus carriers.

3) Effective regimens for the patient with repeated episodes of GABHS pharyngitis include the following:
   a) Clindamycin 20 mg/kg/d ÷ tid × 10 days
   b) Cefuroxime axetil 250 mg bid × 10 days
   c) Penicillin G benzathine IM and rifampin 10 mg/kg (max 600 mg/d) q24h × 8 doses
   d) Rifampin 20 mg/kg (max 600 mg/d) q24h × 4 doses during the last 4 days of a 10-day course of oral penicillin V potassium
4) Prophylaxis with daily penicillin or sulfonamide may be considered for the otherwise normal child who has had "true" recurrent episodes of GABHS pharyngitis, but the efficacy of this technique has not yet been documented in clinical trials.
5) Indications for tonsillectomy include >7 GABHS episodes within 1 year, 5 episodes within each of 2 years, or 3 episodes within each of 3 years, with all episodes consisting of specific clinical findings.

5. Miscellaneous
   a. Culture any symptomatic family members of patients with streptococcal pharyngitis.
   b. A culture of asymptomatic family members generally is not necessary.
   c. In the winter-spring months, as many as 20% of asymptomatic schoolchildren are GABHS carriers.
   d. A routine posttreatment culture is not indicated. Indications include recurring symptoms, a family history of rheumatic fever, "ping-ponging" of streptococcal infections in the family, outbreak in a closed community, and a patient who is being considered for T&A.

G. SINUSITIS

1. 5%-10% of URIs in early childhood are complicated by acute sinusitis, which is suggested by the failure of the URI to improve after 10 days.
2. Predisposing conditions
   a. Anatomic: Nasoseptal deformity, polyps, large adenoids, cleft palate, choanal atresia, intranasal FB
   b. Cystic fibrosis
   c. Immunodeficiency
   d. Ciliary dyskinesia
   e. Allergy
   f. Diving, flying

NOTE: In a teenager with maxillary sinusitis, consider a dental origin.

3. Presentations
   a. Cough (night > day), malodorous breath, low-grade fever, painless periorbital swelling in the morning, anterior/posterior rhinorrhea
   b. High fever, purulent nasal discharge, ± facial pain, ± headache
   c. PE: Boggy, erythematous nasal mucosa; facial tenderness (in older children and adolescents)

4. Bacteriology
   a. Same as otitis media: *S. pneumoniae, H. influenzae, M. (Branhamella) catarrhalis.* In children with chronic sinusitis, up to 50% of isolates may be β-lactamase producers.
   b. *S. pneumoniae* strains that are relatively resistant to penicillin have been recovered from young children with chronic sinusitis.
   c. Anaerobes may play a role in chronic infections, especially in older patients.
   d. An NP culture and TC *do not* correlate with sinus aspirate cultures.

5. Diagnosis
   a. Usually based on clinical picture
   b. Transillumination: Not helpful if <10 years of age
   c. Sinus x-ray studies: Usually sufficient to exclude or confirm the diagnosis in patients with signs and symptoms of acute sinusitis, but routine use is now questionable. X-ray studies are clearly less informative than CT imaging.
      1) Mucosal thickening >4 mm
      2) Air-fluid level
      3) Complete opacification
   d. Ultrasound: May discriminate between mucosal thickening and sinus secretions but is not usually helpful in children
   e. CT scan: Imaging procedure of choice; especially helpful for recurrent, chronic, or complicated cases
   f. Sinus aspiration: "Gold standard," but not routine
      1) Bacterial density >10^4 CFU/mm or >1 organism/HPF on a Gram's stain represents a true infection.
      2) Reserve this technique for treatment failure, immunocompromised patients, those with severe facial pain, and those with orbital and intracranial complications.

NOTE: For patients with chronic/recurrent sinusitis, the work-up may include allergy/ENT consultation, a sweat test (CF), serum immunoglobulin determinations, and nasal mucosal biopsy (ciliary dyskinesia).

6. Treatment
   a. Acute sinusitis: Amoxicillin 40 mg/kg/d ÷ tid × 14 days is ad-

equate for most cases. For hospitalized patients with severe sinusitis, IV cefotaxime plus clindamycin should be considered for initial treatment to cover highly resistant pneumococcal strains.

b. Treatment failures require 14-21 days of therapy.
1) Amoxicillin-clavulanate 40 mg/kg/d ÷ tid
2) Cefuroxime axetil 250 mg bid
3) Erythromycin-sulfisoxazole 50 mg/kg/d erythromycin ÷ qid
4) TMP/SMZ 8 mg/kg/d TMP ÷ bid; some *S. pneumoniae* strains may be resistant to TMP/SMZ

c. Subacute or chronic sinusitis (symptoms >30 days): Treat with one of the previously listed agents for 3-6 weeks.

d. Recurrent sinusitis: A trial of antimicrobial prophylaxis should be considered.

e. Topical decongestants and topical steroids (3-7 days) may reduce mucosal edema and promote patency of ostia. Antihistamines might help a patient with underlying atopy.

f. Surgery (functional endoscopic sinus surgery) is reserved for complicated sinusitis or for patients with chronic or recurrent sinusitis who fail trials of prolonged medical therapy. Surgery should be preceded by a CT scan.

H. UPPER RESPIRATORY INFECTION
1. Supportive measures are the mainstay of therapy.
   a. Rest and fluids
   b. Humidification (cool-mist vaporizer) may soothe inflamed, scratchy nasal and pharyngeal mucosa. Avoid passive smoking and other environmental irritants.
   c. Infants: Buffered saline nose drops + bulb syringe, 2 gtt in each nostril to loosen secretions, then aspirate with nasal aspirator. Use before feeding, bedtime, and prn.

NOTE: It is preferable for parents to obtain buffered saline nose drops at the pharmacy. Homemade solutions are notorious for being made incorrectly, regardless of how simple the recipe, and therefore are strongly discouraged.

   d. Analgesics/antipyretics for malaise and fever prn
2. Antihistamines or sympathomimetics

The efficacy of antihistamines and sympathomimetics has not been demonstrated in controlled studies, but they are often used. They should not be used in children <18 months of age because of hypersensitivity to antihistamine and sympathomimetic effects. Warn patients about drowsiness with antihistamines.

3. Topical decongestants: 0.25% phenylephrine (Neo-Synephrine) nasal drops decrease mucosal swelling and rhinorrhea. Do not use >3-5 days (tachyphylaxis and rhinitis medicamentosa) or in children <6 months of age.
4. Cough medications
    a. Guaifenesin (e.g., plain Robitussin) does not work.
    b. Dextromethorphan is a short-acting cough suppressant and may help, especially with troublesome nighttime coughing.

BIBLIOGRAPHY

Allergic rhinitis

Estelle F, Simons R: Allergic rhinitis: recent advances, *Pediatr Clin North Am* 35:1053, 1988.
Meltzer EO et al: Chronic rhinitis in infants and children: etiologic, diagnostic and therapeutic considerations, *Pediatr Clin North Am* 30:847, 1983.
Naclerio RM: Allergic rhinitis, *N Engl J Med* 325:860, 1991.
Pearlman DS: Chronic rhinitis in children, *Clin Rev Allergy* 2:197, 1984.
Virant PS: Allergic rhinitis, *Pediatr Rev* 13:323, 1992.

Epistaxis

Culbertson M: Epistaxis. In Bluestone CD, Stool SE, editors: *Pediatric otolaryngology,* vol 1, Philadelphia, 1983, WB Saunders.

Foreign bodies

Biehler JL et al: Use of the transmitter-receiver metal detector in the evaluation of pediatric coin ingestions, *Pediatr Emerg Care* 9:208, 1993.
Caravati EM et al: Pediatric coin ingestion: a prospective study on the utility of routine roentgenograms, *Am J Dis Child* 143:549, 1989.
Connors GP et al: Symptoms and spontaneous passage of esophageal coins, *Arch Pediatr Adolesc Med* 149:36, 1995.
Kenna MA, Bluestone CD: Foreign bodies in the air and food passages, *Pediatr Rev* 10:25, 1988.
Litovitz T, Schmitz BF: Ingestion of cylindrical and button batteries: an analysis of 2382 cases, *Pediatrics* 89:747, 1992.

Schunk JE et al: Fluoroscopic Foley catheter removal of esophageal foreign bodies in children: experience with 415 episodes, *Pediatrics* 94:709, 1994.

Schweich PJ: Management of coin ingestion, *Pediatr Emerg Care* 11:37, 1995.

Sheikh A: Button battery ingestions in children, *Pediatr Emerg Care* 9:224, 1993.

Hoarseness

Kenna MA: Hoarseness, *Pediatr Rev* 16:69, 1982.

Otitis media

Barnett ED, Klein JO: The problem of resistant bacteria for the management of acute otitis media, *Pediatr Clin North Am* 42:509, 1995.

Bernard PAM et al: Randomized, controlled trial comparing long-term sulfonamide therapy to ventilation tubes for otitis media with effusion, *Pediatrics* 88:215, 1991.

Bluestone CD: Modern management of otitis media, *Pediatr Clin North Am* 36:1371, 1989.

Cantekin EI et al: Lack of efficacy of a decongestant: antihistamine combination for otitis media with effusion ("secretory" otitis media) in children, *N Engl J Med* 308:297, 1983.

Chang MG et al: *Chlamydia trachomatis* in otitis media in children, *Pediatr Infect Dis J* 1:95, 1982.

Del Beccaro MA et al: Bacteriology of acute otitis media: a new perspective, *J Pediatr* 120:81, 1992.

Hathaway TJ et al: Acute otitis media: who needs posttreatment follow-up? *Pediatrics* 94:143, 1994.

Jung TTK, Rhee CK: Otolaryngologic approach to the diagnosis and management of otitis media, *Otolaryngol Clin North Am* 24:931, 1991.

Kempthorne J, Giebink GS: Pediatric approach to the diagnosis and management of otitis media, *Otolaryngol Clin North Am* 24:905, 1991.

Le CT et al: Evaluation of ventilating tubes and myringotomy in the treatment of recurrent or persistent otitis media, *Pediatr Infect Dis J* 10:2, 1991.

Mandel EM et al: Efficacy of amoxicillin with and without decongestant-antihistamine for otitis media with effusion in children: results of a double-blind, randomized trial, *N Engl J Med* 316:432, 1987.

Otitis media guideline panel: Managing otitis media with effusion in young children, *Pediatrics* 94:766, 1994.

Paradise JL: Managing otitis media: a time for change, *Pediatrics* 96:712, 1995.

Rosenfeld RM et al: Clinical efficacy of antimicrobial drugs for acute otitis media: metaanalysis of 5400 children from thirty-three randomized trials, *J Pediatr* 124:355, 1994.

Schwartz RH et al: Use of a short course of prednisone for treating middle ear effusion: a double-blind crossover study, *Ann Otol Rhinol Laryngol* 89:296, 1980.

Shurin PA et al: Bacterial etiology of otitis media in first 6 weeks of life, *J Pediatr* 92:893, 1978.

Pharyngitis

Bass JW: Antibiotic management of Group A streptococcal pharyngotonsillitis, *Pediatr Inf Dis J* 10:S43, 1991.

Chaudhary S et al: Penicillin V and rifampin for the treatment of group A streptococcal pharyngitis: a randomized trial of 10 days of penicillin vs 10 days penicillin with rifampin during the final 4 days of therapy, *J Pediatr* 106:481, 1985.

Fries SM: Diagnosis of group A streptococcal pharyngitis in a private clinic: comparative evaluation of an optical immunoassay method and culture, *J Pediatr* 126:933, 1995.

Gerber MA et al: Lack of impact of early antibiotic therapy for streptococcal pharyngitis on recurrence rates, *J Pediatr* 117:853, 1990.

Kaplan EG et al: The role of the carrier in treatment failure after antibiotic therapy for group A streptococci in the upper respiratory tract, *J Lab Clin Med* 98:326, 1981.

Klein JO: Management of streptococcal pharyngitis, *Pediatr Infect Dis J* 13:572, 1994.

Krober MS et al: Optimal dosing interval for penicillin treatment of streptococcal pharyngitis, *Clin Pediatr* 29:646, 1990.

Markowitz M et al: Treatment of streptococcal pharyngotonsillitis: reports of penicillin's demise are premature, *J Pediatr* 123:679, 1993.

McCracken GH: Diagnosis and management of children with streptococcal pharyngitis, *Pediatr Infect Dis J* 5:754, 1987.

Pichichero ME, Margolis PA: A comparison of cephalosporins and penicillins in the treatment of group A beta-hemolytic streptococcal pharyngitis: a metaanalysis supporting the concept of copathogenicity, *Pediatr Infect Dis J* 10:275, 1991.

Shulman ST: Streptococcal pharyngitis: diagnostic considerations, *Pediatr Infect Dis J* 13:567, 1994.

Sumaya CU, Ench Y: Epstein-Barr virus infectious mononucleosis in children: clinical and general laboratory findings, *Pediatrics* 75:1003, 1985.

Sinusitis

Duplechain JK, White JA, Miller RH: Pediatric sinusitis, *Arch Otolaryngol Head Neck Surg* 117:422, 1991.

Lazar RH, Younis RT: The management of recurrent sinusitis in children, *Clin Pediatr* 31:30, 1992.

Tinkelman DG, Silk HJ: Clinical and bacteriologic features of chronic sinusitis in children, *Am J Dis Child* 143:938, 1989.

Wald ER: Sinusitis in children, *N Engl J Med* 326:319, 1992.

PULMONARY DISEASES 18

A. APNEA

1. Apnea is defined as the cessation of respiratory airflow, which may result from the following:
   a. Absence of respiratory effort (central)
   b. Obstruction of the airway (obstructive)
   c. Combination of both (mixed)
2. Occasional respiratory pauses of ≤20 seconds may be a normal finding at any age. Apnea that lasts >20 seconds or is accompanied by bradycardia, pallor, hypotonia, or cyanosis is pathologic and warrants evaluation.
3. There is no evidence that apnea alone increases the risk for SIDS or that apnea progresses to ALTEs.
4. Apparent life-threatening event (formerly called "near-miss" SIDS)
   a. An ALTE is defined as an episode that is frightening to the observer and is characterized by some combination of apnea (central or obstructive), color change (cyanosis, pallor, plethora), limpness, choking, and gagging. In most cases, either vigorous stimulation or CPR has been instituted.
   b. The etiology of ALTEs includes acute infection (sepsis, pneumonia, RSV, meningitis), dysfunctional swallowing, GER, seizures, CNS disease, disorders of respiratory control, anemia, poisoning, metabolic disorders, hypercalcemia, and upper airway obstruction. A treatable etiology is found in approximately 30% of the cases.
   c. The infant who has had an ALTE is at significantly increased risk for SIDS, but such cases probably account for only 10% of SIDS deaths.
   d. The infant who has had an ALTE should be hospitalized for observation, monitoring, and evaluation. Unless there is evidence to suggest otherwise, the parents' or caretakers' observations must be accepted as valid and accurate. Parental anxiety should not be minimized. The evaluation includes the following:

1) Careful history: Focus on circumstances of events, perinatal history, family history. Awake apnea suggests seizures or GER/aspiration.
2) PE: Focus on upper airway, cardiac, pulmonary, and neurologic exams. Observe feeding and sleeping patterns.
3) Laboratory studies: Minimum work-up includes CBC, blood glucose, electrolytes, calcium, bicarbonate, ammonia, and SaO_2 while asleep.
4) Based on the initial evaluation, additional work-up may include ABGs, barium swallow, CXR, ECG, EEG, esophageal pH monitoring, metabolic screening, polysomnography, a head CT scan, and upper airway evaluation.

NOTE: Data obtained from polysomnography are not useful in identifying the infant at risk for SIDS and should not be used to determine the need for home monitoring.

5) Provide cardiorespiratory monitoring and parental CPR instruction.

NOTE: A normal evaluation and laboratory work-up does not indicate that a significant event did not occur or that it will not happen again. If no treatable cause is found, the infant requires home monitoring.

6) Be supportive of the family, answer questions patiently, and ensure adequate follow-up. Parents should be included in the decision-making process.

5. Home monitoring
   a. Indications include the following:
      1) ALTE requiring vigorous stimulation or resuscitation (milder ALTE is a relative indication)
      2) Sibling of two or more SIDS victims (monitoring the sibling of one SIDS victim is not officially recommended but is generally unavoidable)
      3) Surviving twin of a SIDS victim
      4) Infant with hypoventilation syndrome
      5) Infant with tracheostomy or O_2-dependent BPD
      6) Apnea and bradycardia associated with dysfunctional swallowing or GER, unless the GER is controlled by medical or surgical treatment
   b. The monitor alarm should be set to sound for a respiratory pause >20 seconds or for the following HR: <1 month, 80 bpm; 1-3 months, 70 bpm; 4-6 months, 60 bpm; >6 months, 50 bpm.
   c. A documented ("smart") monitor with a built-in event recorder can be helpful in distinguishing "true" events from insignificant (e.g.,

loose lead) events. The monitor also provides information on compliance with monitor use.

    d. Use of the monitor can be discontinued if the infant has gone 3 months without a significant event and has demonstrated an ability to tolerate stresses such as infection without apnea or bradycardia alarms.

NOTE: It is now recommended that all infants (except those with GER and craniofacial abnormalities) be placed in the crib to sleep in the supine position.

6. "Factitious" apnea
    a. There is evidence that recurrent episodes of apnea may be related to child abuse (Munchausen by proxy) (see p. 41).
    b. Clues to factitious apnea include the following:
        1) Episodes that begin only in the presence of the parent (caretaker) but are witnessed by other persons called for assistance (often in the hospital setting); may need to be confirmed by covert video surveillance
        2) Evidence of physical abuse
        3) Previous SIDS death in the family
        4) Simultaneous death of twins
        5) History of unexplained disorders in the victim (symptoms do not make sense medically)
        6) Death at an unusual age for SIDS
        7) One of the parents (usually the mother) is medically sophisticated and shows exemplary behavior in the medical setting; may be a discrepancy between family's and medical team's level of concern

B. ASTHMA

1. Diagnosis
    a. In children, recurrent episodes of coughing, wheezing, and dyspnea are almost always a result of asthma. Some children have only chronic/recurrent coughing (cough-variant asthma).
    b. Features suggestive of asthma are periodicity of symptoms, nocturnal attacks, seasonal variation, and the relation of symptoms to allergen exposure or exertion. There is often a personal or family history of atopy.
    c. Pulmonary function testing, including bronchodilator responsiveness, is helpful. Most important is the clinical response to antiasthma therapy.
    d. Airway inflammation is present in almost all patients with asthma,

even during clinical remission; antiinflammatory drugs are the cornerstone of asthma management. A number of triggers such as viral infection, cold air, exercise, allergens, and pollutants (e.g., cigarette smoke) can increase airway responsiveness and trigger acute attacks.

    e. If the response to treatment is poor or if the patient has a productive cough, failure to thrive, choking episodes, or focal lung findings, consider other diagnoses such as FB, vascular ring, laryngeal web, CF, GER, aspiration, laryngotracheomalacia, ciliary dyskinesia, immunodeficiency, enlarged mediastinal nodes or tumor, or congenital lobar emphysema.

2. Management of acute asthma

    a. Estimation of severity of an acute exacerbation is shown in Table 18-1. A prolonged prehospital course implies a significant component of airway inflammation.

    b. Home: For an acute exacerbation, the patient should be instructed to use albuterol by nebulization or an MDI/spacer q20min up to 1 hour (Fig. 18-1).

    c. Emergency department (Fig. 18-2)

        1) History: If the patient is in acute distress, obtain a brief, pertinent history. When did wheezing begin? Precipitating event (e.g., URI, allergen, irritant, exercise, weather change)? Is the child a known asthmatic, or is this a "first-time" wheezer? Any associated illness? Medications? Last dose? Course of previous episodes? Previous hospitalizations? What type of ED or inpatient treatment has usually reversed acute attacks? Consider other diagnoses if this is the first wheezing episode, especially if wheezing is atypical or not responding to therapy or if there is no family history for atopy.

        2) PE: Check all vital signs. Assess the degree of severity; supraclavicular retractions correlate well with the degree of obstruction. Cyanosis? Tightness? (Some patients may have such poor air movement that no wheezing is heard.) Measure pulsus paradoxus (significant bronchospasm produces pulsus paradoxus >15 mm Hg). Evaluate the state of hydration and mental status. Look for a focus of infection.

        3) Laboratory tests: If a patient is taking theophylline, obtain a serum theophylline level. In a cooperative child >6 years of age, measure PEFR; a flow rate <30% predicted often predicts a need for admission. Measure O_2 saturation by pulse oximetry. ABGs should be obtained in a patient with evidence of severe

TABLE 18-1.
Estimation of Severity of Acute Exacerbations of Asthma in Children*

Sign/symptom	Mild	Moderate	Severe
PEFR†	70%-90% predicted or personal best	50%-70% predicted or personal best	<50% predicted or personal best
Respiratory rate, resting or sleeping	Normal to 30% increase above the mean	30%-50% increase above the mean	Increase over 50% above the mean
Alertness	Normal	Normal	May be decreased
Dyspnea‡	Absent or mild; speaks in complete sentences	Moderate; speaks in phrases or partial sentences; infants cry softer and shorter; infant has difficulty suckling and feeding	Severe; speaks only in single words or short phrases; infant's cry softer and shorter; infant stops suckling and feeding
Pulsus paradoxus§	<10 mm Hg	10-20 mm Hg	20-40 mm Hg
Accessory muscle use	No intercostal to mild retractions	Moderate intercostal retraction with tracheosternal retractions; use of sternocleidomastoid muscles; chest hyperinflation	Severe intercostal retractions; tracheostemal retractions with nasal flaring during inspiration; chest hyperinflation
Color	Good	Pale	Possibly cyanotic
Auscultation	End expiratory wheeze only	Wheeze during entire expiration and inspiration	Breath sounds becoming inaudible
Oxygen saturation	>95%	90%-95%	<90%
P_{CO_2}	<35	<40	>40

From National Heart, Lung and Blood Institute, National Institutes of Health: Bethesda, Md, publ no. 91-3042A, June 1991.
*Within each category the presence of several parameters, but not necessarily all, indicates general classification of the exacerbation.
†For children 5 years of age or older.
‡Parents' or physicians' impression of the degree of the child's breathlessness.
§Pulsus paradoxus does not correlate with the phase of respiration in small children.

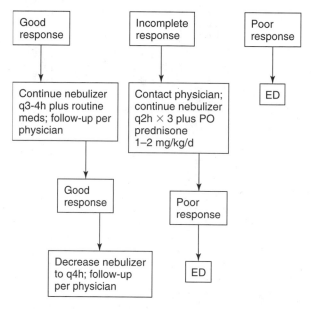

FIG 18-1. Home management of acute asthma exacerbation.

obstruction, a change in mental status, or clinical worsening. Po_2 <50 mm Hg or Pco_2 >40 mm Hg indicates respiratory failure. A normal or slightly elevated Pco_2 in a patient with tachypnea may be a sign of impending respiratory failure.

4) CXR: Not generally helpful and not indicated as a routine procedure. Radiographic findings do not correlate with the severity of the attack. An x-ray examination may be indicated for the following:
   a) Initial episode of wheezing
   b) Temperature >38.5° C
   c) Localized, persistent rales, especially in a child >2 years of age

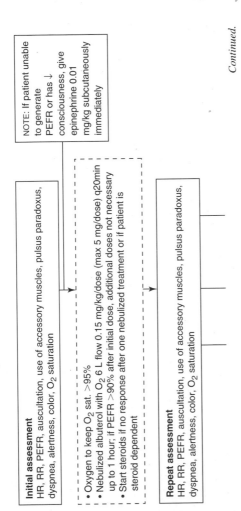

NOTE: If patient unable to generate PEFR or has ↓ consciousness, give epinephrine 0.01 mg/kg subcutaneously immediately

Initial assessment
HR, RR, PEFR, auscultation, use of accessory muscles, pulsus paradoxus, dyspnea, alertness, color, O_2 saturation

• Oxygen to keep O_2 sat. >95%
• Nebulized albuterol with O_2 6 L flow 0.15 mg/kg/dose (max 5 mg/dose) q20min up to 1 hour; if PEFR >90% after initial dose, additional doses not necessary
• Start steroids if no response after one nebulized treatment or if patient is steroid dependent

Repeat assessment
HR, RR, PEFR, auscultation, use of accessory muscles, pulsus paradoxus, dyspnea, alertness, color, O_2 saturation

Continued.

FIG 18-2. Emergency department management of asthma exacerbation. Therapies are often available in a physician's office; however, most acutely severe exacerbations of asthma require a complete course of therapy in an emergency department. *PEFR % baseline is the norm for the patient as established by the clinician. This percentage may be predicted based on standardized norms or on the patient's personal best. (From National Heart, Lung, and Blood Institute, Pub No 91-3042A, Bethesda, Md, June 1991, National Institutes of Health.)

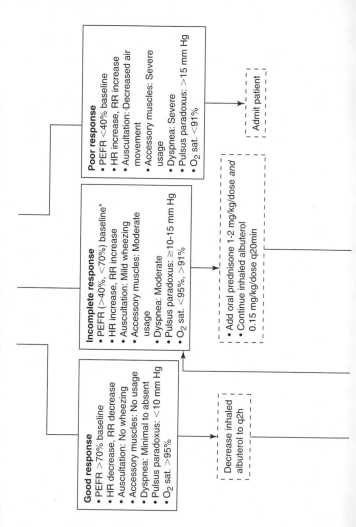

Good response
- PEFR >70% baseline
- HR decrease, RR decrease
- Auscultation: No wheezing
- Accessory muscles: No usage
- Dyspnea: Minimal to absent
- Pulsus paradoxus: <10 mm Hg
- O₂ sat. >95%

Incomplete response
- PEFR (>40%, <70%) baseline*
- HR increase, RR increase
- Auscultation: Mild wheezing
- Accessory muscles: Moderate usage
- Dyspnea: Moderate
- Pulsus paradoxus: ≥10-15 mm Hg
- O₂ sat. <95%, >91%

Poor response
- PEFR <40% baseline
- HR increase, RR increase
- Auscultation: Decreased air movement
- Accessory muscles: Severe usage
- Dyspnea: Severe
- Pulsus paradoxus: >15 mm Hg
- O₂ sat. <91%

- Decrease inhaled albuterol to q2h

- Add oral prednisone 1-2 mg/kg/dose *and*
- Continue inhaled albuterol 0.15 mg/kg/dose q20min

- Admit patient

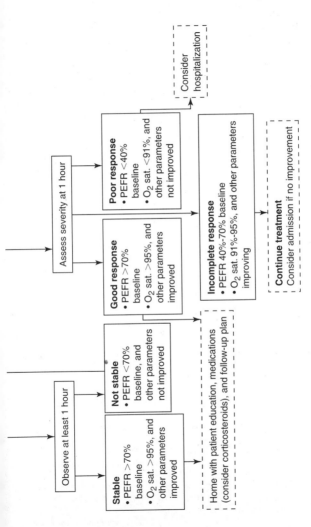

Observe at least 1 hour

Stable
• PEFR >70%
  baseline
• O₂ sat. >95%, and
  other parameters
  improved

Not stable
• PEFR <70%
  baseline, and
  other parameters
  not improved

Home with patient education, medications
(consider corticosteroids), and follow-up plan

Assess severity at 1 hour

Good response
• PEFR >70%
  baseline
• O₂ sat. >95%, and
  other parameters
  improved

Poor response
• PEFR <40%
  baseline
• O₂ sat. <91%, and
  other parameters
  not improved

Incomplete response
• PEFR 40%-70% baseline
• O₂ sat. 91%-95%, and other parameters
  improving

Continue treatment
Consider admission if no improvement

Consider hospitalization

FIG 18-2, cont. For legend see p. 321.

      d) Patient who appears particularly ill or does not respond to treatment as expected

      e) Suspected pneumothorax

   5) Estimation of severity

   6) Management (see Fig. 18-2); if the patient is discharged home, the following steps should be taken:

      a) Outline, at a minimum, a 3-5–day treatment regimen. In most cases this regimen should include a short course of oral corticosteroids (1-2 mg/kg q AM × 5-7 days ± taper).

      b) Ensure that a follow-up appointment has been made.

      c) Consider having the patient perform daily PEFR measurements at home.

      d) Review discharge medications and provide education regarding the avoidance of asthma triggers.

   7) Dosages of drugs for acute exacerbations (Table 18-2)

      a) In children with acute asthma and impending respiratory failure, there is evidence that continuous nebulization of a β_2-agonist results in more rapid improvement compared with intermittent nebulizations.

      b) Anticholinergic (ipratropium bromide) nebulizations play a minimal role in the treatment of an acute asthma exacerbation. They may provide an additional 20%-25% improvement in FEV_1 over β_2-agonists alone but are not shown to improve clinical outcome. However, combination therapy may be indicated for patients with severe obstruction.

  d. Hospital (Fig. 18-3)

3. Management of chronic asthma

  a. Mild

   1) Intermittent brief (<1 hour) episodes of coughing, wheezing, dyspnea, and tightness up to two times/wk; usually asymptomatic between episodes

   2) Brief (<½ hour) wheezing, coughing, and dyspnea with activity

   3) Infrequent (<2 times/month) nocturnal coughing/wheezing

   4) FEV_1 or PEFR >80% baseline when asymptomatic

   5) Treatment

      a) Asymptomatic: Pretreatment prn with 1-2 puffs β_2-agonist and/or cromolyn for exposure to exercise, allergens, or other triggers

      b) Symptomatic <5 yr: Nebulized or oral β_2-agonist prn

      c) Symptomatic >5 yr: Inhaled β_2-agonist with a spacer device q4-6h prn for duration of episode

Text continued on p. 331.

TABLE 18-2.
Dosages of Drugs in Acute Exacerbations

Drug	Available form	Dosage	Comment
Inhaled β_2-agonist			
Albuterol			
Metered-dose inhaler	90 µg/puff	2 inhalations every 5 min for total of 12 puffs, with monitoring of PEFR or FEV_1 to document response	If not improved, switch to nebulizer; if improved, decrease to 4 puffs every hour
Nebulizer solution	0.5% (5 mg/ml)	0.1–0.15 mg/kg/dose up to 5 mg q20min for 1–2 hr (minimum dose 1.25 mg/dose)	If improved, decrease to 1–2 hr; if not improved, use by continuous inhalation
		0.5 mg/kg/h by continuous nebulization (maximum 15 mg/h)	
Metaproterenol			
Metered-dose inhaler	650 µg/puff	2 inhalations	Frequent high-dose administration has not been evaluated; metaproterenol is not interchangeable with β_2-agonists albuterol and terbutaline
Nebulizer solution	5% (50 mg/ml)	0.1–0.3 ml (5–15 mg); do not exceed 15 mg	
	0.6% unit dose vial of 2.5 ml (15 mg)	As above 5–15 mg; do not exceed 15 mg	

Continued.

TABLE 18-2 (cont.)

Drug	Available form	Dosage	Comment
Terbutaline Metered-dose inhaler used in nebulizer Injectable solution	200 µg/puff 0.1% (1 mg/1 ml) solution in 0.9% NaCl solution for injection Not FDA approved for inhalation	2 inhalations q5min for a total of 12 puffs	Not recommended because not available as nebulizer solution; offers no advantage over albuterol, which is available as a nebulizer solution
Inhaled anticholinergic			
Ipratropium bromide (Atrovent) Metered-dose inhaler Nebulizer solution	18 µg/puff 0.02% (2.5 ml)	1-2 inhalations 3 times/d; up to 6 inhalations/24 h 250-500 µg 3-4 times/d	Not indicated for the initial treatment of acute episodes of bronchospasm
Systemic β-agonist			
Epinephrine HCl	1:1000 (1 mg/ml)	0.01 mg/kg up to 0.3 mg subcutaneously q20 min for 3 doses	Inhaled β_2-agonist preferred
Terbutaline	(0.1%) 1 mg/ml solution for injection in 0.9% NaCl	Subcutaneous 0.01 mg/kg up to 0.3 mg q2-6h as needed; IV 10 µg/kg over 10 min loading dose; maintenance: 0.4 µg/kg/min; increase as necessary by 0.2 µg/kg/min and expect to use 3-6 µg/kg/min	Inhaled β_2-agonist preferred

Methylxanthines

Theophylline	Aminophylline (80% anhydrous theophylline)	Loading dose* (if theophylline concentration is known): Every 1 mg/kg aminophylline gives 2 μg/ml increase in serum concentration	
		Loading dose* (if theophylline concentration is unknown): No previous theophylline—6 mg/kg aminophylline; previous theophylline—3 mg/kg aminophylline	
		Constant infusion rates*: Infusion rates to obtain a mean steady-state concentration of 15 μg/ml	
		Age	
		1-6 mo	0.5 mg/kg/h aminophylline
		6 mo-1 yr	1.0 mg/kg/h aminophylline
		1-9 yr	1.5 mg/kg/h aminophylline
		10-16 yr	1.2 mg/kg/h aminophylline

Corticosteroids

Outpatients	Oral prednisone, prednisolone, or methylprednisolone	1-2 mg/kg/d in single or divided doses	Reassess at 3 days because only a short burst may be needed; no need to taper dose
Emergency department or hospitalized patients	Methylprednisolone IV or PO	1-2 mg/kg/dose q6h for 24 hr, then 1-2 mg/kg/d in divided doses q8-12 h	Length depends on response; may need only a few days

*Check serum concentration approximately 1, 12, and 24 hours after starting the infusion.

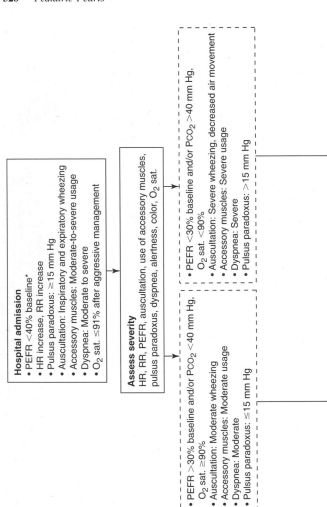

Hospital admission
- PEFR <40% baseline*
- HR increase, RR increase
- Pulsus paradoxus: ≥15 mm Hg
- Auscultation: Inspiratory and expiratory wheezing
- Accessory muscles: Moderate-to-severe usage
- Dyspnea: Moderate to severe
- O_2 sat. ≤91% after aggressive management

Assess severity
HR, RR, PEFR, auscultation, use of accessory muscles, pulsus paradoxus, dyspnea, alertness, color, O_2 sat.

- PEFR >30% baseline and/or PCO_2 <40 mm Hg.
  O_2 sat. ≥90%
- Auscultation: Moderate wheezing
- Accessory muscles: Moderate usage
- Dyspnea: Moderate
- Pulsus paradoxus: ≤15 mm Hg

- PEFR <30% baseline and/or PCO_2 >40 mm Hg.
  O_2 sat. <90%
- Auscultation: Severe wheezing, decreased air movement
- Accessory muscles: Severe usage
- Dyspnea: Severe
- Pulsus paradoxus: >15 mm Hg

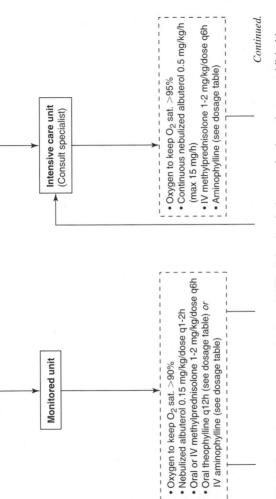

Continued.

FIG 18-3. Hospital management of asthma. *PEFR % baseline is the norm for the patient as established by the clinician. This percentage may be predicted based on standardized norms or the patient's personal best. (From National Heart, Lung, and Blood Institute, Pub No 91-3042A, June 1991, Bethesda, Md, National Institutes of Health.)

Monitored unit

• Oxygen to keep O_2 sat. >90%
• Nebulized albuterol 0.15 mg/kg/dose q1-2h
• Oral or IV methylprednisolone 1-2 mg/kg/dose q6h
• Oral theophylline q12h (see dosage table) *or* IV aminophylline (see dosage table)

Intensive care unit (Consult specialist)

• Oxygen to keep O_2 sat. >95%
• Continuous nebulized albuterol 0.5 mg/kg/h (max 15 mg/h)
• IV methylprednisolone 1-2 mg/kg/dose q6h
• Aminophylline (see dosage table)

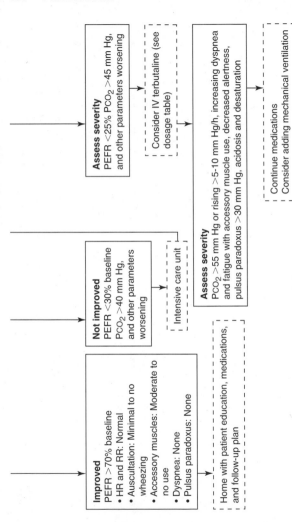

Assess severity
PEFR <25% PCO$_2$ >45 mm Hg,
and other parameters worsening

Consider IV terbutaline (see
dosage table)

Assess severity
PCO$_2$ >55 mm Hg or rising >5-10 mm Hg/h, increasing dyspnea
and fatigue with accessory muscle use, decreased alertness,
pulsus paradoxus >30 mm Hg, acidosis and desaturation

Continue medications
Consider adding mechanical ventilation

Not improved
PEFR <30% baseline
PCO$_2$ >40 mm Hg,
and other parameters
worsening

Intensive care unit

Improved
PEFR >70% baseline
• HR and RR: Normal
• Auscultation: Minimal to no
  wheezing
• Accessory muscles: Moderate to
  no use
• Dyspnea: None
• Pulsus paradoxus: None

Home with patient education, medications,
and follow-up plan

FIG 18-3, cont. For legend see p. 329.

    b. Moderate
       1) Symptoms >1-2 times/wk
       2) Exacerbations that may last several days
       3) Occasional need for emergency care
       4) FEV_1 or PEFR 60%-80% of baseline when asymptomatic
       5) Treatment
          a) Inhaled or nebulized β_2-agonist prn or tid/qid + cromolyn 2 puffs or ampule bid-qid
            or
          b) Inhaled or nebulized β_2-agonist prn-tid/qid + sustained-release theophylline (serum concentration 5-15 µg/ml) or oral β_2-agonist
          c) If symptoms persist, may substitute inhaled corticosteroid for cromolyn or theophylline

NOTE: There is no clear-cut benefit of nedocromil sodium (Tilade) over cromolyn sodium.

    c. Severe
       1) Continuous symptoms
       2) Limited activity level
       3) Frequent exacerbations
       4) Frequent nocturnal symptoms
       5) Occasional need for emergency treatment and hospitalization
       6) FEV_1 or PEFR <60% baseline
       7) Treatment
          a) Inhaled or nebulized β_2-agonist prn-tid/qid
            +
            Inhaled corticosteroid 2-4 puffs bid-qid
            ±
            Cromolyn 2 puffs bid-qid
            ±
            Sustained-release theophylline, especially for nocturnal symptoms (serum concentration 5-15 µg/ml) and/or oral β_2-agonist
          b) May consider oral alternate-day AM corticosteroid at the lowest dose that stabilizes symptoms and peak flow
    d. Drug dosages for maintenance therapy (Table 18-3)
    e. Alternative treatment strategies that may have a steroid-sparing effect have been used in patients with severe, oral steroid–dependent asthma and include a macrolide antibiotic (troleandomycin), methotrexate, oral gold (auranofin), and cyclosporin. None of these agents have demonstrated a marked therapeutic effect, and all are

TABLE 18-3.
Drug Dosages for Maintenance Therapy*

β_2-Agonists

Inhaled
Examples: Albuterol, metaproterenol, bitolterol, terbutaline, pirbuteral
  Mode of administration:
    Metered-dose inhaler, 2 puffs q4-6h
    Dry powder inhaler, 1 capsule q4-6h
    Nebulizer solution, albuterol 5 mg/ml, 0.1-0.15 mg/kg in 2 ml of
      saline q4-6h, maximum 5.0 mg or metaproterenol 50 mg/ml, 0.25-
      0.50 mg/kg in 2 ml of saline q4-6h, maximum 15.0 mg
Oral
  Liquids
    Albuterol, 0.1-0.15 mg/kg q4-6h
    Metaproterenol, 0.3-0.5 mg/kg q4-6h
  Tablets
    Albuterol, 2- or 4-mg tablet q4-6h
    Metaproterenol, 10- or 20-mg tablet q4-6h
    Terbutaline, 2.5- or 5.0-mg tablet q4-6h

Cromolyn sodium

Metered-dose inhaler, 1 mg/puff; 2 puffs bid-qid
Dry powder inhaler, 20 mg/capsule; 1 capsule bid-qid
Nebulizer solution, 20 mg/2 ml ampule; 1 ampule bid-qid

Theophylline

Liquid
Tablets, capsules
Sustained-release tablets, capsules
Dosage to achieve serum concentration of 5-15 µg/ml

Corticosteroids

Inhaled†
  Beclomethasone, 42 µg/puff 2-4 puffs bid-qid
  Triamcinolone, 100 µg/puff 2-4 puffs bid-qid
  Flunisolide, 250 µg/puff 2-4 puffs bid
Oral‡
  Liquids
    Prednisone, 5 mg/5 ml
    Prednisolone, 5 mg/5 ml, 15 mg/5 ml
  Tablets
    Prednisone, 1, 2.5, 5, 10, 20, 25, 50 mg
    Prednisolone, 5 mg
    Methylprednisolone, 2, 4, 8, 16, 24, 32 g

---

*Premixed solutions are available. It is suggested that the per/kg dosage recommendations be followed.
†Consider use of spacer devices to minimize local adverse effects.
‡For acute exacerbations, doses of 1-2 mg/kg in single or divided doses are used initially and then modified. Reassess in 3 days because only a short burst may be needed. There is no need to taper a short (3- to 5-day) course of therapy. If therapy extends beyond this period, it may be appropriate to taper the dosage. For chronic dosage, the lowest possible alternate-day AM dosage should be established.

associated with a high prevalence of side effects. They are of limited use in very select patients.

4. Exercise-induced asthma
    a. Exercise-induced asthma may occur in almost all patients with asthma. However, in some patients exercise may be the only trigger.
    b. The diagnosis is suggested by coughing, SOB, chest pain or tightness, wheezing, or endurance problems during exercise.
    c. It can be documented by an exercise challenge; a 15% or greater decrease in FEV_1 or PEFR within 10 minutes after exercise confirms the dianosis.
    d. Management
        1) An inhaled β_2-agonist or cromolyn immediately before exercise is helpful for up to several hours. After 2 hours and if exercise continues, this treatment may be repeated prn.
        2) In a patient with breakthrough symptoms, may pretreat with a combination of β_2-agonist 2 puffs and cromolyn 2 puffs.
        3) Inhaled steroids have little effect on exercise-induced asthma unless they are used for several weeks.
        4) Teachers and coaches should be alerted to the child's problem and management.

5. Adjuncts to therapy
    a. Environmental control
        1) Obtain a careful history of the relationship between attacks and allergen exposure. Skin tests and RASTs may be helpful.
        2) If sensitive, avoid outdoor allergens (ragweed, trees, grass, molds) and stay indoors with the windows closed in an air-conditioned environment. Air purifiers and ventilation systems may be helpful.
        3) Control indoor allergens, primarily house dust (Table 18-4) and molds; control roaches; remove animals from the home or at least from the patient's bedroom.
        4) Avoid tobacco smoke, pollutants, wood stoves, and chemicals.
    b. Allergen-specific immunotherapy: Indicated in highly selected patients when one or more allergic triggers have been identified and the patient's symptoms cannot be controlled by medication and environmental measures
    c. Education: Probably *the most* important component of successful asthma management; every patient and family should be provided with the following:

TABLE 18-4.
House Dust Mite Control Measures

Essential

Encase mattress in an airtight cover.
Either encase pillow or wash it weekly.
Wash bedding in 48.8° C water weekly.
Avoid sleeping or lying on upholstered furniture.
Remove carpets that are laid on concrete.

Desirable

Reduce indoor humidity to <50%.
Remove carpeting from bedroom.
Chemical agents to kill mites or alter mite antigens.

1) An understanding of asthma
2) A program to monitor symptoms, peak flow, and medication usage
3) A prearranged action plan for exacerbations
4) Written guidelines

C. BRONCHIOLITIS

1. Bronchiolitis is an acute, viral-induced inflammatory process of the small airways that causes airway hyperreactivity, edema, and inflammation. The peak age is 2-9 months; most cases occur November-March.
2. Cause: The majority of cases are secondary to RSV infection, but adenovirus infection is associated with increased morbidity and mortality (bronchiolitis obliterans).
3. Clinical presentation: Acute onset of respiratory distress with coughing, wheezing, tachypnea, retractions, rales, nasal discharge, irritability, and variable fever. Apnea may occur in up to 20% of all cases.
4. PE: Assess the degree of respiratory distress. Tachypnea? Flaring? Retractions? Cyanosis? Hydration? Decreased air entry, lethargy, and cyanosis are *bad* signs. There is good correlation between the severity of retractions and the degree of hypoxia.
5. Laboratory tests: Not usually helpful. CXR shows hyperinflation. ABGs are indicated in patients with severe distress or evidence of incipient respiratory failure.
6. Predictors of severe disease include the following:
   a. Toxic appearance
   b. History of prematurity (<34 weeks' gestation), chronic cardiorespiratory disease

  c. O_2 saturation <95% (single best predictor of severity)
  d. Age <3 months
  e. Atelectasis on CXR
  f. Respiratory rate >70
7. Treatment
  a. Most patients can be treated at home.
    1) Oral or inhaled albuterol (0.5% solution, 0.15 mg/kg/dose in 2 ml saline q2-4h) should be tried.
    2) There is some evidence that a combination of oral steroids and inhaled β_2-agonists may be effective.
  b. Indications for hospitalization include severe respiratory distress, hypoxia, dehydration, age <2 months, and underlying cardiopulmonary disease.
    1) Maintenance IV fluids
    2) Humidified O_2 by nasal cannula or oxygen hood to maintain O_2 saturation >95%
    3) Inhaled albuterol q1-4h plus IV steroid
    4) The role of the antiviral agent ribavirin is controversial; it may be used in infants with severe bronchiolitis and underlying congenital heart disease, immunodeficiency, or severe chronic lung disease (CF, BPD).
    5) CPAP administered nasally or by endotracheal tube can help correct severe hypoxia; mechanical ventilation is indicated in patients with respiratory failure.
    6) Strict isolation precautions are mandatory in the hospital setting.
8. Course
  a. Major symptoms last 2-3 days and are followed by slow resolution over 10-14 days.
  b. Among patients requiring hospitalization, 25%-50% develop recurrent episodes of wheezing.

D. CHRONIC COUGH
A chronic cough is defined as a cough that persists >1 month. A prolonged cough is abnormal at any age but is of particular concern in a young infant.
1. Cause varies by age group, but there is much overlap.
  a. Infants: Congenital malformations (TEF, vascular ring, laryngeal cleft), dysfunctional swallowing, reflux/aspiration, bronchial hyperreactivity (especially postviral infection), pertussis, *Pneumocystis* organisms, *Chlamydia* organisms, CF, interstitial pneumonia
  b. Toddlers and preschool-age children: FB aspiration, cough-variant asthma, recurrent viral URIs

    c. Adolescents: Smoking, psychogenic (habitual) cough ("honking" cough only during waking hours in an otherwise well-appearing adolescent)

    d. All ages: Cough-variant asthma, sinusitis/postnasal drip, allergy, infection (TB, pertussis, mycoplasma), CF, passive smoke exposure, recurrent viral URIs, ciliary dyskinesia

2. History: Often the best clue to diagnosis. Duration? Timing (season, day, night, feedings)? Degree of illness? Associated features? Character (Table 18-5)? Precipitating events? Family history? Sputum production? Wheezing? Growth pattern? Exercise tolerance? Immunizations? Environmental exposures? Allergies?

3. PE: General health, growth parameters, evidence of atopy, chest wall deformity, rales, wheezing, decreased breath sounds (localized findings with FB), digital clubbing (CF, bronchiectasis)

4. Laboratory studies: Guided by results of the history and PE. Watchful waiting and reevaluation are often indicated before embarking on costly laboratory/radiographic work-ups.

    a. X-ray examination
       1) CXR: Infection, anomalies, CF, FB
       2) Barium esophagram: Vascular ring, GER
       3) Sinus CT scan: Sinusitis
       4) Fluoroscopy: FB

    b. PPD, serologic tests, cultures: Infection

    c. Sweat test: CF

    d. Immunoglobulins, T-cell studies, HIV testing: Immunodeficiency

    e. Cineradiographic swallowing study: Dysfunctional swallow, aspiration

    f. Pulmonary function tests (including bronchoprovocation): Reactive airway disease

    g. Bronchoscopy: Diagnostic procedure of choice for FB

TABLE 18-5.
Clues to Etiology From Characteristics of Cough

Paroxysmal with cyanosis or choking: Pertussis, *Chlamydia* organisms, *Mycoplasma* organisms, CF

Short, dry, wheezing: Cough-variant asthma, lower respiratory tract infection

Harsh, barking: Tracheal irritation, compression of intrathoracic airways

Wet, productive: Resolving infection, suppurative lung disease, CF

Bizarre, barking: Psychogenic (habit)

5. Treatment is directed at the specific cause.
   a. Cough-variant asthma, often in the absence of wheezing, is the most common cause of chronic cough in children. It may be precipitated by viral illness, cold air, exercise, irritants, and allergens and is often worse at night. With high suspicion of cough-variant asthma, a trial of bronchodilator is useful.
   b. Psychogenic cough is often related to secondary gain or school phobia and is a therapeutic challenge. Options include suggestion, sheet-wrapping of the chest, hypnosis, behavior modification, and lidocaine nebulizations.
   c. There is little role for cough suppressants; codeine and dextromethorphan have been shown to be ineffective in children.

E. CROUP

1. Viral laryngotracheobronchitis is the most common cause of acute stridor in young children. There is an acute onset of biphasic or inspiratory stridor, a "barking" cough, hoarseness, retractions, variable fever, and variable respiratory distress; it usually follows URI. The child often appears well between coughing episodes. The usual course is 3-7 days.
   a. Etiology: Parainfluenza, RSV, adenovirus, influenza A
   b. Usually occurs in fall-winter; peak age 6 months–3 years
   c. PE: Assess the degree of distress, hydration, general activity, air entry, retractions, mental status (agitation, restlessness), tachycardia out of proportion to fever, and cyanosis.
   d. Laboratory tests: Not usually helpful. An AP neck x-ray study may show subglottic narrowing (steeple sign) but is not indicated in all cases. ABGs are indicated only with clinical deterioration. Respiratory rate is the best predictor of hypoxia. Pulse oximetry may be helpful but is not as reliable as careful, serial clinical assessments.
   e. Differential diagnosis: Epiglottitis, peritonsillar abscess, bacterial tracheitis, FB, retropharyngeal abscess, subglottic stenosis, infectious mononucleosis, angioneurotic edema
   f. Management: Calm the child (and family); avoid painful procedures.
      1) Provide humidification with cool mist ± O_2 based on oximetry results.
      2) RE (0.25 ml of 2.25% solution in 2.5 ml normal saline) may be nebulized q2h; peak effect in 30 minutes; duration 60-90 minutes; often followed by rebound. RE should be used only in

hospitalized patients; it does not alter the natural history but may decrease the need for an artificial airway.

NOTE: Nebulized L-epinephrine (5 ml of 1:1000 solution) is just as effective as RE.

3) Where available, an inhaled steroid (budesonide) has been shown to be effective.
4) In a patient who has more than mild symptoms, give IM dexamethasone 0.6 mg/kg; dose may be repeated in 1-2 days.
5) Do *not* use sedation.
6) Indications for admission include dehydration or evidence of respiratory compromise (e.g., cyanosis, fatigue, hypotonia, Pco_2 >45, Po_2 <70).
7) Intubation (nasotracheal) or tracheostomy is rarely necessary.
8) Endoscopy is indicated for atypical, severe, or recurrent cases of LTB or for the child who fails extubation.

2. **Spasmodic croup**

Spasmodic croup is an acute onset of a "barking" cough and inspiratory stridor with or without a preceding URI in a previously well afebrile child. It often occurs at night. Symptoms usually abate promptly but may recur for several nights.

a. Cause: Probably viral, but may represent an "allergic" response to a viral agent
b. Management: Cool mist, reassurance; IM dexamethasone may be helpful but is seldom necessary.

3. **Bacterial tracheitis**

Bacterial tracheitis is also known as pseudomembranous croup or membranous laryngotracheitis. URI/cough is followed by an abrupt onset of fever, stridor, barking cough, toxic appearance, and respiratory distress. There is leukocytosis with a shift to the left; there is accompanying pneumonia in 50% of the cases.

a. Cause: *Staphylococcus aureus* (most common), *Haemophilus influenzae*
b. Diagnosis: Established at laryngoscopy/bronchoscopy; airway obstruction secondary to thick, tracheal secretions; adherent membrane over inflamed, friable mucosa. An x-ray examination of the airway may show irregular tracheal densities with scalloping and narrowing of the trachea.
c. Management
   1) Continuous monitoring in intensive care unit
   2) Endoscopic removal of thick tracheal secretions or membranous exudate

   3) Appropriate parenteral antibiotic therapy (e.g., IV cefuroxime)
   4) Respiratory support; intubation often necessary

F. EPIGLOTTITIS (Tables 18-6 and 18-7)

A true pediatric emergency! The initial goal is to establish and maintain a good airway. A physician skilled in airway management *must* accompany the patient *at all times.*

1. Classic presentation
   a. Fulminant course in a previously well child
   b. Stridor, respiratory distress (within hours of onset), sore throat, muffled voice, dysphagia (refuses to drink), high fever. The typical appearance is a child in a toxic condition who prefers to sit (do not make the patient lie down!), head forward (tripod position), open mouth, drooling, anxious appearance; coughing is not a prominent feature.
   c. Age at onset: Range 7 months-10 years (average age 3 years). Infants <2 years of age may have a less fulminant course that may be confused with viral croup.
   d. Cause: *H. influenzae* type B; the blood culture is positive in 80% of the cases.
   e. Differential diagnosis: Croup, pharyngitis, bacterial tracheitis, retropharyngeal abscess, angioneurotic edema. Croup does *not* have such a rapid evolution and has more coughing and hoarseness;

TABLE 18-6.
Clinical Guidelines: Epiglottitis vs. Croup (Laryngotracheobronchitis)

	Epiglottitis	Croup
Age	May affect all ages, peak 3-5 yr	Younger children, 3 mo–3 yr
Etiology	Bacterial *(H. influenzae)*	Viral (parainfluenza)
Site of inflammation	Supraglottic	Subglottic
Onset of respiratory symptoms	Usually rapid (30 min–6 hr)	Slow (1-4 days)
Symptoms		
Appearance	Anxious, ill, toxic	Often nontoxic
Position	Upright, forward	Variable
Temperature	Usually high (>39° C)	Normal to high
Respiratory distress	Usually present	Variable
Retractions	Usually late finding	Progressive
Voice/cough	Muffled/often absent	Hoarse/"seal bark"
Mouth	Open, jaw forward, may drool	Closed, nasal flaring

TABLE 18-7.
Frequency of Symptoms in Combined Series of Epiglottitis Patients

Symptom	Frequency (%)	Symptom	Frequency (%)
Fever	85	Dysphagia	40
Respiratory distress	80	Drooling	37
Retractions	59	Cyanosis	33
Stridor	54	Cough	25
Sore throat	46	Hoarseness	23

stridor may be similar to epiglottitis. Although croup may be severe, the child is not usually in the degree of distress that is seen with epiglottitis.

2. Initial management: Minimize disturbance, keep child calm, and avoid attempts to visualize the pharynx or epiglottis. Laboratory tests are not usually helpful or indicated.

   a. If the child has the classic presentation, ENT and/or anesthesiology should be notified and the child transported to the OR for direct inspection of the supraglottic larynx and nasotracheal intubation. A tracheostomy is rarely needed.

   b. If the presentation is not straightforward and if the child is not in severe distress, immediately obtain an x-ray examination *(lateral view)* of the neck with the patient *erect (not* supine) and call ENT and/or anesthesiology.

NOTE: The lateral neck x-ray study is normal in 20% of cases of epiglottitis.

   c. *All* patients with documented epiglottitis need an artificial airway regardless of the degree of distress at the time of evaluation because they can decompensate quickly; the airway should be placed in the OR.

   d. If a patient is clinically *suspected* of having epiglottitis, the following protocol is followed:

      1) *Examination of the pharynx is prohibited once epiglottitis is suspected.* Minimize disturbance; keep the patient upright; unobtrusively administer facial O_2 (blow-by); *do not* draw blood or place IV lines; do not give PO fluids.

      2) The patient should never be left without a physician in attendance. Parents often are helpful in relieving the child's anxiety. *Do not* crowd the child.

3) When the child is transported for any reason, he or she should be accompanied by a parent and a physician capable of securing an airway. Airway equipment should be on hand (resuscitation bag, laryngoscope, ETT, and 14-gauge angiocatheter for emergency tracheotomy). The patient should be transported in the *upright* position, with *minimum disturbance,* and with oxygen unobtrusively administered.

e. Treatment should include an antibiotic effective against β-lactamase–producing strains of *H. influenzae* (e.g., IV cefotaxime, ceftriaxone); there is no role for steroids.

NOTE: Do not forget rifampin prophylaxis for appropriate family members/contacts.

G. FOREIGN-BODY ASPIRATION

1. Presentation of lower airway FB
   a. Signs and symptoms include wheezing, coughing, stridor, dyspnea, and evidence of chest infection; there may be hemoptysis. A choking episode is observed in only 50%-80% of cases, which often leads to a delay in diagnosis.
   b. The usual age is 6 months–3 years. Males are affected twice as often as females.
   c. The most common object is a peanut; hot dogs, balloons, toy parts, and balls are also common.
   d. Always suspect an FB if pneumonia does not resolve completely or recurs after antibiotic therapy is stopped.
2. Diagnosis
   a. The history is crucial but is often not obtained or appreciated. There may be a long latent period between aspiration and the signs and symptoms of infection.
   b. The diagnostic triad includes coughing, localized wheezing, and locally diminished or absent breath sounds but is not present in up to 50% of patients.
   c. CXR may show air trapping, mediastinal shift, atelectasis, or pneumonia but is normal in up to one third of all cases; a radiopaque object is seen in ≈15% of cases.

NOTE: Left-sided aspiration is almost as common as right-sided aspiration.

   d. Inspiratory and expiratory x-ray studies and fluoroscopy may be helpful. However, if suspicious of FB and the initial evaluation results are normal, refer the patient for bronchoscopy.

3. Management
   a. Rigid bronchoscopy is the procedure of choice.
   b. Because of the possibility of airway obstruction, chest physio-
      therapy should *not* be performed before endoscopy.
NOTE: There may be more than one FB. The endoscopist needs to look
on both sides.

H. HEMOPTYSIS (Table 18-8)

1. Although a rare event, hemoptysis can be life threatening; it may be
   confused with hematemesis.
NOTE: Always think of a pulmonary source of bleeding in children with
unexplained hematemesis.
2. Differential diagnosis
   a. In children, the most likely causes are infection and aspirated FBs.
   b. In infants and young children, need to consider tumors, autoim-
      mune disease, bronchiectasis, AV malformations, cysts, child
      abuse, and hemosiderosis (hemoptysis, infiltrates, iron deficiency
      anemia).
3. Evaluation
   a. Obtain a careful history of underlying illness, fever, coughing,
      sputum, stridor, wheezing, joint pain, weight loss, family illness,
      trauma, choking episodes, medication use, exposure to toxins, and
      travel.
   b. Always start the exam at the top; the nasopharynx or oral cavity is
      often the source of bleeding.
   c. Check skin for hemangiomata, telangiectases, and signs of trauma.
   d. CXR is the test with the highest yield. However, a normal x-ray
      study does not rule out a pulmonary source of bleeding. Except in
      cases of blood-tinged sputum or mild bleeding, a patient with
      hemoptysis should be admitted. Bronchoscopy is necessary if
      initial evaluation results are normal.
4. Treatment of hemoptysis is management of the underlying disorder.

TABLE 18-8.
Comparison of Hemoptysis with Hematemesis

	Hemoptysis	Hematemesis
Color	Bright red	Dark red
pH	Alkaline	Acid
Appearance	Frothy	± Food particles
Symptoms	Cough	Nausea, retching

I. PNEUMONIA

1. History: May be *acute* or *subacute* onset, fever ± chills, coughing, difficult or rapid breathing ± pain on inspiration, malaise. Ask about exposure to TB, immunization status, previous pneumonia, and HIV risk factors.

2. PE: All vital signs
   a. Tachypnea is a very sensitive clinical sign but may be associated with other disorders (e.g., DKA, salicylate poisoning, FB, bronchiolitis, asthma).
   b. Rales are often present but may be absent depending on the type of pneumonic process.
   c. Sputum production is rare in young children (i.e., <6 years of age).
   d. Shallow breathing or splinting secondary to pleuritic pain occurs.
   e. There are localized findings of decreased breath sounds and dullness to percussion.
   f. Look for other sites of infection (e.g., OM, conjunctivitis).

3. Laboratory
   a. CXR: Infiltrate may not be present early in illness. Infiltrates may be lobar, segmental, nodular, miliary, interstitial, or perihilar. Other significant findings include pleural effusion, pneumatoceles (can be seen with many bacteria, not just *S. aureus*), and cavitations. In most cases the CXR cannot differentiate among bacterial, viral, mycoplasma, and chlamydia pneumonias. A CXR is not indicated in all patients with suspected pneumonia; most are diagnosed clinically.
   b. TB skin test: Indicated in patients with chronic or complicated pneumonia, those with a positive family history, and for other high-risk groups (e.g., immigrants from southeast Asia)
   c. CBC: WBC count may be higher in bacterial vs. viral pneumonias, but there is a great deal of overlap, and the results do not usually alter treatment. Moderate eosinophilia may be present in chlamydia, parasitic, allergic, or hypersensitivity pneumonias.
   d. Blood culture: Not obtained routinely. It is positive in only 5%-10% of patients with presumed bacterial pneumonia. Consider the clinical setting (e.g., age, fever, WBC count, toxic appearance).
   e. Cold agglutinins: Used as a screening test for *Mycoplasma pneumoniae* but does not discriminate well between mycoplasma and viral infections
   f. CIE: Serum or urine CIE or slide agglutination tests for pneumococcal and *H. influenzae* antigens can help establish a bacterial etiology but are not practical in most outpatient settings.

g. Chlamydia studies: Conjunctival scraping or NP swab may be Giemsa stained or cultured (special media required) for *Chlamydia* organisms. A fluorescent antibody microscopy of NP secretions correlates well with culture results.

h. Cultures: In most cases an NP culture is worthless; a culture and Gram's stain may be helpful if a good sputum (not saliva) specimen is obtained.

i. Tracheal aspirate: Rarely used in children; probably better than sputum but still may be contaminated with upper respiratory secretions

j. Pleural effusions: Should be tapped. The fluid should be sent for culture, AFB, Gram's stain, chemistry studies, and cytologic tests.

k. A lung puncture, open-lung biopsy, or bronchoalveolar lavage may be helpful in highly select, complicated cases.

l. CRP: In general, an elevated CRP is indicative of bacterial infection, but there is considerable overlap with other conditions.

4. Etiology: Conclusive evidence is difficult to obtain in children. Etiology may be suspected on the basis of clinical presentation and community outbreaks. Among pediatric outpatients with pneumonia, approximately 10%-20% result from a bacterial agent; most result from viral agents such as influenza, parainfluenza, adenovirus, and RSV (especially in infants). In approximately 10% of children there is coexistent viral and bacterial infection. In older children (>8 years of age) and adolescents, *M. pneumoniae* and *Chlamydia pneumoniae* are common etiologic agents.

a. Bacterial: Acute onset of symptoms with significant fever and lobar consolidation suggests bacterial pneumonia. Most common organisms (based on lung punctures and blood cultures) are *Streptococcus pneumoniae* and *H. influenzae*. *S. aureus* should be considered in young or debilitated infants, especially if effusions or pneumatoceles are present. Streptococcal pneumonia may be associated with a scarlatiniform rash; the blood culture and pleural fluid cultures may be positive, but TC is often negative. It may run a fulminant course.

b. Viral: Viral causes include adenovirus, influenza, parainfluenza, and RSV. In older children there is usually a nonproductive cough and systemic symptoms such as myalgias, headaches, coryza, fatigue, and general malaise. In infants, wheezing is often a prominent feature.

c. *Chlamydia* organisms: *Chlamydia trachomatis* may be responsible for 15%-30% of afebrile pneumonias in early infancy. The typical patient is afebrile with a staccato cough, peripheral eosinophilia, and diffuse interstitial infiltrates. Half of the patients have conjunctivitis.

d. *Mycoplasma* organisms: Common in school-age children and young adults. Infection is characterized by a gradual onset, low-grade or absent fever, interstitial infiltrates, and greater severity of symptoms.

e. Fungal, protozoal, and TB infections must be considered in chronic pneumonia.

f. In general, viral and bacterial causes cannot be reliably distinguished on the basis of the clinical picture, laboratory results, or radiographic findings. In addition to investigating the cause, consider the underlying disease process predisposing the patient to chronic, persistent, or recurrent pneumonias, such as immune compromise (congenital, AIDS-related, iatrogenic), CF, TEF, GER, FB, lobar emphysema, and bronchogenic cysts. Remember that not all infiltrates are infectious (e.g., metastases, lymphoma).

5. Treatment: Whom to admit

a. Infants <2 months of age should be hospitalized and treated with antibiotics after an appropriate sepsis evaluation. Antibiotic choice varies with the patient's clinical presentation and with the physician's differential diagnosis. Consider coverage for streptococci, *H. influenzae,* pneumococci, staphylococci, *Escherichia coli,* and *Chlamydia* organisms. Any patient who appears very ill, has significant respiratory compromise (hypoxia), or is toxic should certainly be admitted. In addition, patients with progression of pneumonia during outpatient treatment, the presence of other complicating factors, or unreliable parents should be admitted.

b. Outpatient treatment is appropriate for most children with mild-to-moderate symptoms. Prudent clinical practice involves treating pneumonia as if it were bacterial and not performing an extensive laboratory evaluation. Initial therapy with amoxicillin 25-50 mg/kg/d ÷ tid or amoxicillin plus clavulanate potassium (Augmentin) 25-40 mg/kg/d ÷ tid is appropriate. For the patient with moderate-to-severe symptoms or failure to respond after 48 hours, treatment with IV cefotaxime 200-300 mg/kg/d ÷ q6h or q8h or IM ceftriaxone 50-75 mg/kg/d in 1-2 divided doses is appropriate. For those with a penicillin allergy, for children >8 years of age, and for young infants with suspected chlamydia infection, treatment with erythromycin 50 mg/kg/d alone or in combination with sulfisoxazole × 10-14 days is appropriate initial therapy.

NOTE: There is an emerging problem with *S. pneumoniae* isolates that show intermediate or high-level resistance to penicillin. Many of these strains may show a pattern of multiple drug resistance. Vancomycin remains uniformly effective. Cefotaxime and ceftriaxone achieve high serum (but not CSF) concentrations that are effective against most penicillin- and cephalosporin-resistant isolates. For community-acquired pneumonia, cefotaxime is appropriate initial treatment, with the addition of clindamycin 40 mg/kg/d ÷ q6h for the severely ill patient. Initial therapy should be modified once pneumococcal sensitivities are known.

   c. Recently introduced alternatives for the treatment of community-acquired pneumonia are azithromycin and clarithromycin. These antibiotics are structurally similar to erythromycin but have excellent activity against many gram-negative bacteria (*H. influenzae, Moraxella catarrhalis*) as well as gram-positive organisms, *Legionella pneumophila, Mycoplasma* organisms, and *Chlamydia* organisms. Because azithromycin has a very long elimination time, a teenager can be treated with 500 mg on day 1, followed by 250 mg once daily on days 2-5 or 500 mg once daily × 3 days for a mycoplasma infection.

   d. Antiviral agents, ribavirin, amantadine, acyclovir, and ganciclovir should be considered for highly select patients, especially those with an immunodeficiency.

   e. General supportive care: Rest, antipyretics as necessary, hydration. Cough suppressants are not recommended for pneumonia; expectorants do not work.

   f. Follow up patient in 1-2 days.
      1) If improved, see patient again at the completion of therapy. Uncomplicated bacterial pneumonia should improve in 24-48 hours.
      2) Consider inadequate therapy, incorrect diagnosis (FB?), or noncompliance if no improvement or progression of the process occurs.
      3) Follow-up CXR: Usually not necessary unless patient has persistent symptoms, recurrent pneumonia, or FTT. In one study, 20% of children had residual infiltrates 3-4 weeks after acute pneumonia (although clinically better), whereas 100% had a negative x-ray study within 3 months.
      4) Remember to perform a TB skin test on the patient if one has not recently been placed.

BIBLIOGRAPHY

Apnea

Bruhn FW et al: Apnea associated with respiratory syncytial virus infection in young infants, *J Pediatr* 90:382, 1977.

Herbst JJ et al: Gastroesophageal reflux in the "near-miss" sudden infant death syndrome, *J Pediatr* 92:73, 1978.

Keens TG, Ward SLD: Apnea spells, sudden death, and the role of the apnea monitor, *Pediatr Clin North Am* 40:897, 1993.

Kravitz RM, Wilmott RW: Munchausen syndrome by proxy presenting as factitious apnea, *Clin Pediatr* 29:587, 1990.

NIH consensus development conference on infantile apnea and home monitoring, *Pediatrics* 79:292, 1987.

See CC et al: Gastroesophageal reflux–induced hypoxemia in infants with apparent life-threatening event(s), *Am J Dis Child* 143:951, 1989.

Asthma

Asthma: A follow-up statement from an international paediatric asthma consensus group, *Arch Dis Child* 67:240, 1992.

Ben-Zvi Z et al: An evaluation of the initial treatment of acute asthma, *Pediatrics* 70:348, 1982.

Boulet L-P: Long- versus short-acting β_2-agonists: implications for drug therapy, *Drugs* 47:207, 1994.

Edwards AM, Stevens MT: The clinical efficacy of inhaled nedocromil sodium (Tilade) in the treatment of asthma, *Eur Respir J* 6:35, 1993.

Ellis EF: Asthma: current therapeutic approach, *Pediatr Clin North Am* 35:1041, 1988.

Galant SP et al: The value of pulsus paradoxus in assessing the child with status asthmaticus, *Pediatrics* 61:46, 1978.

Gelber LE et al: Sensitization and exposure to indoor allergens as risk factors for asthma among patients presenting to the hospital, *Am Rev Resp Dis* 147:573, 1993.

Inman MD, O'Bryne PM: Anti-inflammatory therapy in the treatment of asthma, *Curr Opin Pulm Med* 1:50, 1995.

Kattan M et al: Corticosteroids in status asthmaticus, *J Pediatr* 96:596, 1980.

Larsen GL: Asthma in children, *N Engl J Med* 326:1540, 1992.

McFadden ER, Jr: Management of patients with acute asthma: What do we know? What do we need to know? *Ann Allergy* 72:385, 1994.

Murphy SA, Kelly HW: Cromolyn sodium: a review of mechanisms and clinical use in asthma, *Drug Intell Clin Pharmacol* 21:22, 1987.

National Heart, Lung, and Blood Institute: Guidelines for the diagnosis and management of asthma, Pub No 91-3042A, Bethesda, Md, June 1991, National Institutes of Health.

Papo MC et al: A prospective, randomized study of continuous versus intermittent nebulized albuterol for severe status asthmaticus in children, *Crit Care Med* 21:1479, 1993.

Schuh S et al: High- versus low-dose, frequently administered, nebulized albuterol in children with severe, acute asthma, *Pediatrics* 83:513, 1989.

Warner JO: The β_2-agonist controversy: another relevance to the treatment of children, *Eur Respir Rev* 4:21, 1994.

Zwerdling RG: Status asthmaticus, *Pediatr Ann* 15:105, 1986.

Bronchiolitis

Fireman P: The wheezing infant, *Pediatr Rev* 6:247, 1986.

Hall CB et al: Aerosolized ribavirin treatment of infants with respiratory syncytial viral infection, *N Engl J Med* 308:1443, 1983.

Klassen TP et al: Randomized trial of salbutamol in acute bronchiolitis, *J Pediatr* 118:807, 1991.

Outwater KM, Crome RK: Management of respiratory failure in infants with acute viral bronchiolitis, *Am J Dis Child* 138:1071, 1984.

Shaw KH et al: Outpatient assessment of infants with bronchiolitis, *Am J Dis Child* 145:151, 1991.

Tal A et al: Dexamethasone and salbutamol in the treatment of acute wheezing in infants, *Pediatrics* 7:13, 1983.

Wohl ME: Bronchiolitis, *Pediatr Ann* 15:307, 1986.

Chronic cough

Cloutier MM, Loughlin GM: Chronic cough in children: a manifestation of airway hyperreactivity, *Pediatrics* 67:6, 1981.

Ewig JM: Chronic cough, *Pediatr Rev* 16:72, 1995.

Kamel RK: Chronic cough in children, *Pediatr Clin North Am* 38:593, 1991.

Lavigne JV et al: Behavioral management of psychogenic cough: alternative to the "bedsheet" and other aversive techniques, *Pediatrics* 87:532, 1991.

Taylor JA et al: Efficacy of cough suppressants in children, *J Pediatr* 122:799, 1993.

Croup and epiglottitis

Battaglia JD: Severe croup: the child with fever and upper airway obstruction, *Pediatr Rev* 7:227, 1986.

Cressman WR, Myer CM, III: Diagnosis and management of croup and epiglottitis, *Pediatr Clin North Am* 41:265, 1994.

Cruz MN et al: Use of dexamethasone in the outpatient management of acute laryngotracheitis, *Pediatrics* 96:220, 1995.

Cunnningham MJ: The old and new of acute laryngotracheal infections, *Clin Pediatr* 31:56, 1992.

Custer JR: Croup and related disorders, *Pediatr Rev* 14:19, 1993.

Losek JD et al: Epiglottitis: comparison of signs and symptoms in children less than 2 years old and older, *Ann Emerg Med* 19:55, 1990.

Skolnik NS: Treatment of croup: a critical review, *Am J Dis Child* 143:1045, 1989.

Tunnessen WW, Jr, Feinstein AR: The steroid-croup controversy: an analytic review of methodologic problems, *J Pediatr* 96:751, 1980.

Waisman Y et al: Prospective randomized double-blind study comparing L-epinephrine and racemic epinephrine aerosols in the treatment of laryngotracheitis (croup), *Pediatrics* 898:302, 1992.

Foreign-body aspiration

Blazer S et al: Foreign body in the airway, *Am J Dis Child* 134:68, 1980.

Gay BB et al: Subglottic foreign bodies in pediatric patients, *Am J Dis Child* 140:165, 1986.

Healy GB: Management of tracheobronchial foreign bodies in children: an update, *Ann Otol Rhinol Laryngol* 99:889, 1990.

Laks Y, Barzilay A: Foreign body aspiration in childhood, *Pediatr Emerg Care* 4:102, 1988.

Puhakka H et al: Tracheobronchial foreign bodies, *Am J Dis Child* 143:543, 1989.

Hemoptysis

Beckerman RC et al: Familial idiopathic pulmonary hemosiderosis, *Am J Dis Child* 133:609, 1979.

Metz SJ, Rosenstein BJ: Uncovering the cause of hemoptysis in children, *J Respir Dis* 5:43, 1984.

Pyman C: Inhaled foreign bodies in childhood, *Med J Aust* 1:62, 1971.

Tom LWC et al: Hemoptysis in children, *Ann Otolaryngol* 89:419, 1980.

Pneumonia

Broughton RA: Infections due to *Mycoplasma pneumoniae* in childhood, *Pediatr Infect Dis J* 5:71, 1986.

Cherian T et al: Simple clinical signs of acute lower respiratory tract infection, *Lancet* 2:125, 1988.

Denny FW: Acute respiratory infections in children: etiology and epidemiology, *Pediatr Rev* 9:135, 1987.

Gooch M III: Bronchitis and pneumonia in ambulatory patients, *Pediatr Infect Dis J* 6:137, 1987.

Grossman LK et al: Roentgenographic follow-up of acute pneumonia in children, *Pediatrics* 63:30, 1979.

Leibovitz E et al: Once-daily intramuscular ceftriaxone in the outpatient treatment of severe community-acquired pneumonia in children, *Clin Pediatr* 29:634, 1990.

Marks MI: Pediatric pneumonia: viral or bacterial? *J Respir Dis* 3:108, 1982.

McCarthy PL et al: Value of the C-reactive protein test in the differentiation of bacterial and viral pneumonias, *Clin Pediatr* 92:454, 1978.

McCarthy PL et al: Radiographic findings and etiologic diagnosis in ambulatory childhood pneumonias, *Clin Pediatr* 20:686, 1981.

Paisley JW et al: Pathogens associated with acute lower respiratory tract infections in young children, *Pediatr Infect Dis J* 3:14, 1984.

Paisley JW et al: Rapid diagnosis of *Chlamydia trachomatis* pneumonia in infants by direct immunofluorescence microscopy of nasopharyngeal secretions, *J Pediatr* 109:653, 1986.

Ramsey BWS et al: Use of bacterial antigen detection in the diagnosis of pediatric lower respiratory tract infections, *Pediatrics* 78:1, 1986.

Schutze GE, Jacobs RF: Management of community-acquired bacterial pneumonia in hospitalized children, *Pediatr Infect Dis J* 11:160, 1992.

Turner RB et al: Etiologic diagnosis of pneumonia in pediatric outpatients by counterimmunoelectrophoresis of urine, *Pediatrics* 71:780, 1983.

Turner RB et al: Pneumonia in pediatric outpatients: cause and clinical manifestations, *J Pediatr* 111:194, 1987.

SCHOOL HEALTH ISSUES

19

A. PHILOSOPHY

1. Children who attend group child care, Head Start, preschool, or formal school merit special attention because they and the staff at these facilities are affected by their presence in groups. Children are likely to acquire a number of viral and bacterial infections from each other. The staff is also challenged by the numerous infections that circulate and by the accommodations they must make for children with special needs.

2. Before entering into group care or school, a child should receive a thorough health assessment by his or her regular medical provider. If performed properly, this assessment is one of the most important that any child will receive; it is meant to detect potential problems that might interfere with learning or participating in group activities. Especially important are assessments of hearing, vision, language, and development. Any detected abnormalities should be noted and, *if significant,* reported to the caregiver and school.

3. Other important information includes a history of allergies (e.g., allergen, if known; usual symptoms and severity; measures to be taken if an exposure occurs); chronic medical conditions, especially those that might require treatment at child care or school; *all* medications, but especially those that might need to be given while the child is in child care or at school; and any emergency procedures that must be followed.

4. It is also a good idea to include certain screening tests during the preenrollment visit. Screening tests for anemia, lead poisoning, and tuberculosis are helpful if a child has not recently had these tests; in some jurisdictions they are mandated by law.

5. Once the child is in child care or in school, there needs to be a free flow of information between the medical provider and the child-care provider or teacher. An "us vs. them" attitude is not in the best interest of the child or family. If the medical provider detects a problem that

will need to be dealt with by a child-care provider or teacher, he or she should communicate the information in a timely fashion. Parents are to be involved in this process. When a child-care provider or teacher detects a new problem or has a question, he or she should discuss it with the parent and, if necessary, contact the medical provider.

6. When children are in group situations, whether child care or school, the medical provider must be careful to consider the public health implications of a given disease in a child of a given age and in a given situation. A child may need to be excluded from care or school depending on the period of contagiousness of a given disease and the age or developmental level of the child.

B. SPECIFIC ISSUES
1. Abuse
   a. Child-care providers or teachers sometimes are reluctant to report suspected abuse because they fear that they lack expertise. They therefore defer to the medical provider. This strategy is not optimal, especially if there is a time lapse between the caregiver or teacher's initial observation and the assessment by the medical provider.
   b. Medical providers should do their best to cooperate with any initiative taken by the child-care facility or school to safeguard a child or clear up any concerns about marks on a child's body.
2. Behavior problems
   a. A full discussion of behavior problems is provided in Chapter 4.
   b. It is important to remember that the behaviors manifested by a child in a child-care facility or school might not be the behaviors that he or she demonstrates in the medical provider's office or at home. For example, a child with school phobia generally has symptoms only at school. An only child who has trouble getting along with other children may have problems at the child-care facility but not at home, where he or she does not need to deal with competition.
3. Chronic conditions
   a. Asthma, seizures, sickle-cell disease, hemophilia, HIV infection, diabetes, and allergies are discussed elsewhere in this text. Child-care providers and school personnel should be aware of the signs and symptoms of a chronic condition, the precipitating events (e.g., specific allergen exposure), and routine/emergency procedures to be followed in the event of an exacerbation. All information and instructions should be in writing, with one copy in the child's medical records and one copy at the child-care facility or school.

b. When a chronic condition warrants medication, try to space the doses so that they are not needed in school if at all possible. Many child-care providers are not permitted under state regulations to dispense medications, and many school personnel are uncomfortable doing so. Remember, not all schools and certainly not all child-care facilities have a nurse on site each day; therefore try to keep medications to a minimum in such settings. Always provide written instructions, including dosage, route, and time of administration on the forms required by the child-care facility or school. Keep a copy in the child's medical records.

c. If a child has very special needs (e.g., tube feedings, respiratory treatments, catheterizations), be sure to be as explicit as possible when documenting when and how to perform such procedures. Specify the type of treatment, the time of administration, and what should be done if it is unsuccessful. For tube feedings, specify the type of formula, dilution (if warranted), rate of feed (especially if gravity- or pump-driven), and measures to be taken if the feeding cannot proceed (e.g., obstruction to fluid inflow, vomiting, abdominal distension, tube extrusion). Such orders must arrive before the child because many schools will not permit a child to remain if the proper orders are not on file.

d. Specify explicitly what the school or child-care facility needs to do in an emergency. For example, should 911 be called immediately, or should other measures be instituted before the 911 call? Remember, there may not be a health professional on site to make a medical decision; therefore try to anticipate questions. If a child has a seizure disorder, do all seizures or only certain ones warrant a 911 call? If the latter, which ones are they? If a child has asthma, which attacks warrant a 911 call and which warrant other therapies first? Does the staff know the signs of severe respiratory distress? If a child has a propensity to experience respiratory arrests, for whatever reason, what should the staff do while waiting for emergency treatment? If a child has diabetes, which reactions warrant a 911 call and which warrant a call to the parent? Does the staff know the signs and symptoms of hypoglycemia, hyperglycemia, and DKA? If the child has severe allergic reactions or anaphylaxis in response to an allergen, does the child-care facility or school have an EpiPen on hand, and do they know how to use it?

Take nothing for granted! When writing directives for nonmedical personnel, make sure that they both have the recommended equipment and know how to use it. Be as explicit in your instructions as possible, and always encourage questions.

e. If a child has a chronic, terminal condition, do not assume that he or she will die at home or in a hospital. Many children have struggled to attend school for as long as possible, and therefore it is quite possible that such children could die at school. Make sure you know the laws in your state regarding DNR (do not resuscitate). Document the parents' wishes and your orders on any legal forms required. Give guidelines for what *can* be done and what should *not* be done. For example, if a child can receive "blow-by" oxygen but not intubation or CPR, state this. In many jurisdictions, if an ambulance is called the paramedics *will* begin CPR unless the patient is accompanied by DNR documentation. If this procedure is followed in your state, obtain the necessary documentation so that a needless resuscitation is not instituted. For information regarding the laws in your state, call your local Emergency Medical Services or hospice organization.

4. Dermatologic conditions
   a. If a child has an acute or chronic skin condition that is infectious, provide this information in writing to the child-care facility or school. Because child-care or school personnel encounter many children with undefined rashes, they often err on the conservative side and exclude any child with a rash until they are reassured that it is not contagious.
   b. Although skin conditions have been discussed in Chapter 5, the common conditions listed in Table 19-1 warrant exclusion criteria.

5. Giftedness
   a. The definition of *giftedness* includes general intellectual ability, specific academic aptitude, the ability for creative thinking, leadership ability, psychomotor ability, and the ability to excel in the visual or performing arts. Obviously, few individuals possess all of these gifts. However, the definition is important because it highlights the fact that giftedness is not merely having a high IQ.
   b. When parents perceive that their children are gifted, they may knowingly or unknowingly place demands on them. Some parents may be overly critical, overly dominating, overly conscientious, or overly directive.
   c. The parental behaviors listed in Point b may cause a gifted child to become perfectionistic (fear of failure), overly controlling, overly frustrated with his or her own abilities, or overly demanding of others to meet his or her expectations. If they are bored, gifted children may also act out in class and disrupt other students who are trying to learn at their own pace.

TABLE 19-1.
Common Dermatologic Conditions

Spread	Incubation	Infectious period	Exclusion
Head lice			
Head-to-head	17-25 days	When viable nits are present	Until 24 hr after therapy or as long as viable ova remain
Herpes			
Direct contact	3-5 days	Up to 3 wk (without acyclovir)	Until all cutaneous lesions are scabbed
Impetigo			
Direct contact, fomites	1-10 days	As long as draining/weepy lesions are present	As long as draining lesions are present or until 24 hr of therapy (streptococcus) or 48 hr of therapy (staphylococcus)
Scabies			
Human-to-human	14-17 days	As long as mites are present	Until 24 hr after therapy
Tinea			
Direct contact, fomites	2-3 wk for obvious lesions	Months to years if untreated	None once therapy is started; remember, scalp lesions require *oral* therapy
Warts			
Direct contact	1-20 mo (usually 4 mo)	Months to years	None, but try to cover warts

    d. Medical providers should encourage the parent(s) of a child who appears gifted to discuss class placement with the teacher. If the child becomes disruptive when bored, additional challenging assignments can perhaps be provided. Medical providers should caution parents to treat their gifted children age appropriately and not as small adults. Just because a child is gifted intellectually or artistically does not mean that he or she is emotionally mature for his or her age. Although parents should be encouraged to stimulate their children's abilities, every activity need not be stimulating. Gifted children need to relax too.

  e. Referral for counseling might be in a gifted child's best interest if the child appears to be under enormous stress to succeed (whether imposed internally or externally), disruptive, or without friends.

6. Immunizations

  a. All children should be current-for-age on their immunizations at the time they enter child care or school. This information should be documented on the proper form for your jurisdiction. Any religious exemption or medical contraindication for one or more immunizations should be clearly documented.

  b. Some jurisdictions require a second MMR upon entry into elementary school. Follow the laws in your area when considering when to immunize your patients.

7. Infectious illnesses

  a. Most of the conditions listed in Table 19-2 are discussed in greater detail elsewhere.

  b. Special considerations should be taken when an ill child is in child care, preschool, or the early elementary grades or if the child lacks control of body secretions/excretions.

8. Learning problems

There are a number of reasons why some children do not succeed in school or do not work to their capacity. Some of these reasons are outlined as follows:

  a. School readiness

    1) Although most children are ready to begin kindergarten at age 5, others are ready at age 4, and still others are not ready until 6 or 7 years of age. The result of starting a child in school too early may be sub-par performance or outright failure, which leads to retention in a given grade. Reasons such as poor grade achievement, young chronologic age, social immaturity, behavior problems, delayed physical development, and parental wishes are given for a student's failure to be promoted. Generally, retained students are more likely to be younger for their grade, male, and of lower socioeconomic status. Children who were of low birth weight, malnourished in early life, or exposed to drugs, alcohol, or cigarettes in utero are more likely to fail a grade. Children whose families are not supportive of education are also less likely to succeed in school.

Text continued on p. 364.

TABLE 19-2.
Infectious Illnesses

Spread	Incubation	Infectious period	Exclusion
Adenoviral infections			
Respiratory droplets, fecal-oral	2-14 days	Respiratory illness, 2-8 days; GI illness, 0-8 days; conjunctivitis, 14 days	Respiratory illness, none; diarrheal illness, until no further diarrhea; conjunctivitis, 14 days
Campylobacter organisms			
Fecal-oral, contaminated water	1-7 days, usually 2-4 days	2-3 days after onset of therapy; if no therapy, 5-7 wk	Until 2 days after initiation of antibiotics or until no longer symptomatic
Chlamydia trachomatis			
Vertical only	5-14 days (conjunctivitis), 14-60 days (pneumonia)	None (no horizontal transmission)	None
Coronavirus			
Respiratory, aerosols	2-3 days	Several days	None
Coxsackievirus A16 (Hand-foot-and-mouth disease)			
Fecal-oral, oral-oral	4-6 days	Weeks	None
Cryptosporidia			
Fecal-oral, including fomites and contaminated water	5-10 days	2-5 wk or 2 wk after cessation of therapy	Until asymptomatic

Continued.

TABLE 19-2. (cont.)

Spread	Incubation	Infectious period	Exclusion
Cytomegalovirus			
Contact with urine or saliva	1 mo	6-24 mo	None
***Enterobius vermicularis* (Pinworm)**			
Ingestion of eggs	2-8 wk	As long as adult worms are present	Until properly treated
Enterovirus			
Fecal-oral, oral-oral	7-14 days	Weeks	None, except children with poliovirus, who should be excluded until no further symptoms are present
Giardia lamblia			
Fecal-oral, including fomites	1-4 wk	Up to 12-14 mo (as long as cysts are excreted)	With completion of therapy and when no further diarrhea is present
Haemophilus influenzae			
Respiratory	Within 60 days (classroom)	Until 24 hr after initiation of parenteral therapy (invasive disease)	Until well and after receiving oral rifampin
Hepatitis A			
Fecal-oral	15-50 days	Until 10 days after onset of dark urine	At least 10 days after onset of dark urine
Hepatitis B			
Percutaneous, permucosal	6-24 mo	As long as surface antigen-positive	None

Infectious mononucleosis		
Oral-oral, saliva	5-7 wk	Weeks-months	1-2 wk or longer depending on child's degree of illness
Influenza (Flu)		
Respiratory	1-3 days	1-10 days	Until asymptomatic
Meningococcus		
Respiratory, oral-oral	2 days to several weeks	Until at least 1 day after initiation of therapy; remember carrier state	Until asymptomatic
Mumps		
Respiratory	12-25 days (usually 16-18 days)	From 1 week before to 9 days after symptoms	Until 9 days after onset of parotid swelling
Mycoplasma pneumoniae		
Respiratory	2-3 wk	As long as cough is present	Until child is no longer ill
Parainfluenza viruses		
Respiratory, direct contact	3-6 days	3-16 days	Until child is no longer ill
Human parvovirus B19 (Fifth disease)		
Respiratory, direct contact	4-14 days	1-3 days before onset of rash	None
Pneumococcal disease		
Respiratory	Up to 1 mo	Carrier state	Until child is no longer ill
Respiratory syncytial virus		
Respiratory, including fomites	3-7 days	Before symptoms and for 1-3 wk; older children 3-7 days	Until child is no longer ill

Continued.

TABLE 19-2. (cont.)

Spread	Incubation	Infectious period	Exclusion
Rhinoviruses (Common cold)			
Respiratory, including fomites; direct contact	1-2 days	3 wk or as long as nasal symptoms are present	None
Roseola			
Not fully known	5-15 days	Not fully known	Until rash is resolved and child is well
Rotaviral infection			
Fecal-oral, including fomites	1-3 days	Usually 4-5 days	Until no longer vomiting or having diarrhea
Rubella			
Respiratory, direct contact	14-21 days	From 5 days before to 7 days after onset of illness	At least 7 days after onset of rash
Rubeola			
Respiratory, direct contact	10-12 days	Until onset of rash	Until 5 days after onset of rash
***Salmonella* organisms**			
Contaminated food	6-72 hr	Months	Until no further diarrhea
***Shigella* organisms**			
Fecal-oral, including fomites	12-48 hr (usually)	1-4 days (treated), 7-30 days without treatment	Until 5 days of antibiotics or two successive negative stool cultures

Staphylococcal disease			
Direct contact, fomites	1-10 days (usually)	As long as lesions drain	As long as lesions drain or until at least 48 hr of antibiotics
Streptococcal disease			
Direct contact, respiratory spread	12-96 hr (pharyngitis), 10 days (impetigo)	Up to 2 wk	Until at least 24 hr after start of antibiotics and afebrile
Tuberculosis			
Respiratory	2-10 wk	None in young children	None, unless draining wounds; however, children need to be receiving therapy
Varicella			
Respiratory, direct contact	10-21 days	Until all skin lesions have crusted or until 7 days after onset	Until pox are scabbed; if zoster, exclude if lesions cannot be covered; otherwise child can attend school
Yersinia organisms			
Fecal-oral, contaminated food or water	2-11 days (usually)	Weeks, even with antibiotic therapy	As long as child has diarrhea

2) Helpful information for the medical provider includes observations from the child's preschool experience. For example, how does the child compare with his or her peers in child care? Can the child attend to tasks well, or is he or she easily distracted? How does the child get along with other children? How does he or she handle frustrations or learn new tasks? Medical providers can also screen a child by using the Denver Developmental Screening Test, Preschool Readiness Experimental Screening Scale, or Sprigle School Readiness Screening Test. If on these screens a child does not demonstrate the skills needed for school success, he or she should receive a full evaluation by a psychologist or developmental pediatrician. If a specific disability is detected (e.g., speech delay), a referral should be made to a specialist in that area (e.g., speech therapist). Remedial and developmentally appropriate approaches are preferable to retention in the hope that another year will help the child "catch on."

b. School placement

1) Public law 94-142 mandates that children be educated in the least restrictive environment. For many children with disabilities, this goal is realistic. Sometimes it is in a child's best interest to be educated in a facility that is somewhat more restrictive if that degree of restriction helps him or her to learn and interact with others.

2) Some children who have less severe problems might be able to remain in a regular classroom; sometimes special seating is all that is needed for the child to work more optimally toward his or her potential. Other children can remain in a regular classroom with the understanding that they will receive special instruction geared to their disability once or twice a week. Other students might remain in their regular classes but require daily special instruction.

3) Children with ADD/ADHD may benefit from special seating, special instruction, medication, behavioral modification, or a combination of these four techniques. Children with physical impairments should be handled on a case-by-case basis; some are best served in regular schools, whereas the physical impairments of others are so severe that they require special environments. The same is true of children with chronic medical conditions who experience periodic exacerbations. Placement in regular classes is generally preferred, but such children may

need home (or hospital) teaching during periods of exacerbation. Under this classification would also fall children with infectious conditions such as TB, AIDS, and hepatitis, especially if the child has oozing skin lesions or biting behaviors (AIDS and hepatitis B).

4) Children with severe emotional problems may benefit from inclusion in schools developed especially for them. In such schools the staff is trained to manage such children optimally, and environments are planned to minimize the occurrence of physical injuries when the children lose control.

c. School failure

1) Even the best of efforts does not permit all children to smoothly progress from one grade to another. Sometimes it is in the child's best interest to remain in a grade.

2) The medical provider should fully evaluate every child who fails a grade, especially if the child previously was a good or adequate student. In this evaluation, the usual histories (perinatal, medical, developmental, family, and social) are solicited. The child's academic history is also reviewed (e.g., academic achievement, global or specific problem areas, classroom behavior, school attendance, special school services provided, and any psychoeducational testing).

3) The examination should be complete and particularly highlight the child's emotional state, intellectual functioning (with the examiner), neurologic exam, and sensory exam. Vision and hearing should be tested. Any skin markings that might indicate an underlying neurologic abnormality (e.g., café au lait spots, hypopigmented macules) should be noted in addition to the child's level of puberty. A simple mental status exam (e.g., asking the child for three wishes or asking the child to draw himself or herself or his or her family) may yield useful information about the child's mental state.

4) Neurodevelopmental testing such as the Pediatric Early Elementary Examination test may disclose problems in the way a child functions in different areas of development. Neurodevelopmental testing is best performed by a pediatrician with expertise in this area. A full psychoeducational evaluation is crucial in understanding the interplay of emotions, intellect, and learning style/problems in a particular child.

5) The child who fails usually experiences a diminution in self-esteem; family members may contribute to this feeling.

Consideration should be given to individual or family counseling if the medical provider senses that the child and/or family is coping poorly with the school failure.

d. Language disorders

1) Language disorders include a number of disorders such as difficulty in word comprehension, difficulty in oral language production and use, and difficulty in expression or sound production (e.g., stuttering).

2) Referral to a speech pathologist as soon as a disability is discovered gives the child the best chance for optimal learning and coping with his or her deficit.

e. Mathematical disabilities

1) In this society the ability to use numbers meaningfully is important, not only for scientists and computer operators but also for all individuals who must handle their finances or shop wisely in a store. Hence, children who are "no good at math" are at a serious disadvantage for learning to operate optimally in society. Depending on the severity of the disability, such students may require the services of a number of professionals or only math tutoring. To optimize the child's educational potential, such assistance should be provided as soon as the disability is discovered.

2) It is important not to accept explanations for poor math performance such as "I've never been any good at math; why should she be any different?" or "Girls are not supposed to be good at math." Parents should be counseled not to encourage self-fulfilling prophecies for their children's educational failure. The fact that a parent did not excel at a given subject does not mean that his or her child will share the same fate. The gender of the child does not necessarily predict the subjects in which a child will excel or fail.

f. Dyslexia

1) Even more critical than the ability to compute is the ability to read. Between 5% and 15% of school-aged children have dyslexia (reading disability), with boys outnumbering girls by a ratio of 2:1. Although a complete review of the literature on dyslexia is beyond the scope of this text, it is important to note that a variety of etiologies are suggested. A variety of neuropsychologic tests are used to assess dyslexia and are usually performed by a specialist in the field, who should be consulted as early as possible.

2) It is important for the medical provider to perform a PE, with special attention given to the neurologic exam. "Soft" neurologic signs, as well as the "hard" signs of deficiencies or asymmetries of appearance or function, must be noted and reported.

g. Attention deficit disorder/attention deficit hyperactivity disorder
1) *ADD* implies a short attention span, whereas *ADHD* implies a degree of hyperactivity in association with the short attention span. Between 3% and 5% of children have ADD; 80% of boys and 50% of girls with ADD are hyperactive.
2) The hallmarks of ADD/ADHD are inattention, impulsivity, and hyperactivity. The 14 historical criteria listed in Table 19-3 are used to assess whether a child truly has ADD/ADHD; to meet these diagnoses, a child must have 8 of the 14 symptoms for at least 6 months.
3) The PE may be normal except for the neurologic component; especially important is the detection of certain neurologic signs (Table 19-4). Although these signs may be normal in a younger child, they are not so as a child matures. Not every child with ADD/ADHD has all of these signs, but most have a majority of them when carefully evaluated.
4) Several interventions can be tried if the history and PE point to a diagnosis of ADD or ADHD and include special educational interventions, behavior therapies, individual and family counseling, and medication. Medications should be used only in those children whose history or physical parameters meet the criteria of ADD/ADHD.
   a) Stimulants are the most widely used medications for ADD/ADHD in the United States; they are effective for at least 75% of the children who meet the diagnostic criteria for ADD or ADHD. They improve most levels of functioning but may be associated with a number of side effects such as anorexia/weight loss, insomnia/nightmares, irritability or moodiness/agitation, growth impairment, and others. An alteration of the dose or its timing (especially in response to meals) or a switch to a long-acting rather than a short-acting preparation usually resolves most of these side effects. In some cases, however, a medication may need to be discontinued.
      (1) Methylphenidate (Ritalin) is the most commonly used medication and is available both as a short- and

TABLE 19-3.
Criteria for ADD/ADHD

1. Often fidgets with hands or feet or squirms in seat
2. Has difficulty remaining seated when required to do so
3. Easily distracted by external stimuli
4. Has difficulty waiting for his or her turn
5. Blurts out answer before the question is completed
6. Has difficulty following through on instructions
7. Has difficulty sustaining attention in tasks or play
8. Shifts from one uncompleted activity to another
9. Has difficulty playing quietly
10. Talks excessively
11. Interrupts or intrudes on others' activities
12. Does not listen to what is said to him or her
13. Loses things necessary for tasks or activities
14. Engages in physically dangerous activities without considering the possible consequences

TABLE 19-4.
Neurologic Signs of ADD/ADHD

1. Arms drop or spread when extended
2. Arms drop or spread when head is rotated
3. Hopping or one-foot stand that is too short
4. Finger- or foot-tapping that is too slow
5. Choreiform movements
6. Excessive associated and mirror movements
7. Finger-nose-finger dysmetria
8. Inadequate or sloppy tandem gait
9. Disdiadochokinesia
10. Inadequate ability to imitate finger movements
11. Finger agnosia
12. Double simultaneous stimulation-extinction
13. Head movement with extraocular muscle movement
14. Strabismus or inability to converge
15. Inadequate hold of lateral gaze
16. Grimace/inability to raise brow
17. Irregular tongue waggle
18. Slow speed of speech repeating

long-acting preparation. The dose is 0.3-1.0 mg/kg/dose with a usual dose of 5-10 mg bid (max 40 mg/d).

(2) Dextroamphetamine is also used and is available both as a short- and long-acting preparation, but its attraction as a street drug limits its use. The dose is 0.2-0.45 mg/kg/dose (usually 5-10 mg bid [max 20 mg/d]).

(3) Pemoline (Cylert) is available only as a long-acting preparation. The starting dose is 37.5 mg.
b) All drugs should be increased, when necessary, in careful increments. Look for *any* side effects with a clear understanding among parents, school, and the medical provider that there may be a tradeoff between an "acceptable" effect and the side effects of the drug. If a lower dose is better tolerated but does not quite produce "perfect" results, all concerned may need to live with such results.

h. School phobia
1) School phobia, also known as school refusal or school avoidance, is defined as a child's refusal to go to school or a refusal to stay in school for emotional reasons. Approximately 5% of elementary school students and 2% of middle school students have this disorder.
2) Two types of school phobia
a) Anxiety-related type: The child is worried about something at home or school. There is a persistence of the separation anxiety that most children master by 3-4 years of age. There is overdependence on the parent(s), who tend(s) to be child-oriented and concerned about the child experiencing too much stress in life. The children are excellent students. Girls outnumber boys.
b) Secondary-gain type: There are few anxiety symptoms. Children with this type of school phobia tend to have had an illness for which they had to stay home and for which they received much sympathy and attention. The parent of this type of student is often lenient and does not value education. The children are average-to-poor students. Boys outnumber girls.
3) Although *any* symptom can be associated with this disorder, the most common ones are headaches (real or feigned), abdominal pain, diarrhea, vomiting, chest pains, palpitations, dizziness, hyperventilation, and a "sore throat." The child with the anxiety-related type tends to have physiologic symptoms such as diarrhea, whereas the child with the secondary-gain type has a "sore throat," "fever" (often self-induced), or other symptoms that are hard to verify objectively.
4) The following criteria are essential when faced with a student in whom a diagnosis of school phobia is being considered:
a) Recurrent, often vague, physical symptoms

    b) No physical cause found on careful (sometimes repeated) exams

    c) Symptoms that predominate in the mornings of school days and are virtually absent on weekends, school holidays, or summer vacation

    d) More than 5 days of school missed because of *this* problem

5) A complete history is essential and requires not just the usual items. Also investigate events that may be precipitating the phobia such as a change of school, family stress (parental discord, separation, divorce, death, remarriage, birth of sibling, death of sibling), a recent move, academic stress (fear of "failure," even in a bright child), or stress at school (teacher-child mismatch, difficulties with peers, unsafe school environment, or unsafe journey to school). The following items are essential for an adequate evaluation:

    a) Type, duration, frequency, timetable of symptoms; age of onset; parent's idea of cause; feared medical diagnosis (e.g., "What is the worst thing this could be?"); previous evaluation or treatment

    b) Days absent this year and last year, days late, days sent home, parental attitudes about staying home from school, what the child does and where he or she stays when absent

    c) Change in school; difficulties with school work, teacher(s), classmates, other students; problems on school bus or with traveling to school

    d) Peer relations, both at and outside of school

    e) Family relations, stresses, illnesses

    f) Impressions from school nurse (if present) or teacher regarding the child's difficulties/absenteeism

6) The PE should be complete; except for minor abnormalities, it is invariably normal. The normalcy of the exam should be highlighted for the parent(s) *and* child.

7) Keep laboratory tests to a minimum; order only those that will contribute to your impression. A "million dollar" work-up is unnecessary and leads both the parent and child into thinking that there is a real physical problem present.

8) In considering the diagnosis of school phobia, keep in mind that there are other reasons for school absenteeism, such as parental overresponse to minor illnesses, chronic physical disease or learning disability with poor adaptation, truancy, depression, psychosis, substance abuse (child or parent),

pregnancy, family dysfunction, child abuse (child must stay home until bruises are healed), and the need for one child to "babysit" a younger child while the parent works or runs errands.

9) When fairly certain of the diagnosis of school phobia, explain to the parent(s) what the condition is (and is not), that it is not associated with a hidden physical disease, that the child has normal physical findings and laboratory tests (if ordered), that school phobia occurs in normal children with normal parents, and that the condition can be treated.

10) Treatment consists of enlisting parental support in handling the matter firmly (e.g., insisting that if the child is ill enough to stay home from school, he or she needs to be seen by the medical provider, who will send the child to school if the exam is normal). The medical provider should also spend time with the child, sympathizing when appropriate (with the anxious child) and being firm when appropriate (with the secondary-gain child). Children must be told that it is the law that they attend school and that it is the responsibility of parents and medical providers to help them adjust to and thrive in school. The child's teacher, principal, and school nurse (if available) need to be part of the process. In general, drug therapy has no role in the treatment of school phobia.

11) The following children should be referred to a child psychiatrist or psychologist:
   a) Psychotic children
   b) Depressed children
   c) Children incapacitated by fear
   d) Children of parents who exhibit symbiotic parent-child relations
   e) Children requiring psychoactive drug therapy
   f) Adolescents
   g) Children whose physical disease has necessitated prolonged bed rest
   h) Children/families unresponsive to counseling

12) If parents deliberately keep children out of school, a referral to child protective services is in order.

9. Sports
   a. There are two main issues facing the medical provider in terms of school-related sports activities: the preparticipation physical assessment and the treatment of sports-related injuries.

b. In considering the suitability of a given sport for a given student, considerations of the type of sport and the student's health history are crucial. Sports are classified into contact/collision (e.g., football), limited contact (e.g., baseball), and noncontact (e.g., swimming). Noncontact sports can be further subdivided into strenuous (e.g., aerobics), moderately strenuous (e.g., table tennis), and nonstrenuous (e.g., golf).

c. Some students should not be permitted to engage in collision or strenuous sports because of their health history. For example, a child with psychomotor seizures should not be permitted to engage in contact or strenuous sports; a child with an enlarged liver or spleen should not be permitted to engage in contact/collision/ impact sports; a child with a history of two or more concussions (or even one depending on its severity) should avoid contact/ collision/impact sports. The American Academy of Pediatrics has produced an exhaustive list of medical conditions and acceptable sports participation (see Bibliography).

d. The history obtained at the preparticipation assessment should ascertain whether any of the following are present: chronic or recurrent illness; illnesses lasting more than 1 week; hospitalizations/surgeries; missing or enlarged organs; cardiovascular problems; allergies; chest pain or dizziness with exercise; problems with heat; concussion, unconsciousness, or seizure either associated or unassociated with exercise or sports activity; medication use; eyeglasses use; dental appliance in place; history of injuries such as neck, knee, ankle, back, and shoulder; and a family history of early death or early heart attack.

e. The preparticipation exam should be complete and should particularly highlight the following areas: vision, hearing, chest exam with particular attention to adventitial breath sounds and cardiac sounds and rhythms, neurologic exam, and musculoskeletal exam. The examiner is looking for current and potential "trouble spots" that could lead to the disability or death of the young athlete.

f. Once the student begins his or her athletic career, the best way to prevent injuries is through proper conditioning, proper management of injuries, use of protective equipment, and matching of athletes. Proper nutrition must be stressed; inappropriate dieting must be avoided. The use of anabolic steroids must be strongly discouraged. Students with a history of heat-related illnesses should not compete or practice outdoors during hot weather.

g. The management of moderate-to-severe sports injuries should be left to specialists. Unfortunately, it is sometimes difficult to separate minor injuries from more serious ones. The classic RICE (Rest, Ice, Compression, Elevation) is a useful therapy.

1) Resting the injured area is important for the first 24-72 hours because movement can encourage further bleeding into the tissue. It is very difficult for a young athlete to "lay off" a leg or not use an arm, because he or she really wants to participate. If an injured athlete must get around (e.g., to class), crutches or inflatable splints can be used, but rest is preferable. Further evaluation and treatment may be needed if pain, swelling, or tenderness persists after 3 days.

2) Ice therapy is excellent and needs to be applied as soon as possible after the injury. It causes diminution of pain by slowing down nerve impulses and muscle spasms in the area. It also causes vasoconstriction, which leads to decreased bleeding into the tissue and also less edema. Finally, fewer cells break down because of lessened oxygen demand. Ice needs to be applied during the first 48 hours after an injury for approximately 20 minutes tid or qid.

3) Compression is used to decrease edema. Edema prevents cold therapy from reaching deeper levels, interferes with normal joint movement (and thus increases the need for rehabilitation), and can keep torn tissue ends apart so that scar tissue replaces the injured tissue. Elastic bandage compression is an excellent means of limiting edema.

4) Elevation of an injured limb reduces the hydrostatic pressure that drives plasma into the interstitium and decreases the amount of edema by encouraging lymphatic drainage.

5) Analgesics may be needed if pain is moderate or severe. Aspirin should be avoided because it prolongs bleeding time, which makes it more likely that further bleeding into the injured area will occur. Acetaminophen and ibuprofen are better choices for analgesics.

6) When in doubt about a sports injury, ask for help. Have a low threshold for ordering x-ray studies, especially if there is marked swelling, marked tenderness, hemarthrosis, or deformity. Order AP and lateral views and, in the case of long bones, views of the joint above and below the injured area. *Always* review the films with a radiologist if the injury is severe or if the patient has marked symptoms but the x-ray study looks negative.

BIBLIOGRAPHY

School health

AAP Committee on School Health: Guidelines for urgent care in school, *Pediatrics* 86:999, 1990.

Children with health impairments in schools, *Pediatrics* 86:636, 1990.

Dworkin P: School failure, *Pediatr Rev* 10:301, 1986.

Schmitt B: School refusal, *Pediatr Rev* 8:99, 1986.

School health assessments, *Pediatrics* 88:649, 1991.

Giftedness

Landesman S: Defining giftedness, *Pediatr Ann* 14:698, 1985.

Lewis M: Gifted or dysfunctional? *Pediatr Ann* 14:733, 1985.

McGuffog C: Problems of gifted children, *Pediatr Ann* 14:719, 1985.

Learning disorders

Bashin A et al: Language disorders in childhood and adolescence, *Pediatr Ann* 16:145, 1987.

Garnett K, Fleischner J: Mathematical disabilities, *Pediatr Ann* 16:159, 1987.

Jordan N, Levine M: Learning disorders: assessment and management strategies, *Contemp Pediatr* 4:31, 1987.

Levine M, Jordan N: Learning disorders: the neurodevelopmental underpinnings, *Contemp Pediatr* 4:16, 1987.

Nass R: Developmental dyslexia, *Pediatr Rev* 13:231, 1992.

School readiness and placement

Casey P, Evans L: School readiness: an overview for pediatricians, *Pediatr Rev* 14:4, 1993.

Palfrey J, Rappaport L: School placement, *Pediatr Rev* 8:261, 1987.

Schmitt B: School refusal, *Pediatr Rev* 8:99, 1986.

Attention deficit disorder/attention deficit hyperactivity disorder

Adesman A, Wender E: Improving the outcome for children with ADHD, *Contemp Pediatr* 8:122, 1991.

Barkley R, Murphy J: Treating attention deficit hyperactivity disorder, *Pediatr Ann* 20:256, 1991.

Committee on Children with Disabilities, Committee on Drugs: Medication for children with an attention deficit disorder, *Pediatrics* 80:758, 1987.

Culbert T et al: Children who have attentional disorders: interventions, *Pediatr Rev* 15:5, 1994.

Reiff M et al: Children who have attentional disorders: diagnosis and evaluation, *Pediatr Rev* 14:455, 1993.

Schmitt B: The child with a short attention span (ADD), *Contemp Pediatr* 9:57, 1993.

Sports

Committee on Sports Medicine: Recommendations for participation in competitive sports, *Pediatrics* 81:737, 1988.

Committee on Sports Medicine and Fitness: Medical conditions affecting sports participation, *Pediatrics* 94:757, 1994.

Dyment P: Athletic injuries, *Pediatr Rev* 10:291, 1988.

Dyment P: How to make the sports physical exciting, *Contemp Pediatr* 7:93, 1991.

Hergenroeder A: Diagnosis and treatment of ankle sprains, *Am J Dis Child* 144:809, 1990.

Hulse E, Strong W: Preparticipation evaluation for athletics, *Pediatr Rev* 9:173, 1987.

Resser W: Sports medicine, *Pediatr Rev* 14:424, 1993.

Shaw B, Geraldi J: Avoiding the pitfalls in pediatric sports injuries, *Contemp Pediatr* 9:142, 1992.

SEXUALLY TRANSMITTED DISEASES

20

A. GENERAL

The clinical presentation may include urethritis; vulvovaginitis, cervicitis, or dysuria in women; ulcerations on the penis, vulva, or vagina; inguinal lymphadenopathy; PID; epididymitis; proctitis; pharyngitis; arthritis; rash; and conjunctivitis. At least 20 different causative microorganisms are now recognized (bacteria, viruses, fungi, protozoa, arthropods). Some of these microorganisms are listed in the sections that follow.

B. GONORRHEA

1. May be seen at any age; suspect sexual abuse if prepubertal
2. May be asymptomatic (>50% females, 25% males)
3. Culture cervix, urethra, pharynx, rectum, and inflamed joint if the index of suspicion is high.
4. Diagnosis
   a. Gram's stain showing >8 gram-negative intracellular diplococci (more reliable on urethral swab of male; less reliable on endocervical swab of female). Confirm with culture.
   b. Send specimen to laboratory for culture immediately.
5. Screen for syphilis (VDRL, STS) on all patients suspected of having gonococcal infection. Consider other sexually transmitted infections (e.g., HSV, *Chlamydia, Trichomonas* organisms).
6. Treatment (current recommendations reflect the increase in penicillinase-producing strains)
   a. Asymptomatic and uncomplicated gonorrhea infections (vaginitis, cervicitis, urethritis, proctitis, pharyngitis)
      1) Ceftriaxone 125-250 mg IM once (250 mg if ≥45 kg)
         or
      2) Cefixime 400 mg PO once
         or

3) Ciprofloxacin 500 mg PO once
   or
4) Ofloxacin 400 mg PO once
5) Other alternatives
   a) Spectinomycin 2 g IM (covers rectal, urethral, and cervical gonococcal infections)
      or
   b) Ceftizoxime 500 mg IM once
      or
   c) Cefotaxime 500 mg IM once
      or
   d) Cefotetan 1 g IM once
      or
   e) Cefoxitin 2 g IM once
6) None of these regimens treat *Chlamydia* organisms. Always treat for *Chlamydia* organisms when treating for gonococcal infection.
7) Prepubertal children (<45 kg)
   a) Ceftriaxone 125 mg IM once; ceftriaxone 50 mg/kg (max 1 g) IM or IV qd × 7 days for bacteremia or arthritis. Increase to maximum of 2 g/d × 10-14 days for meningitis.
      or
   b) Spectinomycin 40 mg/kg (max 2 g) IM once

NOTE: Follow-up culture is *mandatory*. Obtain it approximately 1 week after treatment is completed. Do not forget to treat contacts and to cover for *Chlamydia* organisms.

b. Disseminated gonococcal infection: Symptoms include dermatitis and arthritis.
   1) Ceftriaxone 1 g IM or IV qd
      or
   2) Cefotaxime 1 g IV q8h
      or
   3) Ceftizoxime 1 g IV q8h
      or
   4) Spectinomycin 2 g IM q12h (if allergic to β-lactams)
   5) All regimens should be continued for 24-48 hours after improvement begins. Treatment is then changed to one of the following drugs to complete a full week of treatment. Always treat presumptively for *Chlamydia trachomatis*.
      a) Cefixime 400 mg PO bid
         or
      b) Ciprofloxacin 500 mg PO bid

C. PELVIC INFLAMMATORY DISEASE (SALPINGITIS)

1. Fever occurs in only 33% of patients. Patients may have lower abdominal pain, vaginal discharge, irregular bleeding, and cervical motion/adnexal tenderness. Risk of subsequent sterility exists. Remove IUD if present.

2. Cause: Often polymicrobial. The most common pathogens are *Neisseria gonorrhoeae, C. trachomatis,* and anaerobic bacteria (most commonly *Peptostreptococcus, Peptococcus,* and *Bacteroides* organisms). Other organisms include *Mycoplasma hominis* and *Ureaplasma urealyticum.*

3. Hospitalize the patient if any of the following are true:
   a. Diagnosis is uncertain.
   b. Surgical emergencies such as ectopic pregnancy and appendicitis are to be ruled out.
   c. There is high suspicion of a pelvic abscess or the presence of an adnexal mass.
   d. Severe illness is present (T >38.3° C; WBCs >20,000).
   e. Patient is pregnant.
   f. Patient cannot follow outpatient regimen (especially if significant nausea or vomiting is present), cannot tolerate PO medications, or cannot come back for follow-up in 48-72 hours.
   g. Patient has not responded to outpatient treatment.
   h. Patient is an adolescent. This procedure is controversial but is safe and ensures that the patient will begin treatment properly.
   i. Patient has HIV infection.

4. Treatment
   a. Outpatient
      1) Cefoxitin 2 g IM once and probenecid 1 g PO once
         or
      2) Ceftriaxone 250 mg IM once
      3) *Both* cefoxitin and ceftriaxone should be followed by PO doxycycline 100 mg bid × 10 days
         or
      4) Ofloxacin 400 mg PO bid × 14 days *plus*
         a) Clindamycin 450 mg PO qid × 14 days
            or
         b) Metronidazole 500 mg PO bid × 14 days
   b. Inpatient (gynecologist should be consulted)
      1) Cefoxitin 2 g IV qid *or* cefotetan 2 g IV q12h, *plus* doxycycline 100 mg IV bid until improvement, followed by PO doxycycline 100 mg bid to complete 14-day course
      2) Alternative is IV clindamycin 900 mg q8h *plus* gentamicin 2

mg/kg once, followed by gentamicin 1.5 mg/kg tid until
improvement, followed by PO clindamycin 450 mg qid *or*
doxycycline 100 mg PO bid to complete 14-day course
c. Miscellaneous
   1) Treat contacts.
   2) Get follow-up culture.

D. FITZ-HUGH–CURTIS SYNDROME
With Fitz-Hugh–Curtis syndrome, infection extends from salpingitis to
the capsule and outer surface of the liver. Consider if patient has RUQ
pain, palpable liver, abnormal LFTs, or adnexal/cervical motion
tenderness. Treatment is as listed in Section C, Point 4b.

E. CHLAMYDIA INFECTIONS
1. May be found in mixed infections
2. Presents with urethritis, cervicitis, salpingitis, Fitz-Hugh–Curtis
   syndrome in females, inguinal lymphadenopathy, epididymitis,
   proctitis in males; may be asymptomatic
3. Diagnosis: Culture in specific media, MicroTrak (direct fluorescent
   staining), ELISA, endocervical Gram's stain >30 WBCs per oil
   immersion field, in males >10 WBCs/HPF in first 15 ml of void
4. Treatment
   a. Adults and adolescents (nonpregnant)
      1) Doxycycline 100 mg bid × 7 days (not in pregnancy)
         or
      2) Azithromycin 1 g PO once
         or
      3) Ofloxacin 300 mg PO bid × 7 days
         or
      4) Erythromycin base 500 mg qid × 7 days
         or
      5) Erythromycin ethylsuccinate 800 mg PO qid × 7 days
         or
      6) Sulfisoxazole 500 mg qid × 10 days (inferior to other regimens)
   b. Pregnancy
      1) Erythromycin base 500 mg PO qid × 7 days
         or
      2) Erythromycin base 250 mg PO qid × 14 days
         or
      3) Erythromycin ethylsuccinate 800 mg PO qid × 7 days
         or

    4) Erythromycin ethylsuccinate 400 mg PO qid × 14 days
       or
    5) Amoxicillin 500 mg PO tid × 7-10 days (if intolerant of erythromycins)
  c. Children <45 kg: Erythromycin 50 mg/kg/d ÷ qid (max 2 g/d) × 10-14 days
  d. Children >45 kg, <8 years of age: Same erythromycin dosages as for adults
  e. Children >45 kg, >8 years of age: Same doxycycline dosages as for adults
5. Treatment for conjunctivitis and pneumonia in infancy
  a. Erythromycin 50 mg/kg/d ÷ qid × 10-14 days
  b. Topical therapy not needed
6. Be sure to contact and treat all sexual partners of the patient (or parent in the case of neonatal chlamydia infection).

F. SYPHILIS

1. Forms
  a. Congenital: Mucocutaneous lesions, "snuffles," rash, bone changes (painful, pseudoparalysis, dactylitis), hepatosplenomegaly, lymphadenopathy, fever, anemia, FTT. Infants may not always manifest symptoms.
    1) Infected infants may be seronegative if maternal infection was late in gestation.
    2) Infants should be treated at birth if maternal treatment was inadequate, unknown, with drugs other than penicillin, or if adequate follow-up cannot be ensured.
    3) Always examine CSF before treatment.
  b. Acquired syphilis
    1) Primary stage: Chancre detectable in adolescents and adults, less common in children
    2) Secondary stage: Rash, condylomata lata
2. Evaluation
  a. Obtain serologic tests for VDRL or RPR, followed by confirmation with FTA-ABS.
  b. CSF: Protein, cells, VDRL. Perform darkfield microscopy for spirochetes.
  c. Scrape any mucosal or cutaneous lesion and perform darkfield microscopy.
  d. Perform bone x-ray examinations as indicated for congenital infection.

3. Treatment
   a. Congenital syphilis
      1) Crystalline penicillin G 50,000 U/kg/dose q12h × first 7 days of life, then q8h for another 3-7 days *or* penicillin G procaine 50,000 U/kg/d IM qd × 10-14 days
      2) If >1 day of therapy is missed, the entire course should be restarted.
      3) If CSF is initially positive, reexamine CSF q6mo until normal. Repeat if CSF serologic test remains positive for 6 months after first therapy, if the blood serologic test remains positive 1 year after treatment, or if there is a fourfold rise in VDRL. The child should be retreated if the CSF cell count is abnormal after 2 years *or* if VDRL-CSF is still reactive after 6 months.
   b. Acquired syphilis
      1) Primary, secondary, or early latent syphilis (<1 year duration): Penicillin G benzathine 50,000 U/kg (max 2.4 million U) IM once
         a) Alternate therapy if penicillin absolutely cannot be used: Doxycycline 100 mg PO bid *or* tetracycline 500 mg PO qid × 2 weeks if child >8 years of age
         b) Need follow-up serologic test: Successful outcome is a negative serologic test by 12 months for primary syphilis, by 24 months for secondary syphilis, and by 48 months for latent syphilis
      2) For syphilis >1 year in duration: Penicillin G benzathine 50,000 U/kg (max 2.4 million U) IM q7d × 3 wk (total 7.2 million U max); alternatively, PO doxycycline 100 mg bid *or* tetracycline 500 mg PO qid × 4 weeks. Repeat if there is not a fourfold decrease in titer by 1 year after treatment or if clinical signs and symptoms persist.

NOTE: Remember: Contact, evaluate, and treat all sexual partners!

      3) For neurosyphilis: Aqueous penicillin G 2-4 million U IV q4h × 10-14 days or penicillin G procaine 2.4 million U IM qd plus probenecid 500 mg qid × 10-14 days. Either regimen is followed by penicillin G benzathine 2.4 million U IM weekly × 3 weeks.
      4) Follow-up and retreatment
         a) All patients with early syphilis and congenital syphilis should have repeat VDRL at 3, 6, and 12 months after treatment.

   b) VDRL will be nonreactive or reactive with a low titer within a year following successful therapy.

   c) The possibility of reinfection should be considered when a patient with early syphilis needs to be retreated. Retreatment should be considered if any of the following are true:

     (1) Clinical signs of syphilis persist or recur.

     (2) There is a fourfold increase in VDRL titer.

     (3) High-titer VDRL fails to show a fourfold decrease in 1 year. Retreat according to the schedules recommended for syphilis of >1 year's duration.

G. HERPES SIMPLEX VIRUS

1. Patient may be asymptomatic or have painful ulcerations on genitalia. Ulcers between vaginal folds and the posterior cervix can be easily missed.

   a. Cytologic tests (e.g., Pap or Tzanck smear) reveal multinucleated giant cells in approximately 75% of culture-positive specimens.

   b. Viral medium is needed for culture.

2. Treatment of primary genital herpes in adolescents

   a. Oral acyclovir 200 mg 5 times/day × 7-10 days (adult dosage)

   b. The use of topical acyclovir is discouraged.

3. Suppression of recurrent genital herpes: Long-term acyclovir 400 mg PO bid *or* acyclovir 200 mg PO 3-5 times/day

H. HEPATITIS B (see also Chapter 8)

1. Clinical: Jaundice, anorexia, vomiting, liver enlargement/tenderness

2. Chemistries: ↑ LFTs and ↑ bilirubin; + serologic findings for hepatitis B; if severe liver disease, PT/PTT may be prolonged

3. Abnormal urine (↑ bilirubin), abnormal stool (acholic)

4. Universal immunization of infants against hepatitis B now recommended

I. HUMAN PAPILLOMAVIRUS INFECTION

1. HPV causes warts known as condyloma acuminata; the incubation period is 1-6 months. Certain types are associated with genital neoplasia. Most cases in infants are secondary to perinatal transmission.

2. The wart has a cauliflower-like appearance (white or strawberry pink-red) and can be located on the genitalia, around the anus, or in and around the mouth. At the time of detection, the lesions may range in size from several millimeters to several centimeters because of confluence of multiple lesions.

3. PE and laboratory tests are necessary to rule out other venereal diseases. Investigate the possibility of sexual abuse.
4. Treatments vary by extent and location of lesions.
   a. Cryotherapy
      or
   b. Podofilox 0.5% solution (patient can apply bid × 3 days, followed by 4 days of no treatment; can have a total of 4 cycles of such therapy)
      or
   c. Podophyllum 10%-25% in compound tincture of benzoin, applied weekly (up to 6 weeks) by a health professional
      or
   d. Tricholoracetic acid 80%-90%, applied weekly (up to 6 weeks) by a health professional, to be followed by talc or baking soda to remove unreacted acid
      or
   e. Electrodesiccation/electrocautery
   NOTE: Podophyllin should *not* be used for internal lesions.
5. Recalcitrant warts and those in the urethra, vagina, or rectum may require cryotherapy with liquid N_2 or laser surgery.

BIBLIOGRAPHY

General

Gittes E, Irwin C: Sexually transmitted diseases in adolescents, *Pediatr Rev* 14:180, 1993.
Johnson J, Shew M: Screening and diagnostic tests for sexually transmitted diseases in adolescents, *Semin Pediatr Infect Dis* 4:142, 1993.
Judson F, Ehret J: Laboratory diagnosis of sexually transmitted infections, *Pediatr Ann* 23:361, 1994.
Quinn T: Recent advances in diagnosis of sexually transmitted diseases, *Sex Transm Dis* 21(2 Suppl):S19, 1994.
Reed B, Eyler A: Vaginal infections: diagnosis and management, *Am Fam Physician* 47:1805, 1993.
Sexually transmitted diseases: treatment guidelines 1993, *MMWR* 42(RR-14):1, 1993.

Gonorrhea

Ingram D: *Neisseria gonorrhoeae* in children, *Pediatr Ann* 23:341, 1994.

Chlamydia

Biro F et al: A comparison of diagnostic methods in adolescent girls with and without symptoms of chlamydia urogenital infection, *Pediatrics* 93:476, 1994.

Grayston JT: *Chlamydia pneumoniae* (TWAR) infections in children, *Pediatr Infect Dis J* 13:675, 1994.

Hammerschlag M: *Chlamydia trachomatis* in children, *Pediatr Ann* 23:349, 1994.

McMillan J: Chlamydia: unsuspected, undiagnosed, untreated, *Contemp Pediatr* 2:14, 1985.

Syphilis

Starling B: Syphilis in infancy and young children, *Pediatr Ann* 23:334, 1994.

Stoll B: Congenital syphilis: evaluation and management of newborns born to mothers with reactive serologic tests for syphilis, *Pediatr Infect Dis J* 13:845, 1994.

Herpes simplex virus

Arvin A, Prober C: Herpes simplex virus infections: the genital tract and the newborn, *Pediatr Rev* 13:107, 1992.

Breese-Hall C: Herpes and the rash of roses, *Pediatr Ann* 19:517, 1990.

Bryson Y et al: Treatment of first episodes of genital herpes simplex virus infection with oral acyclovir, *N Engl J Med* 308:916, 1983.

Douglas J et al: A double-blind study of oral acyclovir for suppression of recurrences of genital herpes simplex virus infection, *N Engl J Med* 310:1551, 1984.

Straus S et al: Suppression of frequently recurring genital herpes, *N Engl J Med* 310:1545, 1984.

Hepatitis B

American Academy of Pediatrics Committee on Infectious Diseases: Update on timing of hepatitis B vaccination for premature infants and for children with lapsed immunizations, *Pediatrics* 94:403, 1994.

Inactivated hepatitis B virus vaccine: a comprehensive strategy for eliminating transmission in the United States through universal childhood vaccination, *MMWR* 40:1, 1991.

Pickering L: Management of the infant of a mother with viral hepatitis, *Pediatr Rev* 9:315, 1988.

Pon E et al: Hepatitis B virus infection in Honolulu students, *Pediatrics* 92:574, 1993.

Shapiro C: Epidemiology of hepatitis B, *Pediatr Infect Dis J* 12:433, 1993.

TRAUMA

21

M. Douglas Baker

A. BITES: HUMAN

1. Determine the circumstances of the attack; examine the skin carefully.
2. Wash the wound immediately; irrigate it copiously with sterile saline; debride. Examine for vascular, muscle, tendon, and nerve damage.
3. Closed-fist injuries (with the wound usually on the first or second metacarpophalangeal joint) may appear benign but can lead to serious morbidity. Joint infection is one of the main concerns. Clean well before suturing and consider using antibiotic prophylaxis.
4. The use of prophylactic antibiotics in human bites is controversial. Bacteria that cause infections include streptococci, staphylococci, anaerobes, and (rarely) aerobic gram-negative organisms. Oral amoxicillin plus clavulanic acid or IV penicillin plus oxacillin is effective in most of these infections. Continued cleansing is important adjunctive therapy.
5. Frequent follow-up q1-3d to check for infection is advisable.
6. Do not forget tetanus prophylaxis.

B. BITES: ANIMAL

1. Determine the circumstances of the attack, the type of animal, and whether the animal is domestic or wild, known to the victim, and current on its rabies shots.
2. Wash the wound (may use benzalkonium [Zephiran]); copiously irrigate lacerations and deeper wounds with sterile saline; debride thoroughly. Examine for vascular, muscle, nerve, and tendon damage.
3. Most lacerations can be sutured after cleansing and debridement. *Do not* suture puncture wounds or deep wounds on the hand, which cannot be adequately cleansed (high risk of infection).
4. Prophylactic antibiotics are controversial; they may be of value in

hard-to-irrigate wounds. Bacteria commonly found in infected bites include *Pasteurella multocida,* streptococci, and staphylococci. Amoxicillin plus clavulanic acid is effective in 95% of the cases. Do not forget tetanus prophylaxis.

NOTE: Sutured dog bites of the head and neck tend to heal especially well and, even in the absence of antibiotics, have a low rate of infection.
5. Frequent follow-up q1-3d is advisable.

C. RABIES POSTEXPOSURE PROPHYLAXIS
1. Rabies is very unusual in domestic cats and dogs but does occur.
2. Rabies is also unusual in rodents (rats, squirrels, hamsters, mice) and lagomorphs (rabbits).
3. Most human rabies comes from contact with carnivorous wild animals (skunks, raccoons, ferrets, woodchucks, coyotes, foxes) and bats.
4. Rabid animals concentrate the rabies virus in their saliva.
5. Unprovoked attacks might indicate that the animal is rabid more than do provoked attacks.
6. Outside of caves and laboratories (airborne transmission), rabies is transmitted only by introducing the virus into open cuts or wounds in the skin or via mucous membranes.
7. The recommendations provided in Table 21-1 are only a guide. In applying them, take into account the animal species involved, the circumstances of the bite or other exposure (e.g., scratches, abrasions, open wounds or mucous membranes contaminated with saliva or other potentially infectious material from a rabid animal), the vaccination status of the animal, and the presence of rabies in the region.

NOTE: RIG and HDCV should never be administered in the same syringe or into the same site.
8. If antirabies treatment is indicated, both RIG and HDCV should be given as soon as possible, regardless of the interval between exposure and treatment.
9. The dose of RIG is 20 IU/kg.
    a. If possible, infiltrate half of the dose around the wound and give the rest IM.
    b. RIG provides passive immunity while the body mounts an active immune response.
    c. If RIG was not given when the HDCV vaccination was begun, it can be given until the eighth day after the first dose of vaccine was given.

TABLE 21-1.
Rabies Postexposure Prophylaxis Guide

Animal type	Evaluation and disposition of animal	Postexposure prophylaxis recommendations
Dogs and cats	Healthy and available for 10-day observation	Do not begin prophylaxis unless animal develops symptoms of rabies*
	Rabid or suspected rabid†	Immediate vaccination and RIG‡
	Unknown (escaped)	Consult public health officials for advice
Skunks, raccoons, bats, foxes, and most other carnivores; woodchucks	Regarded as rabid unless geographic area is known to be free of rabies or until animal proven negative by laboratory tests†	Immediate vaccination and RIG‡
Livestock, ferrets, rodents, and lagomorphs (rabbits and hares)	Consider individually	Consult public health officials; bites of squirrels, hamsters, guinea pigs, gerbils, chipmunks, rats, mice, other rodents, rabbits, and hares almost never require antirabies treatment

From *1994 Red Book: Report of the Committee on Infectious Diseases,* ed 23, Elk Grove Village, IL, 1994, American Academy of Pediatrics.
*During the 10-day holding period, treatment with RIG and vaccine should be initiated at the first sign of rabies in the biting dog or cat. The symptomatic animal should be killed immediately and tested.
†The animal should be killed and tested as soon as possible. Holding for observation is not recommended. Vaccination is discontinued if immunofluorescent test of the animal is negative.
‡RIG, Rabies immune globulin (human).

Thereafter, RIG is unnecessary because presumably an active antibody response to the vaccine has occurred.
10. The dose of HDCV is five 1-ml doses IM (deltoid or anterior part of the thigh; *never* in the gluteal area).
    a. HDCV induces an active immune response that requires approximately 7-10 days to develop and persists for as long as 1 year.
    b. Give the first dose as soon as possible after exposure; give additional doses 3, 7, 14, and 28 days after the first dose.

c. A postvaccination serum specimen for rabies antibody testing is no longer necessary unless the patient is suspected of being immunocompromised (i.e., receiving steroids or immunosuppressive therapy essential for the treatment of another condition).

11. Side effects
   a. HDCV: Side effects are less common than with the duck embryo vaccine previously used. Local reactions are pain, erythema, swelling, or itching in up to 25% of recipients. Systemic reactions are headache, nausea, abdominal pain, muscle aches, and dizziness in up to 20% of recipients. Few serious anaphylactic or systemic reactions have been reported. The rate of neurologic abnormalities after HDCV is approximately 1 in 150,000. Once rabies prophylaxis has been started, do not interrupt or discontinue it because of local or mild systemic reactions. Usually these reactions can be managed with acetaminophen.
   b. If a patient experiences an allergic reaction to HDCV, RVA can be substituted using the same dosage schedule.
   c. RIG is much better than the old equine antirabies serum. Fever and localized pain are the most common side effects.

12. Standard wound care instructions should be given to all patients who sustain an animal bite. Ask parents to report the bite to police. The police usually have the owners or the animal pound watch the animal for signs of rabies for 10 days.

13. Give tetanus prophylaxis if indicated.

D. BURNS

1. Children with first-degree burns (erythema only) may be treated with analgesics, cool compresses, suntan creams and, if itching is a problem, oral antihistamines.

2. Children with second-degree burns (pain, blisters, ± areas of blanching within the burn area) may need to be hospitalized if the burns involve the face, perineum, hands, or feet or if the total body surface area burned is >5% in infants, >10% in children, or >15% in adolescents/adults.
   a. The initial management of second-degree burns includes cleansing the area with saline, trimming broken blisters or ragged skin edges (leaving intact blisters alone), applying 1% silver sulfadiazine (Silvadene) or Xeroform to a more superficial burn, and securing the burn with clean gauze (and elastic netting if necessary for the particular body part).

b. The patient should be seen daily until healing is well underway. Further debridement, if necessary, can be performed at these visits.

c. Burn cleansing and dressing may be done at home. Nonviable tissue should be completely removed before each redressing.

d. Systemic antibiotics should be instituted at the first sign of burn site infection. Remember that a thin rim of erythema at the periphery of the burn is to be expected during healing.

e. Pain relief should be provided by analgesics (acetaminophen, codeine). Parenterally administered narcotics may be more effective than oral agents in hospitalized patients.

f. Once the burn has healed (7-14 days), an emollient should be applied to protect the new, fragile epidermis. Protection against strong sunlight should also be instituted.

g. Do not forget tetanus prophylaxis.

3. For the management of children with extensive second- or third-degree burns, refer to *The Harriet Lane Handbook,* ed. 14.

E. DENTAL TRAUMA

1. The various types of dental trauma are as follows:

a. Concussion: Injury to periodontal ligaments without displacement or mobility of the tooth. There is percussion sensitivity.

b. Subluxation: The tooth is mobile horizontally and is tender to percussion.

c. Displacement: The tooth is intruded into the socket, extruded lingually, or avulsed.

d. Fracture: In an enamel fracture, only an edge is missing. In crown fractures, there are cracks in the enamel but no tooth discoloration. In dentin fractures, there is a yellow discoloration (if the pulp is exposed, a pinkish color is obvious).

e. Mandibular fracture
1) Unilateral: Mandible deviates toward the affected side.
2) Bilateral: Mouth is gaping and malocclusion is present.

f. Maxillary fracture: Involvement of bony processes into which the teeth are embedded. Teeth may be displaced and mobile.

2. Examine the face and lips for obvious traumatic lesions and asymmetries.

a. The mandible and maxilla should be palpated for tenderness.

b. The patient should open and close the mouth so that asymmetric and unstable areas may be appreciated.

    c. The mouth should be examined for bleeding, swelling, or broken teeth.

    d. With the patient biting down, ask if the bite feels normal.

    e. Check each tooth individually for pain and mobility.

3. Concussions and crown and enamel fractures require a timely dental referral.

    a. Subluxations, displacements, and fractures with pulp exposure require an immediate dental referral.

    b. Fractures of the upper or lower jaw require treatment by an oral surgeon.

    c. An avulsed permanent tooth may be reimplanted within 1 hour of the injury; do not reimplant primary teeth. Do not scrub teeth before reimplantation.

F. FROSTBITE

1. In frostbite, freezing of tissues occurs.

    a. The toes, fingers, ears, and nose are commonly involved.

    b. Initially the frostbitten tissue is white, firm, and numb; with progression, cyanosis, mottling, and vesicles appear.

    c. With rewarming, superficially frostbitten areas become red, swollen, and painful. No cyanosis is present, and sensation is normal.

    d. On rewarming, deeply frostbitten areas may be cyanotic, lack sensation, and be excruciatingly painful.

2. Treatment involves rapidly warming affected areas in tepid water (40°-43° C) for 20-40 minutes.

    a. Do not rub; doing so increases tissue injury.

    b. If vesicles or bullae are present, do not rupture them; cover them with gauze.

    c. Plastic surgery consultation and hospitalization are necessary whenever there is deep frostbite.

G. INSECT REACTIONS

1. The reaction to insect bites or stings may be local (redness, pain, swelling at the site) and/or systemic (urticaria, hypotension, wheezing, laryngeal edema, shock). These reactions generally occur within 2 hours of the sting.

    a. Delayed reactions can occur as long as 1 week following the sting and include fever, arthralgias, urticaria and, rarely, neuritis or vasculitis.

b. Always try to identify the stinging insect by the history. Determine if there have been previous systemic (or local) reactions to stings and if there is a history of allergy.

2. Treatment for local reactions includes stinger removal, cleansing, applying ice to the area, and diphenhydramine (Benadryl) (5 mg/kg/d ÷ qid).

   a. If the wound is >24 hours old and appears infected (tumor, rubor, dolor, calor), cephalexin (25-50 mg/kg/d ÷ qid) should be given.

   b. For mild systemic reactions that occur immediately (e.g., generalized urticaria), diphenhydramine 5 mg/kg/d ÷ qid or hydroxyzine (Atarax) 2 mg/kg/d ÷ qid may be given.

   c. For anaphylactic reactions, epinephrine 0.01 mg/kg is given either SQ (preferred, 0.01 ml/kg of 1:1000 solution) or IV (0.1 ml/kg of 1:10,000 solution). The patient may require IV fluids, nebulized albuterol, methylprednisolone 1-2 mg/kg IV, and diphenhydramine 1 mg/kg IV.

H. TICKS

1. The tick attaches itself to the skin, and its saliva can induce tissue destruction. It should be promptly removed by applying steady, slow traction with forceps (or tweezers if at home). Do not squeeze or crush the tick. An ulcer or granuloma may develop if the tick's mouth parts remain after removal; intralesional steroids or excision treats the lesion.

2. Ticks spread RMSF (relapsing fever, rash, headache), Lyme disease (erythema chronicum migrans, polyarthritis, neurologic disease, carditis), and other diseases. Treatment of RMSF is tetracycline 25-40 mg/kg q6h (max 2 g/d) for patients >8 years of age, or IV chloramphenicol 50-100 mg/kg/d (max 4 g/d) Serum drug levels should be checked to decrease the likelihood of toxic reactions to chloramphenicol. The treatment of Lyme disease is discussed on p. 272.

I. SPIDERS

1. Black widow spiders (Lactrodectus mactans) produce a neurotoxin that causes severe muscular cramps and pain and a rigid abdomen within ½ hour after the bite.

   a. Muscle spasms may be relieved by diazepam 0.1-0.2 mg/kg/dose q2-4h (max 0.6 mg/kg) and IV calcium gluconate.

   b. The neurotoxin may also cause an ascending motor paralysis; fever, vomiting, convulsions, and shock may occur.

c. A specific *Lactrodectus mactans* antiserum is useful for high-risk patients who test negative for an allergy to horse serum.

d. Narcotics may be necessary for pain relief.

2. The bite of a brown recluse spider induces redness and swelling at the site in mild cases. In moderate-to-severe cases there is local tissue and vessel damage, necrosis, and systemic reactions such as a generalized rash, urticaria, arthralgias, fever, nausea, vomiting and, occasionally, hemolysis or DIC.

3. The bite of other spiders causes pain, swelling, and pruritus at the site.

4. Tetanus prophylaxis is advisable after any spider bite.

5. Treatment for local reactions consists of diphenhydramine or hydroxyzine.

6. Systemic steroids are indicated for patients with systemic symptoms or with bites in cosmetic or functional areas. In these patients, monitoring for the onset of hemolysis or DIC is mandatory. Plastic surgery is usually necessary for a good cosmetic result in the bite area.

J. LACERATIONS

1. Determine how the injury happened, how long ago, and where (e.g., outdoors, home); the patient's last tetanus shot; other medical problems; and medications.

2. Calm the patient and family. Parents may help to comfort the child by staying nearby.

3. Test the function of muscle, tendon, nerve, and vascular status before administering an anesthetic. *Thoroughly* examine the wound. If it appears complicated or deep, call the appropriate specialist.

4. Sterile technique is mandatory. Wash hands; apply sterile gloves.

5. Place a drainage pad under the wound.

6. Swab the surrounding intact skin with povidone-iodine (Betadine).

7. Administer a local anesthetic ± sedation. Preschool-age children can be safely sedated with intranasal midazolam.

   a. A conventional local anesthetic uses 1% lidocaine (Xylocaine) with a 25-gauge needle.

   b. 1% lidocaine with epinephrine may be used on the face or scalp to decrease bleeding, but never use it on the nose, fingers, toes, or penis.

   c. Always aspirate before injection to avoid injection into a vessel.

   d. TAC (tetracaine, adrenaline, cocaine) or LET (lidocaine, epinephrine, tetracaine) applied via saturated gauze is also effective but cannot be used on end organs or near mucous membranes.

8. After the lesion has been anesthetized, irrigate it *copiously* with

saline and drain adequately. Irrigation with at least 100 ml normal saline per 1 cm laceration is recommended.

9. Explore the wound for deep injury. Remove foreign bodies and dirt. Scrub when necessary. Judiciously debride *all* devitalized tissue.
10. Obtain an x-ray examination of the wound if there is *any* suspicion of residual metal pieces or glass. Metal and glass appear on x-ray study; wood and plastic do not.
11. Suture

NOTE: As needle size increases, radius increases. As suture size increases, caliber decreases.

   a. Use 5-0 or 6-0 nylon on the face; use 5-0 and 4-0 elsewhere, except 3-0 nylon for scalp and knee lacerations in older children.
   b. Use 4-0, 3-0, or 2-0 absorbable polyglactin 910 (Vicryl) sutures for subcutaneous sutures. Rapidly absorbing sutures also can be used on surface areas in which suture removal is difficult.
   c. Avoid dead space.

12. Apply a dressing.
   a. Dress in position for function.
   b. Apply antibiotic ointment.
   c. Apply a three-layer dressing; tape appropriately.
      1) Nonadherent layer (telfa) applied to skin
      2) Absorbent layer of 4 × 4 gauze
      3) Protective layer of gauze and/or elastic netting
   d. An elastic bandage occasionally is needed for immobilization or hemostasis. Care should be taken to avoid excessive compression of the wrapped area.

13. Immobilization is sometimes required if the laceration is in a mobile area. Continue to splint 1-2 weeks after the sutures are out.
14. To avoid edema, advise elevation × 24 hours for lacerations involving the hands and feet.
15. Length of time for sutures to remain in place.
   a. Face: 4-5 days; then may add tape closure
   b. Nonmobile area: 5-7 days; then may add tape closure
   c. Distal site or mobile area: 7-14 days; then may add tape closure
16. Give tetanus prophylaxis, if needed.
17. Antibiotics are not generally used unless the laceration is infection prone (e.g., human bite, cat bite, deep puncture, crush injury).
18. When not to suture
   a. Ideally, wounds should be sutured soon after the injury.
   b. Puncture wounds are usually closed by the time the child comes for medical attention. If so, thoroughly clean the wound with

povidone-iodine; do not reopen. If the wound is slightly open, clean it with saline, and irrigate copiously. *Never* suture a puncture wound (increased risk of infection).

c. Lacerations can be sutured any time before healing is complete. There is concern that suturing older wounds (i.e., 12-30 hours old) may increase the risk of infection. In such cases, aggressive cleansing and antibiotic prophylaxis are advised.

BIBLIOGRAPHY

Bites

Human

Baker MD: Human bites in children, *Am J Dis Child* 141:1285, 1987.

Brook I: Microbiology of human and animal bite wounds, *Pediatr Infect Dis J* 6:29, 1987.

Schweich P, Fleisher G: Human bites in children, *Pediatr Emerg Care* 1:51, 1985.

Animal

Avner JR, Baker MD: Dog bites in urban children, *Pediatrics* 88:55, 1991.

Boenning D et al: Dog bites in children, *Am J Emerg Med* 1:17, 1983.

Brook I: Microbiology of human and animal bite wounds in children, *Pediatr Infect Dis J* 6:29, 1987.

Cummings P: Antibiotics to prevent infection in patients with dog-bite wounds: a meta-analysis of randomized trials, *Ann Emerg Med* 23:535, 1994.

Feder H et al: Review of 59 patients hospitalized with animal bites, *Pediatr Infect Dis J* 6:24, 1987.

Marcy SM: Infections due to dog and cat bites, *Pediatr Infect Dis J* 1:351, 1982.

Trott A: Care of mammalian bites, *Pediatr Infect Dis J* 6:8, 1987.

Rabies prophylaxis

1994 Red Book Report of the Committee on Infectious Diseases, ed 23, p 388, Elk Grove Village, Ill, 1994, American Academy of Pediatrics.

Kaplan MM, Koprowski H: Rabies, *Sci Am* 242:120, 1980.
Mann J: Systemic decision making in rabies prophylaxis, *Pediatr Infect Dis J* 2:162, 1983.

Burns

Coren C: Burn injuries in children, *Pediatr Ann* 16:328, 1987.
Fitzpatrick K et al: Outpatient management of minor burns, *Phys Assist,* 9:16, 1985.
Gellis S, Kagan B: *Current pediatric therapy,* ed 12, Philadelphia, 1986, WB Saunders.
Guzzetta P, Randolph J: Burns in children, *Pediatr Rev* 4:271, 1983.
Herndon DM et al: Treatment of burns in children, *Pediatr Clin North Am* 32:1311, 1985.
Robinson M, Seward P: Thermal injury in children, *Pediatr Emerg Care* 3:266, 1987.

Dental trauma

Berkowitz R et al: Dental trauma in children and adolescents, *Clin Pediatr* 19:166, 1980.
Committee on Early Childhood, Adoption, and Dependent Care: Oral and dental aspects of child abuse and neglect, *Pediatrics* 78:537, 1986.
McTigue D: Management of orofacial trauma in children, *Pediatr Ann* 14:125, 1985.

Frostbite

Paton B: A quick, effective response to hypothermia and frostbite, *Contemp Pediatr* 3:37, 1986.

Insect reactions

Goldberg G: Stings and bites: emergencies and annoyances, *Contemp Pediatr* 2:32, 1985.
Maguire J, Geha R: Bee, wasp, and hornet stings, *Pediatr Rev* 8:5, 1986.

Ticks and spiders

Goldberg G: Stings and bites: emergencies and annoyances, *Contemp Pediatr* 2:32, 1985.

Lacerations

Bonadio W, Wagner V: Efficacy of TAC topical anesthetic for repair of pediatric lacerations, *Am J Dis Child* 142:203, 1988.

Theroux MC et al: Efficacy of intranasal midazolam in facilitating suturing of lacerations in preschool children in the Emergency Department, *Pediatrics* 91:624, 1993.

MISCELLANEOUS DISEASES AND DISORDERS

22

A. AIDS

1. The human T lymphotrophic virus type III (more commonly known as HIV) is the cause of AIDS. HIV infects the helper CD4 T lymphocytes, causing lymphocyte dysfunction with resultant immunodeficiency.

2. Because the virus incorporates its own DNA into the human host DNA, it can remain latent for many years.

3. Most HIV infections in infants and children are secondary to perinatal transmission from infected mothers. Other children, especially those born prematurely and those with hemophilia, have acquired their disease through transfusions with contaminated blood. Shared contaminated IV drug needles and unprotected sexual intercourse are the most common means of HIV spread in adults and adolescents. Younger children have also been infected with HIV after sexual abuse (intercourse) by infected individuals.

4. Infants infected with HIV may have FTT, profound weight loss, developmental delay, or persistent oral candidiasis. Hepatosplenomegaly, generalized lymphadenopathy, chronic diarrhea, fever, malaise, and recurrent infections should also raise suspicions about HIV. Persistent parotitis and lymphoid interstitial pneumonia are peculiar to childhood AIDS.

5. The most common presentation of AIDS in older children, adolescents, and adults is *Pneumocystis carinii* pneumonia.

6. Opportunistic infections (e.g., CMV, herpesvirus) are common.

7. The PE must be complete. AIDS is a multisystem disease, and there are often multiple abnormal physical findings.

8. Laboratory tests to support a clinical diagnosis include an ELISA screen for HIV antibodies (with the Western blot test to confirm a positive ELISA). Infants can have passively transferred maternal

antibodies and test falsely positive well into the second year of life. An HIV culture and/or PCR can be used to document true infection, even as early as 2-3 months of age.

9. Other tests to assess immune function include a CBC with differential, CD4 count, CD4/CD8 (T cell) ratio, T-cell function tests, and serum immunoglobulins. Remember, CD4 counts normally vary by age and are highest during infancy. LFTs and a CXR are also helpful.

10. Therapy

a. Antiretroviral drugs interfere with viral replication; they suppress rather than kill the virus. Indications for use are symptomatic disease or CD4 counts (cells/cc): <1750 if <1 year of age, <1000 if 1-6 years, and <500 if >6 years. The approved antiretroviral drugs for children are zidovudine (AZT), didanosine (ddI), and lamivudine (3TC).

1) AZT is indicated for use in HIV-infected children >3 months of age who have HIV-related symptoms or are asymptomatic but have abnormal laboratory values indicating significant HIV-related immunosuppression. AZT is also used during pregnancy to reduce the chance of viral transmission from mother to fetus. When used during pregnancy, it is important to continue AZT therapy in the neonate for 6 weeks after birth at a dosage of 2 mg/kg/dose PO q6h.

a) The AZT dosage in HIV-infected children is 360-720 mg/m^2 ÷ tid.

b) Because AZT is myelosuppressive, the CBC must be monitored often. Hepatic function should also be monitored often.

(1) Reduce the AZT dosage if the Hgb is <8.0 g/dL or for declines >2.0 g/dL from baseline.

(2) Discontinue AZT and other myelosuppressive drugs if the absolute neutrophil count is <500/c^2. Restart AZT at 120 mg/m^2/dose when the count increases to >500/cc.

(3) The dosage may be increased to 180 mg/m^2/dose if hematologic values exceed these thresholds after 1 month of reduced dosage.

(4) Another antiretroviral agent should be used if the neutrophil count cannot be maintained at >500 cells/cc, especially if a granulocyte colony-stimulating factor is used.

2) In children ddI is an alternative to AZT. Its advantage is that it is not myelosuppressive. It is used when a child cannot tolerate

AZT or clinically worsens while on AZT; it is also used in combination with AZT when lower doses of AZT are indicated because of associated side effects. Improvements in clinical, virologic, and immunologic parameters may be sustained in a number of patients who receive ddI for several years.

a) The dosage is 100 mg/m^2 PO q12h given on an empty stomach.

b) The use of ddI has been associated with pancreatitis and peripheral retinal depigmentation, usually unassociated with visual impairment in 5% of those receiving dosages $\geq$270 mg/m^2/d. Peripheral neuropathy may also occur.

c) Children receiving ddI should have monthly serum amylase and lipase determinations, an ophthalmology evaluation before and q6mo therafter or as needed, and prompt evaluation if there is any tingling, numbness, or pain in the hands or feet.

d) Combination AZT/ddI therapy has been used with success. It is especially useful when higher doses of AZT alone lead to toxicity.

3) Lamivudine (3TC) has recently been approved for use in combination with zidovudine. Experience with pediatric patients is currently limited. It should not be used in any patient with pancreatitis or at risk to develop it.

a) The dosage is 4 mg/kg (max 150 mg) bid.

b) Its use in children has been associated with pancreatitis; monitoring serum amylase is essential.

c) The dosage is governed by the creatinine clearance, which also should be assessed periodically.

b. Infections must be aggressively treated. IV immune globulin (400 mg/kg/dose q28d) may be useful in patients with recurrent serious bacterial infections.

c. TMP/SMZ is used for prophylaxis against infection with *P. carinii*. Initiation of prophylaxis is based on CD4 counts.

1) Prophylaxis should be initiated if CD4 counts (cells/cc) are <1500 if <1 year of age, <750 if 1-2 years, <500 if 2-6 years, and <200 if >6 years.

2) Because of sulfa toxicity in neonates, TMP/SMZ is used only in infants >6 weeks of age. All infants of HIV-positive mothers should be treated with this drug from 6 weeks to 12 months of age to prevent infection with *P. carinii* because infants in the first year of life are at particular risk for infection by this

organism. Prophylaxis should continue until the child is known
to be HIV negative; if the child is HIV positive, continuation
of the drug is determined by clinical status, history of *P. carinii*
infection, and CD4 counts.

3) If this drug seems to be responsible for neutropenia, alternate
prophylaxis (e.g., dapsone or pentamidine) should be given.

d. VZIG must be administered if exposure to varicella occurs.
Acyclovir is indicated for clinical varicella and severe herpes
infections.

e. Avoid OPV in infants, children, and their contacts; primary
immunization against polio is with IPV.

f. DTP, *Haemophilus influenzae* type B, pneumococcus, influenza,
and MMR vaccines should be given at the usual schedules and
intervals.

g. TB screening should be carried out on schedule. An anergy
skin-test panel is helpful in interpreting PPD test results, especially
in patients with low CD4 counts.

h. Involve social services and religious support systems (if present)
as early as possible to assist the family and patient.

i. The best way to "cure" AIDS is to prevent it. Persons who are
engaging in sexual intercourse and do not know their partner's
HIV status should use condoms; abstinence is preferable and is the
only certain way to prevent the sexual transmission of HIV. Other
ways to prevent AIDS include the cessation of IV needle sharing
and *universal* testing of blood and blood products for HIV.
Because AZT has been shown to reduce transmission of the virus
from mother to fetus, AZT therapy is indicated in pregnant women
who are HIV-positive.

B. CHEST PAIN

1. Chest pain is a relatively uncommon presenting complaint in young
children but becomes more common as children age. It can be
functional, herald serious disease, or have a significance somewhere
in between.

2. Important historical information includes the following:

a. The onset, duration, recurrence, location, radiation, and quality
(sharp vs. dull) of the pain

b. Relationship to rest, exercise, and eating

c. Precipitating factors

d. Actions or medications that worsen or improve the pain

e. History of similar pain or of being awakened from sleep by pain

    f. Other concomitant symptoms: Diaphoresis, nausea, vomiting, dyspnea, coughing, wheezing, vertigo, syncope, palpitations, skin color changes

    g. Presence of fever, respiratory symptoms, and myalgias (especially if pain is acute)

    h. Symptoms of indigestion

    i. The possibility of foreign-body aspiration

    j. A history of trauma

    k. A history of a heart murmur, cardiac disease or surgery, sickle-cell disease, chronic respiratory disease

    l. Psychosomatic symptoms (is child under stress?)

    m. Medication or illicit drug use

    n. Family history of angina, cardiac disease, death (especially if recent) from cardiac causes

3. The PE should be complete, with special emphasis on the following:

    a. Vital signs

    b. General appearance: Frightened, in pain, indifferent

    c. Skin: Cyanosis, pallor

    d. Respiratory exam: Rate, depth, symmetry of respirations; splinting; rales; wheezes; area of decreased breath sounds

    e. Cardiac exam: PMI, rate, regularity of rhythm, murmurs, rub, gallop, assessment of pulse equality and strength, palpation of chest and neck for thrills, auscultation of neck for bruits (remember to auscultate with the patient in both the supine and sitting positions)

    f. The chest wall: Areas of tenderness, asymmetry, inflammation; palpation of ribs, intercostal spaces, upper abdomen, and vertebral bodies to determine direct or referred areas of tenderness

4. Causes of chest pain

    a. Cardiac: Suggested by pain associated with exercise, palpitations, color change, syncope, vertigo

      1) Ischemia: Squeezing pain, tachypnea, tachycardia, gallop, rales, wheezing, CHF, shock

      2) Left ventricular outflow obstruction: Especially pain precipitated by exercise when cardiac oxygen demand is not met by the supply; aortic valve or subvalvular stenosis (harsh systolic murmur varying little with maneuvers that alter ventricular filling); idiopathic hypertrophic subaortic stenosis (murmur softens during Valsalva's maneuver; pansystolic murmur with S4; ECG *may* show septal Q wave)

      3) Coronary artery disease: Compression, fistula secondary to collagen-vascular disease or Kawasaki disease; systolic/

continuous murmur, gallop; ECG may show infarction or ST-T wave changes

4) Mitral valve prolapse: Usually asymptomatic; midsystolic click or late systolic murmur (altered by position); ECG may show T-wave changes, U wave, tachycardia

5) Dissecting aortic aneurysm: Acute, sharp, "tearing" pain

6) Arrhythmias: Palpitations, chest pain, dizziness; may be tachycardia, bradycardia, or varying rhythms

7) Pericardial infection, inflammation, or infiltration by tumor: Sharp pain exacerbated by inspiration, cough, movement; friction rub heard on auscultation; ECG may show ST elevation and low QRS voltage

b. Pulmonary

1) Pneumonia: Rales, decreased breath sounds, tachypnea, cough, respiratory distress

2) Asthma (exercise induced): May have pain in the absence of wheezing

3) Pleurisy: Sharp pain aggravated by cough/inspiration

4) Pneumothorax: Sharp pain, dyspnea, area(s) of decreased breath sounds

5) Pulmonary infarction: Intense pain, respiratory distress; may be cyanosis and shock

c. Gastrointestinal

1) Esophageal reflux: Substernal pain that is worse after eating or when supine, aerophagia, belching

2) Esophagitis: Similar pain as in reflux but may be more intense

3) Hiatal hernia

4) Mallory-Weiss syndrome: Acute onset, substernal pain; blood commonly in vomitus or stool

5) Gastric spasm, inflammation, ulcer: Lower chest or epigastric pain elicited by direct palpation

6) Duodenal ulcer

7) Biliary/pancreatic disease

d. Mediastinal diseases

1) Pneumomediastinum

2) Tumors

3) Mediastinitis

e. Chest wall disorders

1) Costochondritis: Tender costochondral junctions

2) Trauma: May be able to reproduce pain with palpation over affected area

3) Breast development

4) Slipping rib syndrome

f. Emotional

1) Pain is vague, fleeting, and localized over the heart or left arm.

2) Pain is not precipitated by exercise; it may occur at rest.

3) Other psychosomatic symptoms may be present.

g. Precordial catch syndrome

1) Sharp pain below left sternal border or left breast without radiation

2) Relieved by change of position, chest massage, or deep inspiration

h. Miscellaneous

1) Chest wall zoster

2) Malignancies

3) Hemoglobinopathies

4) Collagen-vascular diseases

5) Spinal root irritations

6) Drug abuse (especially inhaled cocaine)

5. Laboratory tests should be dictated by the history and physical findings as follows:

a. If a cardiac cause for pain is suspected (e.g., pain with exercise, palpitations, color change, syncope), an ECG, ECHO, and prompt referral to a cardiologist are in order.

b. If a pulmonary cause is likely, a CXR and preexertional and postexertional pulmonary function testing may be useful.

c. Even after a complete evaluation, a specific cause is not found in 30%-50% of the cases.

6. Treatment is directed toward the underlying cause of the chest pain.

C. DAY-CARE ISSUES

1. Many infants and preschool-age children are in substitute care arrangements during part of every work day. Day-care arrangements should be part of each child's history.

2. Day-care attendance (e.g., Who cares for the child? Where? For how many hours each day? Are other children present?) should be documented for the following presenting complaints/diagnoses:

a. Sepsis (contacts may need prophylaxis)

b. Meningitis (contacts may need prophylaxis)

c. Epiglottitis (contacts may need prophylaxis)

d. Streptococcal pharyngitis (contacts with pharyngitis need evaluation)

    e. Otitis media (recurrent)

    f. Bacterial diarrhea (contacts may need evaluation)

    g. Food poisoning (ill contacts need evaluation)

    h. Hepatitis (contacts may need prophylaxis)

    i. Lice (contacts need observation)

    j. Scabies (contacts need observation)

    k. Pinworms (contacts need observation)

    l. HSV-1 (children with skin lesions need evaluation)

    m. Impetigo (children with skin lesions need evaluation)

    n. Tinea (children with skin lesions need evaluation)

    o. Chickenpox (children with skin lesions need evaluation)

    p. Conjunctivitis (symptomatic children need evaluation)

    q. Injury that is poorly explained or does not fit the description given

    r. Question of abuse (physical, sexual, emotional)

3. Entities such as pneumonia, otitis media, sinusitis, croup, and bronchiolitis may also be related to day-care attendance. URI and acute GE are common in day-care settings.

D. FAILURE TO THRIVE

1. FTT is defined as weight <3rd percentile *or* <80% of ideal weight *or* weight that decreases by at least two percentile lines on a growth chart. The height and head circumference usually are not affected as much as the weight.

    a. There is an equal race and sex incidence.

    b. Most patients are younger than 24-36 months of age.

    c. FTT may be the reason for presentation or may be an "incidental" finding when the child has an acute illness.

2. Important historical information includes the following:

    a. Prenatal, birth, neonatal histories, especially maternal exposure to drugs, cigarettes, infectious agents, and risk factors for HIV

    b. Sleep, bowel, and bladder habits

    c. Developmental history: Is delay present? If so, is it global or local?

    d. Feeding history: "Average" day diet recall, type of formula used and how it is prepared, amount of formula/milk ingested per day, amount and types of other fluids ingested per day, amount and types of solids ingested per day

    e. Presence of "meal battles," feeding difficulties, tongue thrusting, choking, diaphoresis, color changes, regurgitation

    f. How child is fed: Can the child feed himself or herself? Can the child drink from a cup?

g. Presence of infectious disease symptoms (which ones?), chronic medical conditions, long-term medication use

h. Medical history

i. Review of systems

j. Family history, especially heights/weights of parents, siblings, grandparents

k. Social history: Child's affect and behavior, parental history of abuse or FTT, family's financial and living conditions, parents' social supports, parents' bond with child, other caretakers of child; was this child planned?

3. A complete, meticulous PE is *mandatory!*

a. Particular attention should be given to growth parameters; weight, height, and head circumference should be measured and plotted against the child's age.

1) Weight, height, and head circumference <3rd percentile: Usually in utero insult; however, may represent severe, prolonged caloric deprivation

2) Weight and height <3rd percentile, head circumference normal: Endocrinopathies, structural dystrophies, constitutional short stature

3) Weight <3rd percentile, height and head circumference normal: Caloric deprivation (poor intake vs. poor utilization), nonorganic FTT

b. Child's appearance: Clean vs. dirty, small vs. scrawny, fearful vs. too trusting, clinging, avoiding mother, avoiding eye contact

c. Skin: Dirty, rashes, chronic conditions such as eczema, signs of abuse

d. Muscle mass: Decreased, with little fat

e. Head: Asymmetries; overriding/separated sutures; size, shape, texture of fontanelle; flattened or balding occiput; signs of trauma; transilluminate infant's head

f. Mouth: Tongue thrust, enlarged tongue, teeth (number, condition)

g. Cardiopulmonary: Any abnormality

h. Abdomen: Organomegaly, protuberance

i. Extremities: Length relative to length of trunk

j. Neurologic/developmental assessment

4. Causes

a. Organic (30%-40% of cases)

1) GI (40% of all organic FTT): Most commonly clefts, chalasia, gastroesophageal reflux, celiac disease, Crohn's disease, Hirschsprung's disease, cystic fibrosis, liver disease

2) Renal: Remember renal tubular acidosis in addition to more obvious diseases
3) CNS: 20% of all organic FTT
4) Endocrine: Diabetes mellitus, diabetes insipidus, thyroid disease (hyperthyroidism or hypothyroidism), adrenal disorders, hypopituitarism (congenital or acquired)
5) Chronic infections (e.g., HIV) and toxin exposure (e.g., lead poisoning)

b. Nonorganic (perhaps 75%-90% of all FTT cases in some series; may be as low as 10%-15% depending on population)

1) May be "hyperalert" with minimal vocalization vs. a heightened response to strangers
2) Pale, loss of muscle mass
3) May have tonic immobility (flexed)
4) History of feeding problems; difficult temperament; being unplanned/unwanted, the youngest; parental history of abuse, FTT, depression; lack of involved father; distant/overwrought mother; lack of social supports; poor preventive health care (delinquent immunizations); history of multiple medical providers
5) If such patients are hospitalized, two thirds improve away from home; however, they may require *3-4 weeks!*
6) Usually decreased growth hormone and serum iron parameters, delayed bone age

5. Evaluation

a. Immediate hospitalization is advisable if abuse/neglect is suspected, if the child is ill, or if treatable organic disease is present. Probably should hospitalize any child with FTT within 1-2 months of growth deceleration.

b. Investigate organic and nonorganic causes simultaneously (preferably with a supportive, multidisciplinary approach).

c. Perform a complete history/physical/developmental assessment.

d. Initial laboratory tests: CBC with differential, serum electrolytes, BUN, creatinine, and glucose; U/A and culture; stool exam for reducing substances and fat; PPD; ± CXR

e. Other tests as dictated by history/PE: Radiographic assessment of GI tract, GU tract; ECG; bone age (unreliable if very young); sweat test; and HIV testing. The less evident an organic cause is at presentation, the less likely laboratory tests are to find one. One study examined 185 children with FTT who received 2607 laboratory tests; only 10 (0.4%) established a diagnosis and only 26 (1.0%) supported a diagnosis.

    f. Calorie count/observed feeding trial

6. Treatment is directed toward the underlying cause. Children with nonorganic FTT and their parents merit family counseling/psychotherapy. Unfortunately, only 33% of children are normal at follow-up 5-10 years later, and 50% are delayed or experience learning/personal problems.

E. HYPERTENSION

1. BP measurement is a necessary part of the PE.

    a. In neonates, infants, and toddlers, BP may be more easily measured by an oscillometric method than by auscultation.

    b. The manual method is preferred in older children and adolescents.

        1) The child is seated with the right arm at heart level.

        2) The blood pressure cuff is wrapped around the upper part of the arm; the bladder should encircle the arm and cover it at a minimum two thirds of its length. The cuff is inflated to approximately 2 mm Hg above the point at which the radial pulse disappears.

        3) The cuff is deflated slowly and deliberately while observing the manometer (aneroid or mercury).

        4) Auscultation over the brachial artery reveals the onset of an audible tapping sound (systolic pressure, Korotkoff I sound); further deflation and auscultation reveal a muffled sound (Korotkoff IV) and, finally, its disappearance (Korotkoff V).

        5) Because there is debate as to which sound (IV or V) truly represents diastole, both are recorded (e.g., 110/70/64).

        6) Because some children have heart sounds audible throughout the cuff's deflation, the Korotkoff IV sound has been used in age- and sex-appropriate BP standards.

2. Inaccurate BP measurements occur when the cuff size is incorrect (especially too small); when the patient is moving, crying, or upset; or when the equipment is not calibrated correctly. Observer bias also occurs.

3. A healthy child is said to have high normal BP when he or she has either a systolic or diastolic pressure between the 90th and 95th percentiles for age and sex. If a child's systolic or diastolic pressures equal or exceed the 95th percentile on three separate occasions, he or she has persistently elevated blood pressure (hypertension). Thus

multiple measurements are needed to confirm the diagnosis of hypertension.

4. Causes
   a. Renal: Acute glomerulonephritis, hemolytic-uremic syndrome, nephrosis, lupus, trauma, obstructive uropathy, congenital disorders (polycystic renal disease, dysplasia, hypoplasia), tumors, lead nephropathy, mercury poisoning, radiation nephritis, S/P GU surgery/renal transplant/renal rejection, end-stage renal disease
   b. Vascular: Renal arterial disease, renal vein thrombosis, renal artery stenosis, aortitis, aortic coarctation either in the thoracic or abdominal areas
   c. Endocrine: Primary hyperparathyroidism, primary hyperthyroidism, pheochromocytoma, neuroblastoma, Cushing's syndrome, adrenogenital syndrome (11-hydroxylase and 17-hydroxylase deficiencies), primary aldosteronism
   d. Chemical agents: Therapy with sympathomimetics, steroids, or oral contraceptives; amphetamine or cocaine abuse
   e. Miscellaneous: Collagen-vascular disease, poliomyelitis, Guillain-Barré syndrome, dysautonomia, porphyria, hypercalcemia, Stevens-Johnson syndrome, burns, malignancies, SBE, increased intracranial pressure, neurofibromatosis
   f. Primary hypertension occurs in the absence of conditions known to elevate blood pressure. Both genetics and environment (e.g., high salt intake) may play a role in its genesis. Many children are asymptomatic; symptoms when present include frontal headaches, epistaxis, and nervousness. Obesity may be present in as many as 50% of the children.

5. When a child has a persistently elevated BP, important historical information includes the following:
   a. The child's birth history
   b. Presence of chronic conditions/chronic or recurrent symptoms (headache, epistaxis)
   c. Long-term use of medications
   d. Growth pattern
   e. Urinary tract infections or disorders
   f. Diet history
   g. Family history of hypertension or its complications (renal disease, myocardial infarction, stroke)
   h. Lifestyle and stressors
   i. Hospitalizations and surgeries

6. The PE must be complete because many causes of secondary

hypertension have characteristic physical findings. Check for the presence of an abdominal bruit or café-au-lait spots. Special emphasis is placed on the BP measured in both arms and one leg (to R/O coarctation) and in the right arm with the patient in the supine, sitting, and standing positions. A fundoscopic exam (an abnormal exam indicates that hypertension has been present >1 year) and a complete cardiac exam are mandatory.

7. Laboratory tests are dictated by the history and physical findings. A routine U/A and serum creatinine, BUN, electrolytes, uric acid, and CBC determinations are useful screens. If the patient is obese, a fasting cholesterol (and its fractions) and high- and low-density lipoprotein levels are also useful. In any child for whom drug therapy is considered, a baseline ECHO is needed to assess chronicity of the hypertension. A CXR, renal ultrasound, renal imaging, head CT scan, and peripheral plasma renin activity assessment should also be considered.

8. Management (children and adolescents)
   a. Secondary hypertension: Treat the underlying condition, if possible. Drug therapy might be necessary to control the hypertension.
   b. Primary hypertension
      1) Weight loss to achieve ideal weight
      2) Proper exercise
      3) Limited salt intake
      4) Avoidance of medications with sympathomimetics; avoidance of alcohol and tobacco
      5) Try to maintain a positive attitude with regard to stressors and patience with therapy.

NOTE: Hypertension in children and adolescents was previously initially treated with diuretics and, if diuretic therapy was unsuccessful, β-adrenergic blockers. Angiotension-converting enzyme inhibitors (ACE drugs) and calcium channel blockers are now available and are considered first-line drugs.

      6) ACE drugs (most notably captopril) interfere with the enzymatic conversion of angiotensin I to angiotension II, a major vasoconstrictor. Thus they cause vasodilation and decreased vascular resistance, with more pronounced effects in preterm infants.
         a) The dosage of captopril is 1.5 mg/kg/d (max 6 mg/kg/d) for children and 0.03-0.15 mg/kg/d (max 2 mg/kg/d) for neonates. These dosages can be divided q6-12h. An initial dosage for adolescents is 25 mg bid or tid, which may be

increased gradually to 50 mg. Captopril should be given 1 hour before meals. The onset of action is 60 minutes, with the maximal effect in 1-1½ hours.

b) Serum BUN, creatinine, and potassium should be monitored during therapy for any patient with renal disease who is treated with captopril.

7) Calcium channel blockers (nifedipine) inhibit the inward flux of Ca across the cell membrane of smooth muscle cells of resistance arterioles, thereby diminishing vascular smooth muscle tone. Thus they are potent vasodilators.

a) The dosage of nifedipine is 0.25 mg/kg/d (max 3 mg/kg/d) ÷ tid or qid unless an extended-release preparation is used. The onset of action is 10-15 minutes, with the maximal effect in 1-1½ hours.

b) Common side effects are headaches, palpitations, and flushing.

8) Diuretics can be useful in hypertensive patients with renal disease. They produce an increase in urine volume and Na excretion, which results in decreased extracellular and plasma volume, body weight, and cardiac output.

9) β-Adrenergic–blocking drugs (such as propranolol) were at one time used as first-line therapy for hypertension. However, side effects associated with their use (bradycadia, exacerbation of asthma symptoms, CNS effects, sleep disturbances, altered glucose and lipid metabolism) and the efficacy of ACE drugs and calcium channel blockers has rendered β-blockers less desirable as long-term therapy for hypertension.

10) A hypertensive crisis (abrupt, marked elevation in BP) can occur in renal disease, hemolytic-uremic syndrome, renal vascular disease, pheochromocytoma, renin-secreting tumors, and severe CNS disease. Symptoms include headaches, epistaxis, diplopia, seizures, CHF, facial palsy, edema, and hypertensive retinopathy. The primary goal of drug therapy is to reduce BP at a rate that minimizes complications while ensuring adequate blood supply to vital organs. The following is a list of useful drugs:

a) Nifedipine (0.25-0.5 mg/kg PO) can be used in asymptomatic children who can take drugs orally. When used for emergency therapy, either the drug should be removed from the capsule and administered by syringe, or the child should bite through the capsule. The onset of action is

20-30 minutes. The duration of action is approximately 6 hours.

b) Labetalol 0.2-1.0 mg/kg/dose IV can be given by repeated bolus injections, but a continous infusion (0.4-1.0 mg/kg/hr gives a steadier response. The onset of action is within 5 minutes. The duration of action is during its infusion.

c) Sodium nitroprusside (0.5-8 µg/kg/min IV) can be used to emergently treat severe hypertension in children with normal to only moderately decreased renal function. The onset of action is 30-60 seconds, but BP begins to rise again within seconds of discontinuing the drug.

F. KAWASAKI DISEASE

1. KD is an acute vasculitis of unknown etiology. Patients are usually <5 years of age (peak incidence 18-24 months) with a male-female ratio of 1.5:1. There is a 0.15% mortality rate in the subacute or early convalescent stage, usually from cardiovascular complications.

2. The diagnosis is based on a constellation of characteristic clinical signs and symptoms and laboratory abnormalities. There is a triphasic clinical course.

   a. Acute febrile stage (days 1-15): Fever plus at least four of the five asterisked features should be present to establish the diagnosis. The fever is high and spiking (>40° C) and only temporarily responsive to antipyretics. Fever should be present for at least 5 days before a diagnosis of KD is confirmed, but the disease should be considered earlier if other characteristic features are present.

      *1) Conjunctival injection usually occurs within 2-3 days of fever onset; it is bilateral, painless, nonpurulent, and especially marked in the bulbar conjunctivae.

      *2) Oral mucosal findings occur within 1-3 days of fever onset and involve reddened fissured lips, a reddened oropharynx, and a "strawberry" tongue.

      *3) Rash occurs with the onset of fever and takes several forms (erythematous, irregular plaques that are partially confluent; morbilliform eruption; scarlatiniform; urticarial). The rash occurs principally on the face and trunk but may be accentuated in the perineum; it is *never* vesicular, bullous, petechial, purpuric, or crusting.

      *4) Extremity changes occur within several days of the onset of fever. The palms and soles develop diffuse erythema, often accompanied by indurative edema and tenderness; the skin of the dorsum of the hands and feet can appear shiny and stretched.

NOTE: Not all patients have edema; it is more common in infants.

*5) Lymphadenopathy is the least common major feature; it is usually not generalized but is often a solitary cervical node (>1.5 cm in diameter) that is often tender but rarely fluctuant.

6) Behavior changes: Irritability, lethargy, mood lability

7) Abdominal pain, diarrhea, vomiting, liver inflammation, anorexia, mild jaundice, hydrops of the gallbladder

8) GU signs and symptoms (sterile pyuria, urethritis, hematuria)

9) Cough, rhinorrhea

10) Joint involvement (late in first stage)

11) Cardiovascular involvement (perivasculitis and microvasculitis of coronary arteries, pancarditis), tachycardia

12) Significant laboratory findings: Elevated ESR and CRP, pyuria, elevated WBC count with shift to the left, CSF mononuclear pleocytosis, thrombocytosis (end of this stage), negative cultures

NOTE: Patients with fever and fewer than four of the starred parameters can be considered for therapy with IV immune globulin, as can those with fewer than 5 days of fever if other signs are characteristic.

b. Subacute stage (days 14-21): Fever, rash, and lymphadenopathy subside. Conjunctivae may still be red; oral mucosal changes are still present. Peripheral extremities begin to desquamate, starting periungually and moving proximally between days 10 and 20. Anorexia and mood changes are still present.

1) Joint involvement: Arthralgias/arthritis in large joints (knees, hips, elbows). Effusion(s) may be present.

2) Cardiac disease: Improving pancarditis; coronary arteries demonstrate persistent panvasculitis and may demonstrate areas of thrombosis. Coronary artery aneurysms develop in 20% of untreated patients. Clinically, there may be tachycardia, a gallop, muffled heart sounds, minor ECG changes (prolonged PR interval, ST-T wave changes). More severely ill children may have cardiomyopathy with CHF, pericardial effusion, and mitral valve insufficiency. Sudden death may result from aneurysm rupture or coronary artery occlusion.

3) Significant laboratory findings: Test results abnormal in the first stage are usually still abnormal; thrombocytosis (usually 600,000-1,000,000); mild anemia; elevated AST, CPK, and LDH (if myocarditis)

c. Convalescent stage (up to 3 months after onset): Eyes, oral mucosa, extremities, mood, joint symptoms, and appetite are improving or normal. Early in this stage, coronary artery inflammation is still present; sudden death is still a threat. Most abnormal laboratory values have normalized by the end of this stage.

3. Differential diagnosis in early stage
   a. KD may be confused with measles, group A streptococcal infection (scarlet fever), Epstein-Barr virus, leptospirosis, drug eruption, erythema multiforme, Stevens-Johnson syndrome, toxic shock syndrome (staphylococcus), acrodynia, JRA, SLE, RF, and serum sickness.
   b. Discrete intraoral lesions, purulent conjunctivitis, exudative pharyngitis, splenomegaly, and generalized adenopathy are distinctly uncommon in patients with KD and, when present, suggest an alternate diagnosis.

4. Risk factors have been identified to detect children most likely to develop coronary aneurysms or thrombosis. Children with ≤5 factors generally do well; those with >9 are at high risk.
   a. Male gender
   b. Age <1 year
   c. Duration of initial fever >15 days
   d. Recrudescent rash
   e. WBCs >30,000
   f. Westergren sedimentation rate >100
   g. Presence of cardiomegaly
   h. Presence of arrhythmias
   i. Recrudescent fever
   j. Evidence of myocardial infarction
   k. Prolonged QR interval
   l. Hemoglobin <10
   m. Elevated ESR >5 weeks

5. Management
   a. Acute stage
      1) Appropriate work-up to rule out sepsis, meningitis (if indicated), treatable infections
      2) Baseline CBC, ESR, CRP, U/A; consider liver/cardiac enzymes, CXR, ECG
      3) Immune globulin at a dose of 2 g/kg should be given as a single IV infusion over 10-12 hours as soon as possible after the diagnosis has been established. Retreatment with IV immune globulin may be needed for those with persistent fever or symptoms. The prevalence of coronary abnormalities is only 2% among patients treated with aspirin and IV immune globulin.

4) Give aspirin 80-100 mg/kg/d ÷ qid until the patient is afebrile for 24 hours (some recommend this dose until the fourteenth day of illness) followed by 3-5 mg/kg once daily for 2 months.
5) The child may need to be hospitalized for IV immune globulin; if not hospitalized, the child needs to be seen 2-4 times/week.
6) If an outpatient develops cardiac symptoms or abnormalities, he or she should be hospitalized immediately.
7) Do not use steroids! They increase platelet counts and are associated with a higher incidence of coronary aneurysms.
8) A two-dimensional ECHO may be indicated during the acute phase in some patients but is usually obtained 4-8 weeks after the onset of symptoms. ECHO detects proximal coronary artery dilation and aneurysms with high sensitivity and specificity.
b. Subacute stage
1) After day 14, the aspirin dosage should be reduced to 3-5 mg/kg/d given as a single daily dose.
2) Clinical status, CBC, platelet count, and ECG should be serially monitored.
3) Repeat ECHO (compare with initial one).
4) Provide supportive therapy.
5) If patient has CHF, provide appropriate therapy.
6) Perform a coronary angiogram if the child has an infarction or coronary vessel damage.
c. Convalescent stage
1) Aspirin therapy is stopped if no abnormalities are found on ECHO at 4-8 weeks; follow-up is individualized.
2) Children with evidence of aneurysms should have serial ECHOs to assess aneurysm change. Patients who develop giant coronary aneurysms (internal diameter ≥8 mm) are at the greatest risk for coronary thrombosis, stenosis, and myocardial infarction.
3) Long-term therapy for high-risk children with cardiac abnormalities includes low-dose aspirin, either alone or with dipyridamole.
4) Children with increasing cardiac symptoms or vessel involvement may require coronary artery bypass grafting.

G. LEAD POISONING
1. Sources of lead
a. Lead-based paint (the most common high-dose source of lead exposure for children). Window wells and sills are areas with high concentrations of lead dust.

      b. Soil and dust

      c. Drinking water

      d. Parental occupations and hobbies (furniture refinishing, making stained glass, working in a smelter or battery factory)

      e. Air (much lower now that lead has been removed from gasoline)

      f. Food

      g. Imported ceramic objects, especially if used to hold foods or fluids for consumption

      h. Cosmetic eye decorations containing kohl

2. High-risk children

      a. Children 6-72 months of age who live in or are frequent visitors to deteriorated housing built before 1960

      b. Children 6-72 months of age who live in old houses with recent, ongoing, or planned renovation

      c. Siblings, housemates, and playmates of children with lead poisoning

      d. Children 6-72 months of age who live near lead smelters, battery recycling plants, or other industries likely to result in atmospheric lead release

      e. Children 6-72 months of age whose parents or other household members participate in a lead-related occupation or hobby

3. Symptoms of lead poisoning

      a. Children with elevated lead levels may be asymptomatic.

      b. Mild-to-moderate lead poisoning may be associated with learning/behavior problems, fatigue, malaise, anorexia, irritability, headache, abdominal pain, sporadic vomiting, and constipation.

      c. Severe poisoning is associated with clumsiness, ataxia, paresis, sensorium changes, vomiting, coma, convulsions, and signs of increased intracranial pressure. The possibility of lead encephalopathy should be considered in the differential diagnosis of children presenting with coma and convulsions of unknown etiology.

      d. Consider the possibility of lead poisoning in the child with developmental delay, FTT, ingestions, and parasitic infestation.

4. Screening

      a. Universal screening for lead poisoning is recommended starting at age 6 months in highest-risk children and at age 12-15 months in lower-risk children. Low-risk children should be rescreened at 24 months. High-risk children should be screened every 6 months until age 3 and every 12 months between 3 and 6 years of age unless they have had repeated blood-lead levels in the normal range. A 5-point questionnaire can be administered at well-child–care visits beginning at age 6 months to classify a child's risk for lead exposure. Follow-up screening is based on risk assessment and initial blood-lead results. Children with developmental delay and frequent hand-to-mouth activity may be at increased risk.

b. Blood lead has replaced the EP as the primary screening method. Unless contamination of capillary blood samples can be prevented, lead levels should be determined on venous samples whenever practical. All capillary specimen results should be considered presumptive and must be confirmed on a venous sample.

c. In patients with elevated blood-lead levels, an x=ray study of the abdomen can provide information about ingested lead paint chips, and x-ray studies of the long bones can provide information about the chronicity of the poisoning.

d. All children with blood-lead levels ≥20 μg/dL should be tested for iron deficiency, preferably with serum iron, iron-binding capacity, and serum ferritin.

5. Interpretation of blood-lead test results and follow-up recommendations: Classification is based on blood-lead concentration (Table 22-1).

6. Treatment

Several drugs are used in the treatment of lead poisoning. They bind or chelate lead and deplete the soft and hard (skeletal) tissues of lead. All have potentially serious side effects and must be used with caution. The effect of chelation on neurodevelopmental toxicity in asymptomatic children is controversial. Chelation therapy may be dangerous if the child is not removed from lead exposure.

a. Blood lead 25-44 μg/dL (asymptomatic): Chelation is controversial at this blood-lead level. The calcium EDTA mobilization (challenge) test has been used but is technically difficult and probably not a good predictor of the body burden of lead. Chelation therapy may be of benefit if blood-lead levels remain in this range after aggressive environmental measures.

b. Blood lead 45-69 μg/dL (asymptomatic): Chelation therapy may be carried out with calcium EDTA. Give for 5 days at a dosage of 50 mg/kg/d IV by continuous infusion or in two divided doses per day through a heparin lock over 30-60 minutes; it can also be given IM if mixed with procaine. Monitor renal and hepatic function and serum electrolytes. A second course of treatment may be needed if the blood-lead level rebounds to 45 μg/dL within 7-14 days after treatment. It is important to remove the child from the lead environment.

TABLE 22-1.
Interpretation of Blood-Lead Concentrations in Children

Class	Blood-lead concentration (µg/dL)	Comment
I	≤9	A child in Class I is not considered to be lead-poisoned.
IIA	10-14	Many children (or a large proportion of children) with blood-lead levels in this range should trigger community-wide childhood lead poisoning–prevention activities. Children in this range may need to be rescreened more often.
IIB	15-19	A child in Class IIB should receive nutritional and educational interventions and more frequent screening. If the blood-lead level persists in this range, environmental investigation and intervention should be done.
III	20-44	A child in Class III should receive environmental evaluation and remediation and a medical evaluation. Such a child may need pharmacologic treatment for lead poisoning.
IV	45-69	A child in Class IV needs both medical and environmental interventions, including chelation therapy.
V	≥70	A child with Class V lead poisoning is a medical emergency. Medical and environmental management must begin immediately.

NOTE: Because of dose-related renal toxicity, calcium EDTA should never be given to patients with renal impairment or in the absence of adequate urine flow. When using calcium EDTA, monitor U/A, serum BUN, and creatinine.

    c. Blood lead ≥70 µg/dL (asymptomatic): Chelation therapy should be carried out using both calcium EDTA (50 mg/kg/d by IV infusion) and BAL (25 mg/kg/d ÷ q4h by deep IM injection) × 5 days. The first dose of BAL should always precede the first dose of calcium EDTA by at least 4 hours. Renal and hepatic function and serum electrolytes need to be monitored. A second course of therapy with calcium EDTA alone may be required if the blood-lead level rebounds to 45-69 µg/dL within 5-7 days after treatment. If the rebound is ≥70 µg/dL, BAL plus calcium EDTA should be used.

NOTE: BAL should not be used in children who are allergic to peanuts or peanut products. Medicinal iron should not be administered during

BAL therapy. Except in life-threatening situations, BAL should not be used in children with G-6-PD deficiency (may induce hemolysis).

    d. Symptomatic lead poisoning

       1) Refer the patient to a pediatric center that has expertise in the treatment of lead poisoning.

       2) The patient needs chelation with calcium EDTA plus BAL and careful monitoring.

    e. An alternate therapy for asymptomatic patients with a blood-lead level of 45-69 μg/dL is succimer (2,3 dimercaptosuccinic acid; DMSA; Chemet). Succimer is an orally active heavy metal chelating agent approved in 1991 for the treatment of lead poisoning in children.

       1) Succimer should be administered only in a lead-free environment because it may increase GI absorption of lead.

       2) A treatment course lasts 19 days. Start with a dosage of 10 mg/kg (350 mg/m^2) q8h × 5 days and then reduce dosage to 10 mg/kg q12h for an additional 2 weeks. There is approximately a 60% reduction in blood-lead concentration during treatment.

          a) A child with a history of constipation should have an enema before starting treatment.

          b) Young children who cannot swallow capsules can be given succimer by separating the capsule and sprinkling the beads on soft food or by putting them in a spoon and following with a fruit drink. Succimer can be used in children with G-6-PD deficiency and can be given concomitantly with iron. It is contraindicated in children with an allergy to sulfa or mercaptan.

          c) Maintain adequate hydration; use with caution in patients with compromised renal function.

       3) Adverse events

          a) Such events are uncommon but include malaise, nausea, vomiting, diarrhea, anorexia, rash, reversible neutropenia, and transient increases in serum transaminases and alkaline phosphatase.

          b) Serum transaminases should be monitored before initiating treatment and at least weekly during treatment. Also monitor U/A, CBC, serum BUN, and creatinine.

       4) Follow-up

          a) Blood-lead levels should be monitored weekly until stable. Rebound elevations of 60%-70% are common secondary to redistribution of lead from bone stores; levels plateau 2-3 weeks after discontinuing treatment. Repeated courses of succimer, usually at 4-week intervals, may be necessary. The end point of therapy is a post-rebound blood-lead level of <15 µg/dL.

b) The safety of uninterrupted dosing for longer than 3 weeks has not been established and is not recommended.

7. Interventions to reduce lead exposure
   a. Whenever possible, remove child from lead source
   b. Prevent access to peeling paint or chewable surfaces. Move cribs and playpens away from surfaces containing lead paint. Stabilize or cover lead paint. Put furniture in front of leaded areas to block accessibility.
   c. Wet-mop floors and wet-clean window sills and wells weekly with high-phosphate (5%-8%) solution.
   d. Avoid dry dusting, sweeping, and vacuuming hard surfaces.
   e. Wash child's hands and face before meals.
   f. Wash toys and pacifiers often.
   g. Encourage regular meals and shakes low in fat and high in iron, calcium, phosphorus, and fiber.
   h. Use cold water for cooking; run water for 2-3 minutes in the morning before using.
   i. When a dwelling is being abated for lead, the child should be temporarily relocated to avoid exposure to lead dust.

H. LYMPHADENOPATHY

1. General guidelines

In the evaluation of a child with lymphadenopathy, the following points can be helpful in the differential diagnosis:
   a. Size: Nodes under 3 mm in diameter are normal. Up to 12 years of age, cervical and inguinal nodes up to 1 cm and epitrochlear nodes up to 0.5 cm may be normal. Nodes >2 cm may indicate a granulomatous disease or tumor.
   b. Node location
      1) Hodgkin's disease: Supraclavicular and lower neck
      2) Cat-scratch disease: Preauricular, axillary, inguinal, epitrochlear
      3) Reactive hyperplasia: Inguinal, submental, posterior cervical
      4) Atypical mycobacterium: Upper cervical, submandibular, preauricular

NOTE: Generalized adenopathy usually results from generalized disease.

c. Duration: Not too helpful in suggesting a diagnosis. Biopsy is indicated if the node increases after a 2-week follow-up *or* has not decreased after 4-6 weeks.
d. Consistency
1) Matted or fixed nodes: Neoplasm or granulomatous disease
2) Tender nodes with overlying erythema: Bacterial adenitis; the more tender the node, the less ominous the prognosis
e. Age
1) <4 years: Reactive hyperplasia, atypical mycobacterium
2) >8 years: Reactive hyperplasia, cat-scratch disease, Hodgkin's disease (especially in teenagers)
f. Associated signs and symptoms: Liver/spleen enlargement, prolonged fever, and weight loss suggest a serious systemic illness (malignancy).
2. History
a. Exposure to TB, cats? Medication history (e.g., phenytoin [Dilantin])?
b. The most common cause of cervical adenopathy in children is bacterial or viral infection in the ENT area.
c. Generalized adenopathy (two or more noncontiguous lymph node groups) usually results from reactive hyperplasia and is by far the most common diagnosis in children who undergo biopsy.
d. If the patient is febrile >1 wk, rule out mononucleosis, CMV, toxoplasmosis, and KD.
3. Work-up
a. History, PE, CBC, ESR, PPD, monospot test, TC, viral titers, chest x-ray study
b. The role of needle aspiration is controversial; the most significant treatable conditions are best diagnosed by open biopsy.
4. Timing of lymph node biopsy. In general, indications for biopsy include the following:
a. Unexplained fever and weight loss
b. Fixation of node to overlying skin or underlying tissue
c. Supraclavicular location
d. Abnormal chest x-ray study (strongest predictor of serious disease)
e. Increase in size of node after several weeks of observation
5. The following scoring system may be useful in adolescents:

Abnormal CXR	5 points
Lymph node >2 cm	3 points
ENT symptoms	−3 points
Constant	−2 points

    a. If score is >0, biopsy probably will lead to treatment.

    b. If score is <0, watch; biopsy probably will not alter treatment.

    c. The greater the score, the more likely it is to be correct.

    d. Even after biopsy, a specific cause may be established in only 40% of children. The most common histologic diagnoses are reactive hyperplasia, neoplastic disease, and granulomatous disease.

NOTE: Approximately 20% of children who initially have a nondiagnostic biopsy eventually develop a specific pathologic process. Patients need close follow-up.

6. Specific causes of lymphadenopathy

    a. Atypical mycobacterium

        1) Usually mycobacterium avium complex; acquired from environmental sources. Human contact does not play a role in transmission.

        2) It commonly occurs between 1 and 6 years of age.

        3) Nodes arc unilateral, firm, mobile, and without tenderness but may be fluctuant. The usual location is preauricular, upper anterior cervical, and submandibular.

        4) Systemic and pulmonary manifestations are uncommon.

        5) The CXR is negative. The PPD is negative or weakly positive, but NTM-specific antigens, particularly PPD-B, can be diagnostically helpful.

        6) Diagnosis: Confirmed by positive AFB culture from node but is present in only 50% of cases. A positive AFB smear and characteristic histopathology are helpful but not diagnostic.

        7) Treatment: Total excision; anti-TB drugs are ineffective. Avoid I&D or needle aspiration (may lead to chronic draining sinus tract).

    b. Lymphoma

        1) >8 years of age; usually teenagers

        2) Rubbery, matted or fixed, nontender nodes

        3) Supraclavicular and lower cervical location

        4) Liver/spleen enlargement, fever, weight loss, anemia, abnormal CXR (mediastinal or hilar adenopathy)

        5) Diagnosis: Biopsy

    c. Cat-scratch disease

        1) Unilateral, subacute regional lymphadenitis; parotid, preauricular, axillary, epitrochlear, inguinal; suppurative in 15% of cases; may be accompanied by malaise, fatigue, low-grade fever

        2) History of cat (often kitten) exposure; crusted papule or vesiculopustule at inoculation site distal to node

3) Negative laboratory results for other causes of lymphade-nopathy

4) May be positive cat-scratch skin test, but antigen is not standardized or licensed

5) Biopsy of node shows multiple nonnecrotizing granulomas and microabscesses; positive Warthin-Starry silver stain

6) Etiologic agent: *Rochalimaea henselae*

7) Diagnosis: Suggested by clinical features; can be confirmed by demonstrating elevated antibody titer to *R. henselae* or the presence of *R. henselae* DNA (by PCR) in purulent material aspirated from suppurative node

8) Treatment: Most cases resolve spontaneously within several months. Rifampin, ciprofloxacin, TMP/SMZ, and gentamicin may be effective but are indicated only in patients with severe disease. Avoid I&D of nodes because it may lead to chronic draining sinus tract.

NOTE: Other presentations of cat-scratch disease include Parinaud's oculoglandular syndrome, erythema nodosum, encephalopathy, osteolytic lesions, and multiple hepatic abscesses. Patients with hepatic abscesses have prolonged fever, abdominal pain, hepatomegaly, ± splenomegaly, ± regional lymphadenopathy, and scattered hyperechoic hepatic lesions on CT scan or ultrasound.

    d. Viral

1) Any age

2) Discrete, mobile, soft consistency; no redness or warmth; may be tender

3) Upper anterior cervical, posterior cervical, generalized

4) Associated fever, malaise, URI symptoms; liver/spleen enlargement

5) Diagnosis: Serologic studies

NOTE: CMV and toxoplasmosis may be indistinguishable from Epstein-Barr virus infection.

I. MYOSITIS

Excruciating pain in the calf muscles in association with signs and symptoms of a viral illness is seen in children secondary to Asian influenza B infection. The muscles are tender to palpation, and the children often refuse to bear weight or walk. It usually resolves in several days. Treatment consists of acetaminophen and warm baths. The CPK level may be extremely elevated. The condition may (rarely) be

associated with widespread muscle necrosis with myoglobinuria and •
acute tubular necrosis.•

J. STINGING INSECT REACTIONS (bees, yellow jackets, wasps,
    hornets, fire ants)
1. Small local reaction
    a. Small scattered hives with erythema, pain, and pruritus; lasts
       several hours
    b. Treatment: Cold compress. Carefully remove stinger (honeybee)
       by scraping the sting site with the edge of a credit card.
2. Large local reaction
    a. Swelling at sting site >5 cm; may involve entire extremity.
       Reaction peaks at 48-72 hours and may last as long as 1 week.
    b. Treatment: Ice, oral antihistamine, analgesic, oral prednisone burst
       if severe swelling
3. Mild systemic reaction
    a. Generalized urticaria, erythema, pruritus, and angioedema (in
       children, 70% of systemic reactions to stings are cutaneous)
    b. Treatment: SQ epinephrine 1:1000 0.01 ml/kg up to 0.3 ml, may
       repeat in 15 minutes; PO antihistamine
    c. Skin testing and immunotherapy are not indicated.
    d. Patient should have an epinephrine kit available for self-injection
       (Epipen, AnaKit), especially when away from access to medical
       care. However, among children with a generalized cutaneous
       reaction, the reaction with another sting is almost never more
       severe than the previous reaction.
    e. Careful instructions regarding insect avoidance
4. Life-threatening systemic reaction
    a. Laryngeal edema, bronchospasm, hypotension; often accompanied
       by cutaneous manifestations
    b. Treatment: SQ epinephrine 1:1000 0.01 ml/kg up to 0.3 ml,
       oxygen, volume expanders, pressor agents, airway support, inhaled
       β_2-agonist
    c. Steroids are not generally effective (delayed onset of action) but are
       usually given by IV route.
    d. Patient should be referred to an allergist for skin testing and
       possible venom immunotherapy.
    e. Patient should always carry an epinephrine self-injector (Epipen,
       AnaKit). Patient, family, and caregivers such as school personnel
       should be carefully instructed in the use of the injector device.

5. Unusual reactions following insect stings include serum sickness, vasculitis, encephalitis, nephritis, and Guillain-Barré syndrome.
   NOTE: In general, stinging insect reactions are rarely fatal in children, and severe reactions tend to diminish over time.

K. SUBSTANCE ABUSE
1. Recognizing the adolescent substance abuser
   a. More than 50% of teenagers have some experience with an illicit drug by the time they are high-school seniors. The majority have some experience with alcohol and other drugs. Many experience adverse consequences, and some progress to dependence.
   b. Substance abuse is underidentified by health professionals. Adolescents rarely present with chemical dependency as a primary or secondary complaint. The clinical signs and symptoms of dependency are often not appreciated unless a thorough history with specific questions is conducted. The signs and symptoms of withdrawal are unusual in individuals who use drugs in an episodic fashion. However, acute overdoses and adverse reactions are a major problem. Every adolescent who seeks care, regardless of the chief complaint, should be asked about alcohol and drug abuse.
   c. Risk factors for substance abuse
      1) Family history of alcoholism and other drug use
      2) History of family conflict or verbal, physical, or sexual abuse
      3) Antisocial behavior (conduct disorders), rebelliousness
      4) Academic underachievement
      5) Developmental disabilities
      6) Low self-esteem, alienation
      7) Friends who use drugs
      8) Early first use of drugs
   d. The classic picture includes personality change, poor family interactions, deteriorating school performance, and withdrawal from positive environmental factors (e.g., church, sports, extracurricular activities).
   e. There is often a progression from beer or wine and tobacco to liquor to marijuana to cocaine or heroin. Multiple drug use is the rule for the majority of substance-abusing adolescents.
   f. Consider substance abuse in the adolescent who has any of the following:
      1) Behavior that is unexplained or out of the ordinary (e.g., depression, emotional change)
      2) Fatigue, nonspecific symptoms, or psychosomatic complaints

      3) Injuries related to a fall, fighting, motor vehicle accident, or near-drowning

      4) Attempted suicide. Half to two thirds of young individuals who commit suicide have a history of substance abuse (usually multiple drugs over many years).

   g. Drug screening may be helpful but is only one part of a comprehensive clinical assessment. Indications include the following:

      1) Psychiatric symptoms

      2) Runaways, delinquents

      3) Mental-status or performance changes

      4) Acute-onset behavior changes

      5) Recurrent accidents

      6) Unexplained somatic symptoms

      7) Monitoring of abstinence in a known abuser

2. General approach to patient with an acute drug abuse reaction

   a. Establish an airway and support ventilation (if indicated).

   b. Start IV and support cardiac output, as needed.

   c. If patient is obtunded, give IV or IM naloxone 2.0 mg/dose q2-3min × 3-4 prn.

   d. Hypoglycemia should be considered in any adolescent with obtundation or seizures and confirmed whenever possible by rapid bedside testing. If hypoglycemia is suspected, treat immediately (before lab confirmation) with 50% dextrose 25-50 ml IV.

   e. Patients who remain obtunded or comatose despite these interventions should be examined for internal injuries, including head and neck trauma.

   f. Extreme agitation in an acutely intoxicated adolescent can threaten patient safety and interfere with appropriate therapy. In this situation, IV diazepam 0.1-0.3 mg/kg or midazolam 0.05-0.1 mg/kg can be given (the specific reversal agent flumazenil can be given in the event of an iatrogenic overdose).

   g. Gastric decontamination

      1) Activated charcoal: 50-100 g bolus orally or via NG tube

      2) Cathartic

   h. Initial evaluation

      1) Talk to patient, friends, parents, associates, paramedics. Was the usage recreational, episodic, experimental, or habitual? Was the overuse intentional or accidental?

      2) Complete PE: Closely monitor vital signs; check for associated

trauma; establish neurologic flow sheet and Glasgow Coma Scale score.

   3) Check patient's clothing for clues to the ingested substance; identify any recovered substances; utilize local poison control center.

  i. Obtain urine and blood for toxicology screens; it is important to know what the screen does and does not pick up.

  j. Depending on the initial work-up, obtain CBC, ABGs, electrolytes, blood glucose, BUN, creatinine, LFTs, serum ketones, U/A, and ECG. Measure serum acetaminophen levels in all patients with intentional overdoses, regardless of drug class, to permit early treatment with NAC if serum levels are in the toxic range.

  k. Need to evaluate for STDs and HIV infection (if indicated).

  l. Provide reassurance and psychologic support; restraint and force should be avoided if at all possible.

  m. Any patient with drug-induced cardiorespiratory compromise, seizures, or extreme agitation requires hospitalization.

3. Specific acute drug abuse reactions
  a. Alcohol
    1) Clinical manifestations
      a) Mental status: Aggressive, belligerent behavior; impaired mentation; sleepiness; slurred speech
      b) PE: Ataxia, incoordination, impaired mentation, hypertension, hypotension, hypothermia, respiratory depression, arrhythmias, tachycardia. Look for signs of associated trauma and aspiration. CNS effects are proportional to the concentration of alcohol in the blood.
      c) Withdrawal syndrome: Anxiety, insomnia, irritability. Severe withdrawal (convulsions, delirium, hallucinations) is rarely seen in adolescents.
    2) Treatment: Supportive care and correction of metabolic abnormalities (hypoglycemia, acidosis). Hypoglycemia is a particular consideration for diabetic patients.
  b. Anticholinergics: Atropine, belladonna, benztropine, henbane, jimsonweed seed, procyclidine, propantheline bromide, scopolamine, trihexyphenidyl
    1) Clinical manifestations
      a) Mental status: Amnesia, body image alterations, clouded sensorium, coma, confusion, convulsions, disorientation, drowsiness, restlessness, violent behavior, visual hallucinations

      b) PE: Dilated pupils, dry skin, flushed skin, hyperthermia, tachycardia, decreased bowel sounds, urinary retention

      c) Withdrawal syndrome: GI and musculoskeletal symptoms

  2) Treatment: Supportive care. Physostigmine has serious adverse effects and should be reserved for the treatment of life-threatening manifestations, including coma, respiratory depression, severe hypertension, and uncontrollable convulsions.

c. Cannabis group: Marijuana, hashish, THC, hash oil, sinsemilla

  1) Clinical manifestations

      a) Mental status: Anxiety and anorexia, then increased appetite, confusion, delirium, depersonalization, dreamlike state, fantasy state, euphoria, excitement, hallucinations, panic reactions, paranoia, time-space distortions

      b) PE: Ataxia, dry hacking cough, injected conjunctivae, laryngitis, pharyngitis, postural hypotension, tachycardia

      c) Withdrawal syndrome: Anorexia, anxiety, depression, insomnia, irritability, nausea, restlessness. Acute withdrawal reactions are rare.

  2) Treatment: No specific treatment is indicated. Diazepam may be used for severe anxiety or panic reactions.

d. CNS depressants ("downers"): Barbiturates, benzodiazepines, chloral hydrate, ethchlorvynol, glutethimide, meprobamate, methaqualone, methyprylon, paraldehyde

  1) Clinical manifestations

      a) Mental status: Coma, confusion, delirium, disorientation, drowsiness, slurred speech

      b) PE: Ataxia, convulsions (methaqualone), hyporeflexia, hypotension, hypothermia, hypotonia, incoordination, nystagmus, pulmonary edema, respiratory depression

      c) Withdrawal syndrome: Agitation, anxiety, arrhythmias, convulsions, delirium, disorientation, fever, hallucinations, hyperreflexia, hypertension, insomnia, irritability, sweating, tremors, weakness, cardiovascular collapse

  2) Treatment: Supportive care, maintenance of airway and ventilation, BP support, forced diuresis, alkalinization of urine. Hemodialysis or charcoal hemoperfusion may be indicated with high blood levels of long-acting drugs.

NOTE: Acute withdrawal can be life threatening. The drug dosage may need to be tapered, or phenobarbital or pentobarbital may need to be substituted and the dosage gradually decreased.

e. CNS stimulants ("uppers"): Amphetamine, amphetamine-like antiobesity drugs, Bromo-DMA, caffeine, dextroamphetamine, dimethylpropione, MDA, methylphenidate, phenmetrazine, phenylpropanolamine
   1) Clinical manifestations
      a) Mental status: Agitation, anxiety, coma, decreased appetite, decreased sleep, delirium, hallucinations, hyperactivity, hyperacute or confused sensorium, impulsivity, paranoid ideation, restlessness
      b) PE: Arrhythmias, blurred vision, convulsions, dilated pupils, dry mouth, hyperreflexia, hypertension, hyperthermia, hyperventilation, sweating, tachycardia, tremors
      c) Withdrawal syndrome: Abdominal pain, anxiety, chills, depression, exhaustion, muscle aches, sleep disturbances, tremors, voracious appetite
   2) Treatment: Supportive care; "talking patient down"; haloperidol for aggressiveness, agitation, and hallucinations; diazepam for control of agitation and seizures; forced diuresis. After patient has "crashed," a mild antidepressant (e.g., nortriptyline) can be given.
f. Cocaine
   1) Clinical manifestations
      a) Mental status (see CNS stimulants): Agitation, coma, hallucinations, increased concentration, mood elevation, panic, paranoia, psychosis
      b) PE: Arrhythmia, convulsions, diaphoresis, dilated pupils, epistaxis, hyperpnea, hyperreflexia, hypertension, hyperthermia, myocardial infarction, myoclonus, respiratory failure, sweating, stroke, tachycardia, tremor. Epiglottitis has been reported secondary to smoking cocaine.
      c) Withdrawal syndrome: Depression, irritability
   2) Treatment: Support of ventilation, IV propranolol or nitroprusside for cardiotoxicity, IM haloperidol 2-5 mg q1-8h prn (max 10-30 mg) until psychotic behavior improves, IV diazepam for seizures, cooling blanket for hyperthermia. Observation in a coronary care unit may be indicated for serial monitoring of ECGs and cardiac enzymes.
g. Hallucinogens: DMT, LSD, MDA, mescaline, morning glory seeds, nutmeg, psilocybin
   1) Clinical manifestations
      a) Mental status: Amnesia, anxiety, confusion, convulsions, delusions, depersonalization, depression, drooling, euphoria,

hallucinations, hyperactivity, inappropriate affect, mutism, panic, paranoia, psychosis, synesthesias, time and visual distortions, violent behavior

b) PE: Ataxia, dilated pupils, flushed face, hyperreflexia, hypertension, hyperthermia, nystagmus, tachycardia, tremors

c) Withdrawal syndrome: None

2) Treatment: Supportive care, psychologic support ("talking patient down" in quiet area), mild tranquilizer for extreme anxiety, IM haloperidol for severe agitation, IV diazepam for sedation, cooling blanket for hyperthermia. *Avoid antipsychotic drugs.*

h. Opioids: Codeine, fentanyl, heroin, hydromorphone, meperidine, methadone, morphine, opium, pentazocine, propoxyphene, sufentanil

1) Clinical manifestations

a) Mental status: Coma, euphoria, stupor

b) PE: Constricted pupils, hyporeflexia, hypotension, hypothermia, hypoventilation, pulmonary edema

c) Withdrawal syndrome: Abdominal cramps, anxiety, diarrhea, dilated pupils, gooseflesh, lacrimation, muscle jerks, tachycardia, tremulousness, vomiting, yawning

2) Treatment: IV or IM naloxone 2.0 mg/dose q2-3min × 3-4 prn; positive end-expiratory pressure for pulmonary edema. Clonidine can be used to minimize the discomfort of opiate detoxification.

i. Phencyclidine

1) Clinical manifestations

a) Mental status: Amnesia, anxiety, catalepsy, coma, convulsions, excitement, hallucinations, hyperactivity, impulsiveness, mutism, open-eyed coma, self-destructive or violent behavior, staring spells, stupor, psychosis

b) PE: Ataxia, diaphoresis, drooling, arrhythmia, flushing, hypertension, hyperthermia, hyporeflexia, myoclonus, nystagmus, tachycardia. Always evaluate the patient carefully for signs of trauma.

c) Withdrawal syndrome: None

2) Treatment: Psychologic support, observation in a quiet area (do not "talk down"), IV diazepam for sedation and convulsions, haloperidol 2-5 mg/dose q1-8h prn (max 10-30 mg) for severe agitation until improved, forced diuresis, protection from harm, propranolol for arrhythmias. Admission for psychologic evaluation is often required.

j. Volatile substances: Aliphatic and aromatic hydrocarbons (gasoline, butane, propane, toluene, benzene, xylene), halogenated hydrocarbons (freons, halothane, trichloroethylene), aliphatic nitrites (amyl, *m*-butyl, and isobutyl nitrite), nitrous oxide

    1) Inhalants are often the first consciousness-altering substances used by children. They are popular because of the rapid onset of action, the quality and pattern of the "high," low cost, easy availability, convenient packaging, and the fact that possession is not illegal in most states.

    2) Clinical manifestations

      a) Mental status: Confusion, disorientation, dizziness, euphoria, hallucinations, headache, impulsive behavior, psychosis, somnolence, stupor

      b) PE: Arrhythmias, ataxia, convulsions, coughing, drooling, hyporeflexia, hypotension, peripheral neuropathy, sneezing, tachycardia

      c) Withdrawal syndrome: None

NOTE: Some volatile agents may be associated with acute renal failure, DIC, hemolytic anemia, hypokalemia, methemoglobinemia, and renal tubular acidosis.

      d) Treatment: Support, maintenance of adequate ventilation

4. Occult cocaine exposure

a. Among young children who come to urban emergency rooms, 3%-5% have evidence of unsuspected passive cocaine exposure on a urine toxicology screen.

b. Exposure may be secondary to accidental ingestion, passive inhalation of freebase cocaine vapors, or intentional administration.

c. Cocaine intoxication should be considered in the evaluation of infants and young children with new-onset generalized or focal seizures, arrhythmias, or hypertension.

L. SUICIDE ATTEMPTS

1. Suicide ranks as one of the leading causes of death in adolescents.

2. Suicide attempts (parasuicides) outnumber completed suicides by 50-200:1. The male-female suicide ratio is 3:1.

3. Both suicides and suicide attempts can increase after media reports of a real or fictional suicide victim. Clustering of suicides has occurred in certain communities.

4. Completed suicide attempts are more common in males; violent measures such as firearms are often used.

5. Suicide attempts are more common in females; ingestions (self-poisoning) are often used.
6. Adolescents with chronic conditions can attempt suicide by self-poisoning through overdoses of their medications (e.g., theophylline) or by neglecting to take medications (e.g., insulin).
7. Although an acute event may trigger the suicide act, the following predisposing factors are common:
   a. Parental loss, broken home, or other interpersonal loss
   b. Depression (tearfulness vs. a raging "acting-out") or other major psychiatric disorder
   c. Feelings of anger, rejection, social isolation, or expendability
   d. Few friends/social supports
   e. Failure socially or scholastically
   f. Association with other troubled youths
   g. Previous history of suicide gestures (very important!), especially if high potential of success
   h. Physical illness
   i. History of substance abuse, pregnancy, STD, or psychosocial problems not previously listed
   j. History of prior abuse
   k. Family history of alcoholism, psychiatric disorder, or suicide
   l. Exposure to suicide (personally or via the media, especially if the person who took his or her life was admired)
   m. Easy availability of firearms or drugs in the home
8. When a child or adolescent demonstrates suicidal behavior, take it very seriously!
9. Important historical information includes the following:
   a. Method used (e.g., type and number of pills, weapon and time used)
   b. Whether victim announced the act
   c. Whether victim expresses a wish to die, feels hopeless, has a desire to try again (determine if patient has access to method and a plan), or shows remorse about the attempt
   d. The precipitating incident before the present attempt
   e. Whether the patient has a history of suicide attempts, depression, aggression/acting out, drug/alcohol abuse, psychiatric illness
   f. Whether there is a family history of psychiatric illness or suicide
   g. The patient's interpersonal relationships with parents, siblings, and friends
   h. The patient's functioning in school
   i. The patient's social support systems

10. A complete PE is mandatory, with particular emphasis on skin (needle tracks, marks of inflicted injury), neurologic, and psychiatric assessments.
11. Different treatments are necessary depending on the method of the attempt (e.g., suturing lacerations, gastric decontamination for ingestions, hyperbaric O_2 for CO poisoning).
12. An adolescent who has distanced himself or herself from family and friends, disposed of valued possessions, talked about death or suicide, expressed hopelessness about the future, left a suicide note, or has attempted violent suicide (firearms, hanging, CO exposure) is at extremely high risk for a successful suicide in the future. Individual and family psychotherapy is necessary.
13. Involvement by social work and psychiatry as soon as possible is mandatory.
14. Interviews with family members should be conducted.
15. Admission to either a medical or a psychiatric unit is advisable. If the adolescent shows a high lethality index, keep him or her in a safe and secure environment under one-to-one nursing supervision. If the adolescent refuses voluntary admission, initiate procedures for involuntary hospitalization.

BIBLIOGRAPHY

AIDS

Anderson M, Moore R: HIV and adolescents, *Pediatric Ann* 22:436, 1993.

Centers for Disease Control: Recommendations for prevention of HIV transmission in health-care settings, *MMWR Suppl* 36:2S–18S, 1987.

Centers for Disease Control: Guidelines for prophylaxis against *Pneumocystis carinii* pneumonia for children infected with human immunodeficiency virus, *MMWR* 40:RR2, 1991.

Church J: Clinical aspects of HIV infection in children, *Pediatric Ann* 22:417, 1993.

Cvetkovich T, Frenkel L: Current management of HIV infection in children, *Pediatric Ann* 22:428, 1993.

Edelson P: Childhood AIDS, *Pediatr Clin North Am* 38:1, 1991.

Husson R et al: Zidovudine and didanosine combination therapy in children with HIV infection, *Pediatrics* 93:316, 1994.

Mueller B et al: Clinical and pharmacokinetic evaluation of long-term therapy with didanosine in children with HIV infection, *Pediatrics* 94:724, 1994.

Oleske J et al: Treatment of HIV-infected infants and children, *Pediatr Ann* 17:332, 1988.

Pizzo P, Wilfert C, editors: *Pediatric AIDS: the challenge of HIV infection in infants, children, and adolescents,* Baltimore, 1991, Williams & Wilkins.

Rand T, Meyers A: Role of the general pediatrician in the management of HIV infection in children, *Pediatr Rev* 14:371, 1993.

Rogers M: Pediatric HIV infection, *Pediatr Ann* 17:324, 1988.

Scott G: Clinical manifestations of HIV infection in children, *Pediatr Ann* 17:365, 1988.

Working Group on Antiretroviral Therapy: Antiretroviral therapy and medical management of the HIV-infected child, *Pediatr Infect Dis J* 12:513, 1993.

Chest pain

Brown R: Recurrent chest pain in adolescents, *Pediatr Ann* 20:194, 1991.

Feinstein R, Daniel W: Chronic chest pain in children and adolescents, *Pediatr Ann* 15:685, 1986.

Selbst S: Evaluation of chest pain in children, *Pediatr Rev* 8:56, 1986.

Selbst S et al: Pediatric chest pain: a prospective study, *Pediatrics* 82:319, 1988.

Wiens L et al: Chest pain in otherwise healthy children and adolescents is frequently caused by exercise-induced asthma, *Pediatrics* 90:350, 1992.

Woodward G, Selbst S: Chest pain secondary to cocaine use, *Pediatr Emerg Care* 3:153, 1987.

Failure to thrive

Bithoney W et al: Failure to thrive/growth deficiency, *Pediatr Rev* 13:453, 1992.

Frank D, Zeisel S: Failure to thrive, *Pediatr Clin North Am* 35:1187, 1988.

Frank D et al: Failure to thrive: mystery, myth, and method, *Contemp Pediatr* 8:114, 1993.

Goldbloom R: Growth failure in infancy, *Pediatr Rev* 9:57, 1987.

Sills R, Sills I: Don't overlook environmental causes of failure to thrive, *Contemp Pediatr* 3:25, 1986.

Hypertension

Adelman R: Hypertension in infants, *Pediatr Ann* 18:562, 1989.

Daniels S: Primary hypertension in childhood and adolescence, *Pediatr Ann* 21:224, 1992.

Daniels S et al: Clinical spectrum of intrinsic renovascular hypertension in children, *Pediatrics* 80:698, 1987.

Falkner B: The hypertensive adolescent, *Pediatr Ann* 18:571, 1989.

Farine M, Arbus G: Management of hypertensive emergencies in children, *Pediatr Emerg Care* 5:51, 1989.

Feld L, Springate J: Hypertension in children, *Curr Probl Pediatr* 18:323, 1988.

Gilliman M et al: Use of multiple visits to increase blood pressure–tracking correlations in childhood, *Pediatrics* 87:708, 1991.

Hurley J: A pediatrician's approach to the evaluation of hypertension, *Pediatr Ann* 18:542, 1989.

Ingelfinger J: Noninvasive evaluation of pediatric hypertension, *Pediatr Ann* 18:551, 1989.

Jung F, Inglefinger J: Hypertension in childhood and adolescence, *Pediatr Rev* 14:169, 1993.

Rosner B: Blood pressure nomograms for children and adolescents by height, sex, and age in the US, *J Pediatr* 123:871, 1993.

Sinaiko A: Treatment of hypertension in children, *Pediatr Nephrol* 8:603, 1994.

Task Force on Blood Pressure Control in Children: Report of the Second Task Force on Blood Pressure Control in Children: 1987, *Pediatrics* 79:125, 1987.

Turner ME: What's new in the antihypertensive armamentarium? *Pediatr Ann* 18:597, 1989.

Kawasaki disease

American Heart Association Committee on Rheumatic Fever, Endocarditis, and Kawasaki Disease: Diagnostic guidelines for Kawasaki disease, *Am J Dis Child* 144:1220, 1990.

Burns JC et al: Clinical and epidemiologic characteristics of patients referred for evaluation of possible Kawasaki disease, *J Pediatr* 118:680, 1991.

Committee on Infectious Diseases: Intravenous gamma globulin use in children with Kawasaki disease, *Pediatrics* 82:122, 1988.

Crowley D: Cardiovascular complications of mucocutaneous lymph node syndrome, *Pediatr Clin North Am* 31:1321, 1984.

Fatica N et al: Detection and management of cardiac involvement in the Kawasaki syndrome, *Pediatr Ann* 16:639, 1987.

Gersony W: Diagnosis and management of Kawasaki disease, *JAMA* 265:2699, 1991.

Kato H et al: Kawasaki disease: cardiac problems and management, *Pediatr Rev* 9:209, 1987.

Newburger JW et al: A single intravenous infusion of gamma globulin as compared with four infusions in the treatment of acute Kawasaki syndrome, *N Engl J Med* 324:1633, 1991.

Roberts K: Kawasaki syndrome: in the eye of the beholder, *Contemp Pediatr* 8:126, 1991.

Rowley AH, Shulman ST: Current therapy for acute Kawasaki syndrome, *J Pediatr* 118:987, 1991.

Shulman ST et al: Kawasaki disease, *Pediatr Clin North Am* 42:1205, 1995.

Lead poisoning

American Academy of Pediatrics—Committee on Drugs: Treatment guidelines for lead exposure in children, *Pediatrics* 96:155, 1995.

American Academy of Pediatrics—Committee on Environmental Health: Lead poisoning: from screening to primary prevention, *Pediatrics* 92:176, 1993.

Amitai Y et al: Residential deleading: effects on the blood-lead levels of lead-poisoned children, *Pediatrics* 88:893, 1991.

Faust D, Brown J: Moderately elevated blood lead levels: effects on neuropsychologic functioning in children, *Pediatrics* 80:623, 1987.

Glotzer DE: Management of childhood lead poisoning: strategies for chelation, *Pediatr Ann* 23:606, 1994.

Goldstein G: Neurologic concepts of lead poisoning in children, *Pediatr Ann* 21:384, 1992.

McElvaine M et al: Prevalence of radiographic evidence of paint-chip ingestion amnong children with moderate to severe lead poisoning, *Pediatrics* 89:740, 1992.

Preventing lead poisoning in young children: a statement by the Centers for Disease Control, Atlanta, US Department of Health and Human Services, 1991.

Rabin R: Warnings unheeded: a history of child lead poisoning, *Am J Public Health* 79:1668, 1989.

Tejeda D et al: Do questions about lead exposure predict elevated levels? *Pediatrics* 93:192, 1994.

Weitzman M, Glotzer D: Lead poisoning, *Pediatr Rev* 13:461, 1992.

Lymphadenopathy

Bedross AA, Mann JP: Lymphadenopathy in children, *Adv Pediatr* 28:341, 1981.

Collipp PJ: Cat-scratch disease therapy, *Am J Dis Child* 143:1261, 1989.

Goral S et al: Detection of *Rochalimaea henselae* DNA by polymerase chain reaction from suppurative nodes of children with cat-scratch disease, *Pediatr Infect Dis J* 13:994, 1994.

Huebner RE et al: Usefulness of skin testing with mycobacterial antigens in children with cervical lymphadenopathy, *Pediatr Infect Dis J* 11:450, 1992.

Kew LK et al: Mycobacterial cervical lymphadenopathy: relation of etiologic agents to age, *JAMA* 251:1286, 1984.

Knight PJ et al: When is lymph node biopsy indicated in children with enlarged peripheral nodes? *Pediatrics* 69:391, 1982.

Margileth A: Cervical adenitis, *Pediatr Rev* 7:13, 1985.

Rizkallah MF et al: Hepatic and splenic abscesses in cat-scratch disease, *Pediatr Infect Dis J* 7:191, 1988.

Schaad UB et al: Management of atypical mycobacterial lymphadenitis of childhood: a review based on 380 cases, *J Pediatr* 19:356, 1979.

Slap GB et al: When to perform biopsies of enlarged peripheral lymph nodes in young patients, *JAMA* 252:1321, 1984.

Zangwill KM et al: Cat-scratch disease in Connecticut: epidemiology, risk factors, and evaluation of a new diagnostic test, *N Engl J Med* 329:8, 1993.

Myositis

Dietzman DE et al: Acute myositis associated with influenza B infection, *Pediatrics* 57:255, 1976.

Stinging insect reactions

Graft DF, Schuberth KC: Hymenoptera allergy in children, *Pediatr Clin North Am* 30:873, 1983.

Macguire JF, Geha RS: Bee, wasp and hornet stings, *Pediatr Rev* 8:5, 1986.

Müller U et al: Emergency treatment of allergic reactions to hymenoptera stings, *Clin Exp Allergy* 21:281, 1991.

Reisman RE: Natural history of insect sting allergy: relationship of severity of symptoms of initial sting anaphylaxis to re-sting reactions, *J Allergy Clin Immunol* 90:335, 1992.

Valentine MD: Insect venom allergy: diagnosis and treatment, *J Allergy Clin Immunol* 73:299, 1984.

Substance abuse

Adger H: Problems of alcohol and other drug use and abuse in adolescents, *J Adolesc Health* 12:606, 1991.

American Academy of Pediatrics: A guide to acute medical management of intoxication in adolescents, *Adolesc Health Update* 6:1, 1994.

Bailey GW: Current perspectives on substance abuse in youth, *J Am Acad Child Adolesc Psychiatry* 28:151, 1989.

Felter R et al: Emergency department management of the intoxicated adolescent, *Pediatr Clin North Am* 34:399, 1987.

Kharasch SJ et al: Unsuspected cocaine exposure in young children, *Am J Dis Child* 145:204, 1991.

Kulberg A: Substance abuse: clinical identification and management, *Pediatr Clin North Am* 33:325, 1986.

McDonald DI: Drugs, drinking and adolescence, *Am J Dis Child* 138:117, 1984.

McHugh MJ: The abuse of volatile substances, *Pediatr Clin North Am* 34:333, 1987.

Meeks J: Adolescents at risk for drug and alcohol abuse, *Semin Adolesc Med* 1:231, 1985.

Rosenberg NM et al: Occult cocaine exposure in children, *Am J Dis Child* 145:1430, 1991.

Treatment of acute drug abuse reactions, *Med Lett* 29:83, 1987.

Zarek D et al: Risk factors for adolescent substance abuse, *Pediatr Clin North Am* 34:481, 1987.

Suicide attempts

Brent D: Depression and suicide in children and adolescents, *Pediatr Rev* 14:380, 1993.

Committee on Adolescence: Suicide and suicide attempts in adolescents and young adults, *Pediatrics* 81:322, 1988.

Grossman D: Risk and prevention of youth suicide, *Pediatr Ann* 21:448, 1992.

Hollinger P: The causes, impact, and preventability of childhood injuries in the US: childhood suicide, *Am J Dis Child* 144:670, 1990.

Kjelsberg E et al: Overdose deaths in young substance abusers: accidents or hidden suicides, *Acta Psychiatr Scand* 91:236, 1995.

Pfeffer C: Spotting the red flags for adolescent suicide, *Contemp Pediatr* 6:59, 1989.

Slap G et al: Risk factors for attempted suicide during adolescence, *Pediatrics* 84:762, 1989.

Swedo S et al: Can adolescent suicide attempters be distinguished from at-risk adolescents? *Pediatrics* 88:620, 1991.

Young MA et al: Interaction of risk factors in predicting suicide, *Am J Psych* 151:434, 1994.

INDEX

A

A-2000; *see* Pyrethrin

Abdomen
gastrointestinal bleeding and, 114
palpation of in enuresis, 139
sickle-cell disease and, 179

Abdominal pain, 109-112
in hemophilia, 173, 174
in Henoch-Schönlein purpura, 146-147

Abrasion, corneal, 256

Abscess, brain, 235, 236, 237

Absolute neutrophil count
in neutropenia, 183, 184
in zidovudine therapy, 400

Abuse, 19-26, 354
sexual, 22-24
pediculosis pubis, 67
substance, 426-432

Accessory muscle use in asthma assessment, 319, 321-323, 328-330

Accutane for acne, 60-61

ACE; *see* Angiotensin-converting enzyme

Acetaminophen
for fever, 98, 104, 105
ingestion of, 205-209

Acetone level in diabetic ketoacidosis, 80

N-Acetylcysteine for acetaminophen poisoning, 205-209

Acidosis, metabolic, 13

Acne, 57-61

Acquired immunodeficiency syndrome, 177, 399-402

Acrodermatitis, 58

Acropustulosis, 222

Activated charcoal for gastrointestinal decontamination, 202-203

Acular; *see* Ketorolac

Acute diarrhea, 119

Acute glomerulonephritis, 140-141

Acute otitis media, 298-301

Acyclovir
for herpes, 73, 237, 383
for pneumonia, 346

ADD; *see* Attention deficit disorder

Adenoidectomy for otitis media, 301, 302-303

Adenovirus
in bronchiolitis, 334
in diarrhea, 119
in pharyngitis, 304
in pneumonia, 344
school health and, 359

ADHD; *see* Attention deficit hyperactivity disorder

Adhesion, labial, 162

Administration of drugs at school, 355

Adolescent
acetaminophen poisoning in, 209

441